50% OFF
Online PANCE Prep Course!

by Mometrix

Dear Customer,

We consider it an honor and a privilege that you chose our PANCE Study Guide. As a way of showing our appreciation and to help us better serve you, we are offering **50% off our online PANCE Prep Course**. Many PANCE courses are needlessly expensive and don't deliver enough value. With our course, you get access to the best PANCE prep material, and **you only pay half price**.

We have structured our online course to perfectly complement your printed study guide. The PANCE Prep Course contains **in-depth lessons** that cover all the most important topics, **30+ video reviews** that explain difficult concepts, over **600 practice questions** to ensure you feel prepared, and more than **600 digital flashcards**, so you can study while you're on the go.

Online PANCE Prep Course

Topics Included:

- Task Areas
  - History Taking and Performing Physical Examination
  - Using Diagnostic and Laboratory Studies
  - Formulating Most Likely Diagnosis
  - Clinical Intervention
  - Pharmaceutical Therapies

- Organ Areas
  - Cardiovascular System
  - Dermatologic System
  - Endocrine System
  - Gastrointestinal System
  - Hematologic System

Course Features:

- PANCE Study Guide
  - Get content that complements our best-selling study guide.
- Full-Length Practice Tests
  - With over 600 practice questions, you can test yourself again and again.
- Mobile Friendly
  - If you need to study on the go, the course is easily accessible from your mobile device.
- PANCE Flashcards
  - Our course includes a flashcard mode with over 600 content cards to help you study.

To receive this discount, visit us at mometrix.com/university/pance or simply scan this QR code with your smartphone. At the checkout page, enter the discount code: **pance50off**

If you have any questions or concerns, please contact us at support@mometrix.com.

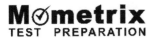

FREE Study Skills Videos/DVD Offer

Dear Customer,

Thank you for your purchase from Mometrix! We consider it an honor and a privilege that you have purchased our product and we want to ensure your satisfaction.

As part of our ongoing effort to meet the needs of test takers, we have developed a set of Study Skills Videos that we would like to give you for <u>FREE</u>. These videos cover our *best practices* for getting ready for your exam, from how to use our study materials to how to best prepare for the day of the test.

All that we ask is that you email us with feedback that would describe your experience so far with our product. Good, bad, or indifferent, we want to know what you think!

To get your FREE Study Skills Videos, you can use the **QR code** below, or send us an **email** at studyvideos@mometrix.com with *FREE VIDEOS* in the subject line and the following information in the body of the email:

- The name of the product you purchased.
- Your product rating on a scale of 1-5, with 5 being the highest rating.
- Your feedback. It can be long, short, or anything in between. We just want to know your impressions and experience so far with our product. (Good feedback might include how our study material met your needs and ways we might be able to make it even better. You could highlight features that you found helpful or features that you think we should add.)

If you have any questions or concerns, please don't hesitate to contact me directly.

Thanks again!

Sincerely,

Jay Willis
Vice President
jay.willis@mometrix.com
1-800-673-8175

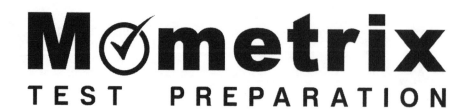

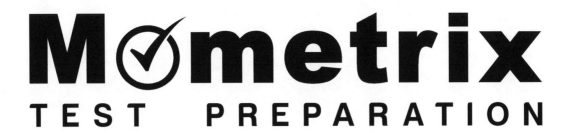

PANCE

Prep Study Guide 2023-2024

750+ Practice Test Questions

Secrets Review Book for the Physician Assistant National Certifying Exam

5th Edition

Written and edited by Mometrix Test Prep

Printed in the United States of America

This paper meets the requirements of ANSI/NISO Z39.48-1992 (Permanence of Paper).

Mometrix offers volume discount pricing to institutions. For more information or a price quote, please contact our sales department at sales@mometrix.com or 888-248-1219.

Mometrix Media LLC is not affiliated with or endorsed by any official testing organization. All organizational and test names are trademarks of their respective owners.

Paperback
ISBN 13: 978-1-5167-2411-6
ISBN 10: 1-5167-2411-9

DEAR FUTURE EXAM SUCCESS STORY

First of all, **THANK YOU** for purchasing Mometrix study materials!

Second, congratulations! You are one of the few determined test-takers who are committed to doing whatever it takes to excel on your exam. **You have come to the right place.** We developed these study materials with one goal in mind: to deliver you the information you need in a format that's concise and easy to use.

In addition to optimizing your guide for the content of the test, we've outlined our recommended steps for breaking down the preparation process into small, attainable goals so you can make sure you stay on track.

We've also analyzed the entire test-taking process, identifying the most common pitfalls and showing how you can overcome them and be ready for any curveball the test throws you.

Standardized testing is one of the biggest obstacles on your road to success, which only increases the importance of doing well in the high-pressure, high-stakes environment of test day. Your results on this test could have a significant impact on your future, and this guide provides the information and practical advice to help you achieve your full potential on test day.

Your success is our success

We would love to hear from you! If you would like to share the story of your exam success or if you have any questions or comments in regard to our products, please contact us at **800-673-8175** or **support@mometrix.com**.

Thanks again for your business and we wish you continued success!

Sincerely,
The Mometrix Test Preparation Team

Need more help? Check out our flashcards at:
http://MometrixFlashcards.com/PANRE

TABLE OF CONTENTS

Introduction

Thank you for purchasing this resource! You have made the choice to prepare yourself for a test that could have a huge impact on your future, and this guide is designed to help you be fully ready for test day. Obviously, it's important to have a solid understanding of the test material, but you also need to be prepared for the unique environment and stressors of the test, so that you can perform to the best of your abilities.

For this purpose, the first section that appears in this guide is the **Secret Keys**. We've devoted countless hours to meticulously researching what works and what doesn't, and we've boiled down our findings to the five most impactful steps you can take to improve your performance on the test. We start at the beginning with study planning and move through the preparation process, all the way to the testing strategies that will help you get the most out of what you know when you're finally sitting in front of the test.

We recommend that you start preparing for your test as far in advance as possible. However, if you've bought this guide as a last-minute study resource and only have a few days before your test, we recommend that you skip over the first two Secret Keys since they address a long-term study plan.

If you struggle with **test anxiety**, we strongly encourage you to check out our recommendations for how you can overcome it. Test anxiety is a formidable foe, but it can be beaten, and we want to make sure you have the tools you need to defeat it.

Secret Key #1 – Plan Big, Study Small

There's a lot riding on your performance. If you want to ace this test, you're going to need to keep your skills sharp and the material fresh in your mind. You need a plan that lets you review everything you need to know while still fitting in your schedule. We'll break this strategy down into three categories.

Information Organization

Start with the information you already have: the official test outline. From this, you can make a complete list of all the concepts you need to cover before the test. Organize these concepts into groups that can be studied together, and create a list of any related vocabulary you need to learn so you can brush up on any difficult terms. You'll want to keep this vocabulary list handy once you actually start studying since you may need to add to it along the way.

Time Management

Once you have your set of study concepts, decide how to spread them out over the time you have left before the test. Break your study plan into small, clear goals so you have a manageable task for each day and know exactly what you're doing. Then just focus on one small step at a time. When you manage your time this way, you don't need to spend hours at a time studying. Studying a small block of content for a short period each day helps you retain information better and avoid stressing over how much you have left to do. You can relax knowing that you have a plan to cover everything in time. In order for this strategy to be effective though, you have to start studying early and stick to your schedule. Avoid the exhaustion and futility that comes from last-minute cramming!

Study Environment

The environment you study in has a big impact on your learning. Studying in a coffee shop, while probably more enjoyable, is not likely to be as fruitful as studying in a quiet room. It's important to keep distractions to a minimum. You're only planning to study for a short block of time, so make the most of it. Don't pause to check your phone or get up to find a snack. It's also important to **avoid multitasking**. Research has consistently shown that multitasking will make your studying dramatically less effective. Your study area should also be comfortable and well-lit so you don't have the distraction of straining your eyes or sitting on an uncomfortable chair.

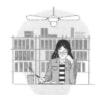 The time of day you study is also important. You want to be rested and alert. Don't wait until just before bedtime. Study when you'll be most likely to comprehend and remember. Even better, if you know what time of day your test will be, set that time aside for study. That way your brain will be used to working on that subject at that specific time and you'll have a better chance of recalling information.

Finally, it can be helpful to team up with others who are studying for the same test. Your actual studying should be done in as isolated an environment as possible, but the work of organizing the information and setting up the study plan can be divided up. In between study sessions, you can discuss with your teammates the concepts that you're all studying and quiz each other on the details. Just be sure that your teammates are as serious about the test as you are. If you find that your study time is being replaced with social time, you might need to find a new team.

Secret Key #2 – Make Your Studying Count

You're devoting a lot of time and effort to preparing for this test, so you want to be absolutely certain it will pay off. This means doing more than just reading the content and hoping you can remember it on test day. It's important to make every minute of study count. There are two main areas you can focus on to make your studying count.

Retention

It doesn't matter how much time you study if you can't remember the material. You need to make sure you are retaining the concepts. To check your retention of the information you're learning, try recalling it at later times with minimal prompting. Try carrying around flashcards and glance at one or two from time to time or ask a friend who's also studying for the test to quiz you.

To enhance your retention, look for ways to put the information into practice so that you can apply it rather than simply recalling it. If you're using the information in practical ways, it will be much easier to remember. Similarly, it helps to solidify a concept in your mind if you're not only reading it to yourself but also explaining it to someone else. Ask a friend to let you teach them about a concept you're a little shaky on (or speak aloud to an imaginary audience if necessary). As you try to summarize, define, give examples, and answer your friend's questions, you'll understand the concepts better and they will stay with you longer. Finally, step back for a big picture view and ask yourself how each piece of information fits with the whole subject. When you link the different concepts together and see them working together as a whole, it's easier to remember the individual components.

Finally, practice showing your work on any multi-step problems, even if you're just studying. Writing out each step you take to solve a problem will help solidify the process in your mind, and you'll be more likely to remember it during the test.

Modality

Modality simply refers to the means or method by which you study. Choosing a study modality that fits your own individual learning style is crucial. No two people learn best in exactly the same way, so it's important to know your strengths and use them to your advantage.

For example, if you learn best by visualization, focus on visualizing a concept in your mind and draw an image or a diagram. Try color-coding your notes, illustrating them, or creating symbols that will trigger your mind to recall a learned concept. If you learn best by hearing or discussing information, find a study partner who learns the same way or read aloud to yourself. Think about how to put the information in your own words. Imagine that you are giving a lecture on the topic and record yourself so you can listen to it later.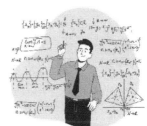

For any learning style, flashcards can be helpful. Organize the information so you can take advantage of spare moments to review. Underline key words or phrases. Use different colors for different categories. Mnemonic devices (such as creating a short list in which every item starts with the same letter) can also help with retention. Find what works best for you and use it to store the information in your mind most effectively and easily.

3

Secret Key #3 – Practice the Right Way

Your success on test day depends not only on how many hours you put into preparing, but also on whether you prepared the right way. It's good to check along the way to see if your studying is paying off. One of the most effective ways to do this is by taking practice tests to evaluate your progress. Practice tests are useful because they show exactly where you need to improve. Every time you take a practice test, pay special attention to these three groups of questions:

- The questions you got wrong
- The questions you had to guess on, even if you guessed right
- The questions you found difficult or slow to work through

This will show you exactly what your weak areas are, and where you need to devote more study time. Ask yourself why each of these questions gave you trouble. Was it because you didn't understand the material? Was it because you didn't remember the vocabulary? Do you need more repetitions on this type of question to build speed and confidence? Dig into those questions and figure out how you can strengthen your weak areas as you go back to review the material.

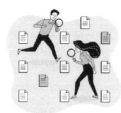 Additionally, many practice tests have a section explaining the answer choices. It can be tempting to read the explanation and think that you now have a good understanding of the concept. However, an explanation likely only covers part of the question's broader context. Even if the explanation makes perfect sense, **go back and investigate** every concept related to the question until you're positive you have a thorough understanding.

As you go along, keep in mind that the practice test is just that: practice. Memorizing these questions and answers will not be very helpful on the actual test because it is unlikely to have any of the same exact questions. If you only know the right answers to the sample questions, you won't be prepared for the real thing. **Study the concepts** until you understand them fully, and then you'll be able to answer any question that shows up on the test.

It's important to wait on the practice tests until you're ready. If you take a test on your first day of study, you may be overwhelmed by the amount of material covered and how much you need to learn. Work up to it gradually.

On test day, you'll need to be prepared for answering questions, managing your time, and using the test-taking strategies you've learned. It's a lot to balance, like a mental marathon that will have a big impact on your future. Like training for a marathon, you'll need to start slowly and work your way up. When test day arrives, you'll be ready.

Start with the strategies you've read in the first two Secret Keys—plan your course and study in the way that works best for you. If you have time, consider using multiple study resources to get different approaches to the same concepts. It can be helpful to see difficult concepts from more than one angle. Then find a good source for practice tests. Many times, the test website will suggest potential study resources or provide sample tests.

Practice Test Strategy

If you're able to find at least three practice tests, we recommend this strategy:

UNTIMED AND OPEN-BOOK PRACTICE

Take the first test with no time constraints and with your notes and study guide handy. Take your time and focus on applying the strategies you've learned.

TIMED AND OPEN-BOOK PRACTICE

Take the second practice test open-book as well, but set a timer and practice pacing yourself to finish in time.

TIMED AND CLOSED-BOOK PRACTICE

Take any other practice tests as if it were test day. Set a timer and put away your study materials. Sit at a table or desk in a quiet room, imagine yourself at the testing center, and answer questions as quickly and accurately as possible.

Keep repeating timed and closed-book tests on a regular basis until you run out of practice tests or it's time for the actual test. Your mind will be ready for the schedule and stress of test day, and you'll be able to focus on recalling the material you've learned.

Secret Key #4 – Pace Yourself

Once you're fully prepared for the material on the test, your biggest challenge on test day will be managing your time. Just knowing that the clock is ticking can make you panic even if you have plenty of time left. Work on pacing yourself so you can build confidence against the time constraints of the exam. Pacing is a difficult skill to master, especially in a high-pressure environment, so **practice is vital**.

Set time expectations for your pace based on how much time is available. For example, if a section has 60 questions and the time limit is 30 minutes, you know you have to average 30 seconds or less per question in order to answer them all. Although 30 seconds is the hard limit, set 25 seconds per question as your goal, so you reserve extra time to spend on harder questions. When you budget extra time for the harder questions, you no longer have any reason to stress when those questions take longer to answer.

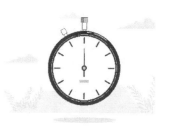

Don't let this time expectation distract you from working through the test at a calm, steady pace, but keep it in mind so you don't spend too much time on any one question. Recognize that taking extra time on one question you don't understand may keep you from answering two that you do understand later in the test. If your time limit for a question is up and you're still not sure of the answer, mark it and move on, and come back to it later if the time and the test format allow. If the testing format doesn't allow you to return to earlier questions, just make an educated guess; then put it out of your mind and move on.

On the easier questions, be careful not to rush. It may seem wise to hurry through them so you have more time for the challenging ones, but it's not worth missing one if you know the concept and just didn't take the time to read the question fully. Work efficiently but make sure you understand the question and have looked at all of the answer choices, since more than one may seem right at first.

Even if you're paying attention to the time, you may find yourself a little behind at some point. You should speed up to get back on track, but do so wisely. Don't panic; just take a few seconds less on each question until you're caught up. Don't guess without thinking, but do look through the answer choices and eliminate any you know are wrong. If you can get down to two choices, it is often worthwhile to guess from those. Once you've chosen an answer, move on and don't dwell on any that you skipped or had to hurry through. If a question was taking too long, chances are it was one of the harder ones, so you weren't as likely to get it right anyway.

On the other hand, if you find yourself getting ahead of schedule, it may be beneficial to slow down a little. The more quickly you work, the more likely you are to make a careless mistake that will affect your score. You've budgeted time for each question, so don't be afraid to spend that time. Practice an efficient but careful pace to get the most out of the time you have.

Secret Key #5 – Have a Plan for Guessing

When you're taking the test, you may find yourself stuck on a question. Some of the answer choices seem better than others, but you don't see the one answer choice that is obviously correct. What do you do?

The scenario described above is very common, yet most test takers have not effectively prepared for it. Developing and practicing a plan for guessing may be one of the single most effective uses of your time as you get ready for the exam.

In developing your plan for guessing, there are three questions to address:

- When should you start the guessing process?
- How should you narrow down the choices?
- Which answer should you choose?

When to Start the Guessing Process

Unless your plan for guessing is to select C every time (which, despite its merits, is not what we recommend), you need to leave yourself enough time to apply your answer elimination strategies. Since you have a limited amount of time for each question, that means that if you're going to give yourself the best shot at guessing correctly, you have to decide quickly whether or not you will guess.

Of course, the best-case scenario is that you don't have to guess at all, so first, see if you can answer the question based on your knowledge of the subject and basic reasoning skills. Focus on the key words in the question and try to jog your memory of related topics. Give yourself a chance to bring the knowledge to mind, but once you realize that you don't have (or you can't access) the knowledge you need to answer the question, it's time to start the guessing process.

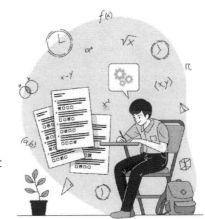

It's almost always better to start the guessing process too early than too late. It only takes a few seconds to remember something and answer the question from knowledge. Carefully eliminating wrong answer choices takes longer. Plus, going through the process of eliminating answer choices can actually help jog your memory.

Summary: Start the guessing process as soon as you decide that you can't answer the question based on your knowledge.

How to Narrow Down the Choices

The next chapter in this book (**Test-Taking Strategies**) includes a wide range of strategies for how to approach questions and how to look for answer choices to eliminate. You will definitely want to read those carefully, practice them, and figure out which ones work best for you. Here though, we're going to address a mindset rather than a particular strategy.

Your odds of guessing an answer correctly depend on how many options you are choosing from.

Number of options left	5	4	3	2	1
Odds of guessing correctly	20%	25%	33%	50%	100%

You can see from this chart just how valuable it is to be able to eliminate incorrect answers and make an educated guess, but there are two things that many test takers do that cause them to miss out on the benefits of guessing:

- Accidentally eliminating the correct answer
- Selecting an answer based on an impression

We'll look at the first one here, and the second one in the next section.

To avoid accidentally eliminating the correct answer, we recommend a thought exercise called **the $5 challenge**. In this challenge, you only eliminate an answer choice from contention if you are willing to bet $5 on it being wrong. Why $5? Five dollars is a small but not insignificant amount of money. It's an amount you could afford to lose but wouldn't want to throw away. And while losing $5 once might not hurt too much, doing it twenty times will set you back $100. In the same way, each small decision you make—eliminating a choice here, guessing on a question there—won't by itself impact your score very much, but when you put them all together, they can make a big difference. By holding each answer choice elimination decision to a higher standard, you can reduce the risk of accidentally eliminating the correct answer.

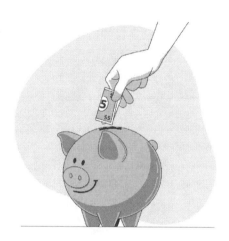

The $5 challenge can also be applied in a positive sense: If you are willing to bet $5 that an answer choice *is* correct, go ahead and mark it as correct.

Summary: Only eliminate an answer choice if you are willing to bet $5 that it is wrong.

Which Answer to Choose

You're taking the test. You've run into a hard question and decided you'll have to guess. You've eliminated all the answer choices you're willing to bet $5 on. Now you have to pick an answer. Why do we even need to talk about this? Why can't you just pick whichever one you feel like when the time comes?

The answer to these questions is that if you don't come into the test with a plan, you'll rely on your impression to select an answer choice, and if you do that, you risk falling into a trap. The test writers know that everyone who takes their test will be guessing on some of the questions, so they intentionally write wrong answer choices to seem plausible. You still have to pick an answer though, and if the wrong answer choices are designed to look right, how can you ever be sure that you're not falling for their trap? The best solution we've found to this dilemma is to take the decision out of your hands entirely. Here is the process we recommend:

Once you've eliminated any choices that you are confident (willing to bet $5) are wrong, select the first remaining choice as your answer.

Whether you choose to select the first remaining choice, the second, or the last, the important thing is that you use some preselected standard. Using this approach guarantees that you will not be enticed into selecting an answer choice that looks right, because you are not basing your decision on how the answer choices look.

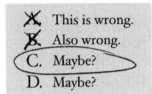

This is not meant to make you question your knowledge. Instead, it is to help you recognize the difference between your knowledge and your impressions. There's a huge difference between thinking an answer is right because of what you know, and thinking an answer is right because it looks or sounds like it should be right.

Summary: To ensure that your selection is appropriately random, make a predetermined selection from among all answer choices you have not eliminated.

9

Test-Taking Strategies

This section contains a list of test-taking strategies that you may find helpful as you work through the test. By taking what you know and applying logical thought, you can maximize your chances of answering any question correctly!

It is very important to realize that every question is different and every person is different: no single strategy will work on every question, and no single strategy will work for every person. That's why we've included all of them here, so you can try them out and determine which ones work best for different types of questions and which ones work best for you.

Question Strategies

☑ READ CAREFULLY

Read the question and the answer choices carefully. Don't miss the question because you misread the terms. You have plenty of time to read each question thoroughly and make sure you understand what is being asked. Yet a happy medium must be attained, so don't waste too much time. You must read carefully and efficiently.

☑ CONTEXTUAL CLUES

Look for contextual clues. If the question includes a word you are not familiar with, look at the immediate context for some indication of what the word might mean. Contextual clues can often give you all the information you need to decipher the meaning of an unfamiliar word. Even if you can't determine the meaning, you may be able to narrow down the possibilities enough to make a solid guess at the answer to the question.

☑ PREFIXES

If you're having trouble with a word in the question or answer choices, try dissecting it. Take advantage of every clue that the word might include. Prefixes can be a huge help. Usually, they allow you to determine a basic meaning. *Pre-* means before, *post-* means after, *pro-* is positive, *de-* is negative. From prefixes, you can get an idea of the general meaning of the word and try to put it into context.

☑ HEDGE WORDS

Watch out for critical hedge words, such as *likely, may, can, sometimes, often, almost, mostly, usually, generally, rarely,* and *sometimes.* Question writers insert these hedge phrases to cover every possibility. Often an answer choice will be wrong simply because it leaves no room for exception. Be on guard for answer choices that have definitive words such as *exactly* and *always.*

☑ SWITCHBACK WORDS

Stay alert for *switchbacks*. These are the words and phrases frequently used to alert you to shifts in thought. The most common switchback words are *but, although,* and *however.* Others include *nevertheless, on the other hand, even though, while, in spite of, despite,* and *regardless of.* Switchback words are important to catch because they can change the direction of the question or an answer choice.

☑ FACE VALUE

When in doubt, use common sense. Accept the situation in the problem at face value. Don't read too much into it. These problems will not require you to make wild assumptions. If you have to go beyond creativity and warp time or space in order to have an answer choice fit the question, then you should move on and consider the other answer choices. These are normal problems rooted in reality. The applicable relationship or explanation may not be readily apparent, but it is there for you to figure out. Use your common sense to interpret anything that isn't clear.

Answer Choice Strategies

☑ ANSWER SELECTION

The most thorough way to pick an answer choice is to identify and eliminate wrong answers until only one is left, then confirm it is the correct answer. Sometimes an answer choice may immediately seem right, but be careful. The test writers will usually put more than one reasonable answer choice on each question, so take a second to read all of them and make sure that the other choices are not equally obvious. As long as you have time left, it is better to read every answer choice than to pick the first one that looks right without checking the others.

☑ ANSWER CHOICE FAMILIES

An answer choice family consists of two (in rare cases, three) answer choices that are very similar in construction and cannot all be true at the same time. If you see two answer choices that are direct opposites or parallels, one of them is usually the correct answer. For instance, if one answer choice says that quantity x increases and another either says that quantity x decreases (opposite) or says that quantity y increases (parallel), then those answer choices would fall into the same family. An answer choice that doesn't match the construction of the answer choice family is more likely to be incorrect. Most questions will not have answer choice families, but when they do appear, you should be prepared to recognize them.

☑ ELIMINATE ANSWERS

Eliminate answer choices as soon as you realize they are wrong, but make sure you consider all possibilities. If you are eliminating answer choices and realize that the last one you are left with is also wrong, don't panic. Start over and consider each choice again. There may be something you missed the first time that you will realize on the second pass.

☑ AVOID FACT TRAPS

Don't be distracted by an answer choice that is factually true but doesn't answer the question. You are looking for the choice that answers the question. Stay focused on what the question is asking for so you don't accidentally pick an answer that is true but incorrect. Always go back to the question and make sure the answer choice you've selected actually answers the question and is not merely a true statement.

☑ EXTREME STATEMENTS

In general, you should avoid answers that put forth extreme actions as standard practice or proclaim controversial ideas as established fact. An answer choice that states the "process should be used in certain situations, if…" is much more likely to be correct than one that states the "process should be discontinued completely." The first is a calm rational statement and doesn't even make a definitive, uncompromising stance, using a hedge word *if* to provide wiggle room, whereas the second choice is far more extreme.

☑ BENCHMARK

As you read through the answer choices and you come across one that seems to answer the question well, mentally select that answer choice. This is not your final answer, but it's the one that will help you evaluate the other answer choices. The one that you selected is your benchmark or standard for judging each of the other answer choices. Every other answer choice must be compared to your benchmark. That choice is correct until proven otherwise by another answer choice beating it. If you find a better answer, then that one becomes your new benchmark. Once you've decided that no other choice answers the question as well as your benchmark, you have your final answer.

11

⊘ Predict the Answer

Before you even start looking at the answer choices, it is often best to try to predict the answer. When you come up with the answer on your own, it is easier to avoid distractions and traps because you will know exactly what to look for. The right answer choice is unlikely to be word-for-word what you came up with, but it should be a close match. Even if you are confident that you have the right answer, you should still take the time to read each option before moving on.

General Strategies

⊘ Tough Questions

If you are stumped on a problem or it appears too hard or too difficult, don't waste time. Move on! Remember though, if you can quickly check for obviously incorrect answer choices, your chances of guessing correctly are greatly improved. Before you completely give up, at least try to knock out a couple of possible answers. Eliminate what you can and then guess at the remaining answer choices before moving on.

⊘ Check Your Work

Since you will probably not know every term listed and the answer to every question, it is important that you get credit for the ones that you do know. Don't miss any questions through careless mistakes. If at all possible, try to take a second to look back over your answer selection and make sure you've selected the correct answer choice and haven't made a costly careless mistake (such as marking an answer choice that you didn't mean to mark). This quick double check should more than pay for itself in caught mistakes for the time it costs.

⊘ Pace Yourself

It's easy to be overwhelmed when you're looking at a page full of questions; your mind is confused and full of random thoughts, and the clock is ticking down faster than you would like. Calm down and maintain the pace that you have set for yourself. Especially as you get down to the last few minutes of the test, don't let the small numbers on the clock make you panic. As long as you are on track by monitoring your pace, you are guaranteed to have time for each question.

⊘ Don't Rush

It is very easy to make errors when you are in a hurry. Maintaining a fast pace in answering questions is pointless if it makes you miss questions that you would have gotten right otherwise. Test writers like to include distracting information and wrong answers that seem right. Taking a little extra time to avoid careless mistakes can make all the difference in your test score. Find a pace that allows you to be confident in the answers that you select.

⊘ Keep Moving

Panicking will not help you pass the test, so do your best to stay calm and keep moving. Taking deep breaths and going through the answer elimination steps you practiced can help to break through a stress barrier and keep your pace.

Final Notes

The combination of a solid foundation of content knowledge and the confidence that comes from practicing your plan for applying that knowledge is the key to maximizing your performance on test day. As your foundation of content knowledge is built up and strengthened, you'll find that the strategies included in this chapter become more and more effective in helping you quickly sift through the distractions and traps of the test to isolate the correct answer.

Now that you're preparing to move forward into the test content chapters of this book, be sure to keep your goal in mind. As you read, think about how you will be able to apply this information on the test. If you've already seen sample questions for the test and you have an idea of the question format and style, try to come up with questions of your own that you can answer based on what you're reading. This will give you valuable practice applying your knowledge in the same ways you can expect to on test day.

Good luck and good studying!

Task Areas

History Taking and Performing Physical Examination

SKIN LESIONS

The following are types of skin lesions:

- **Macule:** small (<1 cm) discolored spot that is neither raised nor depressed against the surrounding skin. A macule also does not affect the skin texture
- **Papule:** small (<1 cm), solid, raised lesion. Coloring may be brown, purple/blue, red, or pink
- **Nodule:** firm, circumscribed lesion that extends into the dermis
- **Vesicle:** small (5 to 10 mm), elevated, fluid-filled (serous), circular lesion that generally ruptures easily then dries to a yellow crust
- **Bulla:** large (>10 mm), elevated, clear fluid-filled, circular lesion; larger than vesicle
- **Pustule:** vesicle with purulent fluid
- **Plaque:** wide, large, well-demarcated, plateau-like, elevated or depressed lesion; may appear red with silvery scaling, as with psoriasis
- **Scale:** accumulation of horny epithelium
- **Urticaria/wheal:** hives; elevated lesions due to edema

BEST LOCATIONS TO AUSCULTATE THE FOUR CARDIAC VALVES

The **S1** or "lub" sound is created by the mitral and tricuspid valves. The **S2** or "dub" sound is created by the aortic and pulmonary valves. Heart sounds are created by the blood flow through the valves, not the valves themselves, so the best auscultation will occur where those reverberated sound waves produce the greatest effect, not at the anatomical point of the heart valve itself.

- **Aortic valve:** Right second intercostal space, right-upper sternal border
- **Pulmonary valve:** Left second intercostal space, left-upper sternal border
- **Mitral valve:** Left fifth intercostal space, medial to left midclavicular line
- **Tricuspid valve:** Xiphisternal junction, lower-left sternal border

MITRAL STENOSIS MURMUR

The best way to detect a **mitral stenosis murmur** is to have the patient roll slightly onto their left side (left lateral decubitus position) and use the bell of the stethoscope over the apex. This allows you to easily detect a **loud S1** followed by low-pitched **rumbling sounds** distinctive to mitral stenosis. These sounds can also be brought on during a stress test or exercise. Exertional dyspnea will also be present. Patches of pink-purple discoloration (mitral facies) in the cheek area may occasionally be present; a bounding jugular pulse may also be visualized. The exam should also assess for heart failure, atrial fibrillation, infection, and embolism.

MESENTERIC ISCHEMIA

There are three major arteries feeding the small and large intestines; when one or more develops restricted blood flow, **mesenteric ischemia** results. The stomach and liver may also be affected. This disease is more common in patients older than the age of 60, in smokers, and in those who have coronary artery disease, peripheral vascular disease, high blood pressure, and elevated cholesterol. Other conditions that may contribute to the development of mesenteric ischemia include chronic low blood pressure, congestive heart failure, aortic dissection, coagulation, and blood vessel disorders. Chronic symptoms often begin as vague complaints; acute problems occur suddenly. Symptoms include severe postprandial pain and bloody diarrhea, and in acute cases caused by a clot, vomiting may also be present.

15

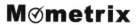

UTERINE FUNDAL HEIGHT DURING NORMAL PREGNANCY

Fundal height is measured from the top of the **pubic bone** to the top of the **uterus**. It's a simple and noninvasive way to help judge the health and growth of the fetus. Variances can indicate a breech or transverse presentation; oligohydramnios, hydramnios, or polyhydramnios; multiple births; or engagement into the pelvis in preparation for birth. Measured in centimeters, **fundal height** should closely correspond to the number of weeks in the pregnancy. The top of the fundus should be palpable above the pubic symphysis at 12 to 15 weeks, at the level of the umbilicus by 20 to 22 weeks, and finally at the level of the xiphisternum by 36 to 38 weeks.

COMMUNICATION REGARDING SEXUAL HISTORY

Be comfortable with your own sexuality, and maintain an objective, nonjudgmental attitude. Clearly specify the **privacy** of information that the patient can expect during and after the interview. Do not assume marital status or orientation. Ask open-ended questions, provide examples that illustrate an acceptance, and signify a "no-wrong-answer" attitude that gives the patient permission to speak freely. Use terms that the patient understands and be clear in your use of terms. **Clarify** any terms the patient uses that might be ambiguous.

HEAVY ALCOHOL USE

Health effects of alcoholism include:

- Anemia and malnutrition (e.g., thiamine and folate deficiency)
- Cancer. Scientists believe that the increased cancer risk is related to the conversion of alcohol into acetaldehyde, a potent carcinogen, in the body. This risk is also increased by smoking. The most common types include mouth, throat, larynx, esophagus, liver, breast, and colorectal.
- Cardiovascular disease, high blood pressure, and abnormal clotting that increase the risk of myocardial infarction or stroke. Atrial flutter can occur with excessive use or withdrawal symptoms.
- Cirrhosis and pancreatitis
- Dementia and other forms of impaired thinking
- Depression
- Seizures, even in the absence of epilepsy. Alcohol can also alter the effectiveness of seizure medications
- Aggravated gout
- Suppressed immune system and nerve damage

COMPREHENSIVE CARDIAC/VASCULAR PATIENT ASSESSMENT

The following are the four basic components of a comprehensive cardiac/vascular patient assessment:

1. **Patient history**: The best source of information about the history of their condition is the patient themselves. Other resources might include past medical records and involved family members.
2. **Physical exam**: Execute a full, head-to-toe and exam including inspection, palpation, percussion, and auscultation methods as appropriate.
3. **Laboratory results**: Typical laboratory tests include cardiac enzymes, clotting function, cholesterol levels, and therapeutic medication levels.
4. **Diagnostic tests**: Diagnostic tests can include x-ray, computed tomography (CT) scan, magnetic resonance imaging (MRI), electrocardiogram (ECG), echocardiography (echo), myocardial perfusion imaging, and cardiac catheterization.

ASSESSMENT OF QUALITIES OF PAIN

The following are qualities of pain that should be assessed in a thorough patient history:

1. **Quality**: Have the patient describe the quality of the pain using words such as *dull, stabbing, sharp, aching, throbbing,* and *burning.*
2. **Severity**: Pain can be rated on a scale of 1 to 10 or by another assessment tool.

3. **Location**: Where on the body is the pain located, and does it radiate or shift?
4. **Timing**: When did the pain begin? Is it constant, or does it come and go with a predictable or random frequency?
5. **Causative factors**: Is the patient able to pinpoint a precipitating event prior to the onset of pain?
6. **Aggravating factors**: Does the quality or severity of pain change with activity, position, stress level, or other varying conditions?
7. **Alleviating factors**: What effects do medications, position, or other noninvasive treatment interventions have on the amount of pain?
8. **Related S/S**: Is the pain accompanied by nausea, dizziness, shortness of breath, or other closely related symptoms?

METHODS OF QUESTIONING TO ENCOURAGE ACCURATE, IN-DEPTH PERSONAL HISTORY

The following are methods of questioning that encourage the patient to give an accurate, in-depth personal history:

- **Encourage open discussion**: Promote patient comfort by encouraging questions and feedback during the interview.
- **Ask open-ended questions**: Ask questions that require more than a "yes" or "no" answer, and give clear permission for the patient to speak freely about their health.
- **Restate and summarize provided information in another way**: This allows you to verify that your understanding of the given information is correct.
- **Focus**: Help the patient to concentrate on identifying their highest healthcare needs or to make connections between healthcare behavior and larger priorities.
- **Order and sequence**: Verify cause and effect and timing of the events given in a patient history.
- **Encourage self-evaluation**: Allow patients to draw their own conclusions regarding information, and do not judge or try to educate at this point.
- **Make observations**: Provide commentary on the patient's physical, mental, and emotional demeanor to help them focus and give permission to discuss further aspects of their health or immediate needs.

CORE PRINCIPLES OF PAIN ASSESSMENT AND MANAGEMENT

All patients have the right to appropriate **assessment and management of pain**. Caregivers should encourage all patients to report their pain and follow through with pain-relieving treatments. Assessments for pain must be appropriate for the individual patient and address all aspects of their pain. Both the patient and family should be included in the assessment process. The most accurate indicator of pain is the **patient's own description**. It is always subjective: The clinician should accept and respect the patient's report of pain. Each person's pain experience is unique and dependent on many contributing factors, such as heredity, energy level, coping skills, and prior experiences. Physiological and behavioral observations should not replace information obtained directly from the patient when it can be communicated. Pain can be present without physiological evidence or cause; pain in such cases should not be immediately assigned to psychological causes. Chronic pain can create an overall lower threshold of tolerance for pain and other stimuli. Unrelieved pain has adverse effects on all aspects of the patient's life.

ORDER OF PROCEDURE FOR PHYSICAL EXAMINATION

The order of procedure for a physical examination is as follows:

- **Inspection**: Visual inspection with the naked eye, and with specialized equipment such as an ophthalmoscope, to view physical features such as height, body mass, skin condition and color, breath frequency and quality, hair distribution, balance, gait, and presence of tremors or physical injuries.
- **Palpation**: Examination by touch for pulses, organ size and location, pain response, temperature, and distinguishable masses.
- **Percussion**: Further touch intervention using the fingers to create sound.

- **Auscultation**: Auditory assessment with and without the assistance of a stethoscope, generally focusing on cardiac, respiratory, and digestive systems. Other useful tools might include the use of Doppler to locate pulses that were difficult to palpate.

This general procedure varies slightly during assessment of the abdomen, placing auscultation before palpation and percussion. Other systems may not require the use of all four examination elements.

DISORDERS ASSOCIATED WITH HISTORY OF SMOKING

The diseases most commonly associated with smoking are **lung cancer** and **chronic obstructive pulmonary disease (COPD)**. Tobacco use is also responsible for an increased risk of mouth, throat, bladder, kidney, liver, stomach, and pancreatic cancers. It decreases blood flow by damaging both peripheral and cerebrovascular vessels, increasing the risk of heart disease, myocardial infarction, and stroke. Respiratory conditions include chronic bronchitis, emphysema, pneumonia, and exacerbation of asthma, as well as respiratory infections and colds. Tobacco use can also cause infertility, miscarriage, stillbirth, and premature and low-birth-weight infants, as well as impotence in men.

MACULAR DEGENERATION

Macular degeneration, also referred to as **age-related macular degeneration (AMD)**, is the leading cause of irreversible vision loss in the patient older than 55 years of age. Risk factors that increase the likelihood of a patient developing AMD include smoking, Caucasian descent, high blood pressure, increased cholesterol levels, and genetics. The **macula**—the most sensitive part of the retina, which provides sharp, central vision—is destroyed. Progression is often very slow and therefore goes undetected for an extended period. If the progression is faster, it is more likely to affect the vision in both eyes. Central vision and the ability to focus on fine detail are lost. This makes it difficult for the patient to drive, recognize facial features, read, or do other close-up work. Therefore, it is important to perform a **fundoscopic exam** (drusen, or yellow deposits, are present early in the disease before any loss of vision) and **visual field testing** on patients during check-ups, especially as they age.

DISORDERS ASSOCIATED WITH OBESITY

A patient who is more than 20% over the highest weight allowance for their height is considered **obese**. In other terms, an adult is considered overweight when their body mass index (BMI) is $25 - 29.9$ kg/m^2. Obesity is defined as a BMI > 30 kg/m^2. Patients with obesity are more at risk—compared to patients within normal weight parameters—for heart disease, high blood pressure, cardiomyopathy, varicose veins, stroke, diabetes, cancer (colon, breast, uterine, kidney and esophageal), gallstones, osteoarthritis, gout, bacterial or fungal skin infections (intertrigo), hirsutism, polycystic ovary syndrome (PCOS), sleep apnea, obesity hypoventilation syndrome, and asthma. These conditions often coexist. **Metabolic syndrome** describes the patient with a grouping of obesity (large abdominal circumference), hypertension, and elevated lipids and blood sugar (fasting blood glucose greater than or equal to 100).

Using Diagnostic and Laboratory Studies

ANION GAP

The anion gap measures the difference between the measured positive cations (Na^+ and K^+) and the measured negative anions (Cl^- and HCO_3^-) in the serum. This gap represents the unmeasured anions in the blood.

$$\text{Anion gap} = (Na^+ + K^+) - (Cl^- + HCO_3^-)$$

Sometimes K^+ is not used in this calculation since its effects are slight. Normal range depends on the lab and is roughly 3–13 mEq/L. **Albumin** is a key unmeasured anion, so the anion gap can be adjusted to reflect this. This is important to consider in the presence of hypoalbuminemia or hyperalbuminemia. The anion gap decreases by 2.5 mEq/L for every 1 g/dL decrease in albumin.

$$\text{Corrected anion gap} = \text{anion gap} + 2.5 \times (\text{normal albumin} - \text{observed albumin})$$

An elevated anion gap usually indicates the presence of **metabolic acidosis**. Also, the anion gap can help determine the cause of metabolic acidosis (anion gap vs. non-anion gap metabolic acidosis).

KOH PREPARATION

Any patient presenting with a scaly rash should undergo a KOH test. A **KOH (potassium hydroxide) preparation** is an inexpensive and noninvasive test used to detect the presence of fungal infections on skin, hair, nails, and vaginal discharge. A minute scraping from the infected area is placed on a microscope slide with KOH and the solvent dimethyl sulfoxide (DMSO). Skin cells will be quickly dissolved, leaving behind only fungal cells that appear as thin branching structures (septate hyphae).

HYDROGEN BREATH TEST

Excess **hydrogen** is produced by intestinal bacteria when there is an overabundance of undigested sugars and carbohydrates present in the small intestine. This hydrogen passes through the small intestine into the main blood supply and then to the lungs to be excreted during exhalation. This excess amount can be measured as a convenient and reliable method to diagnose lactase deficiency, lactose intolerance, bacterial overgrowth in the small intestine, or abnormal rate of digestion. The patient is asked to fast for 12 hours prior to the testing. An initial breath sample is taken by having the patient blow into a balloon. A small amount of sugar is then administered, and the hydrogen levels on the breath are then measured at intervals of 15 minutes for up to 5 hours. Any increase in hydrogen production means that there is a problem with the sugar digestion. An extremely rapid increase may indicate food is traveling through the small intestine too quickly; two separate spikes in hydrogen production may indicate a bacterial infection of the small intestine.

PERTUSSIS

Testing procedures differ between private clinical and public health settings. For the private clinic, the goal is to rapidly diagnose and treat any patient who may be at risk. The **polymerase chain reaction (PCR)** is a rapid method of diagnosis that detects the presence of the DNA sequences particular to *Bordetella pertussis* bacteria without requiring the presence of live bacteria, but still takes 2 days for results. At a public health level, more discrimination against false positives is required by using a culture (gold standard). Typically, both PCR and culture are ordered. Best results are obtained when samples are collected within the first 2 weeks of signs and symptoms (cough) appearing, and testing must be performed before antibiotic treatment begins. Nasopharyngeal swabs or nasal aspirate of mucus is obtained for either PCR or culture (must use proper media). Proper sample collection technique is key. Cultures should be started within 24 hours after collection, and all mucus should be disposed of properly. Culture results take 1–2 weeks. Negative results do not rule out pertussis.

SYPHILIS

Direct visualization of *Treponema pallidum* is possible by preparing a slide from a specimen taken from the suspect lesion. It is then viewed with direct darkfield microscopy, immunofluorescence, immunoperoxidase, or silver staining. Serologic tests include nontreponemal and treponemal tests. The nontreponemal test—also called the Venereal Disease Research Laboratory (VDRL) test—is best for testing for **secondary syphilis**. Specific treponemal testing—the fluorescent treponemal antibody absorption (FTA-ABS) test—can be used for diagnosing **secondary and tertiary syphilis**. Pregnant women, men in same-sex relationships, those infected with HIV, and those with partners testing positive for the disease should be screened for syphilis. Cases of syphilis are reported in every state and tracked by the Centers for Disease Control (CDC).

HYPOTHYROIDISM

The older woman presenting with fatigue, dry skin, constipation, and/or a hoarse voice should be screened for **hypothyroidism**. Thyroid-stimulating hormone (TSH) is the most sensitive test. A high TSH result (4.0 and above) is indicative of a thyroid with reduced function. Other laboratory workups might include triiodothyronine, thyroxine, triiodothyronine uptake, thyroxine-binding globulin, and anti-thyroid peroxidase

19

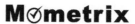

(anti-TPO). Ultrasound of the thyroid may also be considered. Infertility, pregnancy, and mental and cardiac health also require a higher level of monitoring.

SPIROMETRY

Spirometry is an inexpensive and rapid way of assessing the extent and severity of airway obstruction that is causing a patient with asthma, chronic obstructive pulmonary disease (COPD), bronchitis, emphysema, or pulmonary fibrosis to be unable to expire as forcefully or as quickly as a healthy person. These measurements are taken at the time of initial diagnosis and are then monitored periodically to track disease progression. The severity of the breathing restriction is indicated by **decreased forced expiratory volume (FEV1)**, a measure of the amount of air expelled in a single second; **decreased forced vital capacity (FVC)**, a measure of the largest amount of air you are able to expel; and a **decreased FEV1/FVC ratio**. Measurements may also be reevaluated 15 minutes after administration of an inhaled bronchodilator to assess its specific effectiveness.

DIAGNOSTIC STUDIES FOR SUSPECTED PULMONARY EMBOLISM

While the best test may be the pulmonary angiogram, it carries more expense and risk than other options that may be considered first. X-ray cannot diagnose **pulmonary embolism**, but it can rule out other disorders with similar symptoms. Lung scan measures blood flow in the lungs in the nonsmoker. Computed tomography (CT) scan and CT angiography can provide great accuracy in visualizing the lung field. Magnetic resonance imaging (MRI) has even greater accuracy with a comparable raise in expense, but without the effects of the contrast dye used in the CT scan. Ultrasound pulses and echocardiogram may also be helpful, as well as a D-dimer blood test to help detect the clot.

CYSTIC FIBROSIS DIAGNOSIS

Cystic fibrosis is an autosomal recessive disease with mutation of chromosome 7. This particular chromosome is responsible for the transport of chloride across membranes. Failure to move chloride appropriately results in increased lung secretions and eventual fibroid and cyst formation. The immunoreactive trypsinogen (IRT) blood test is a standard screening procedure for newborns. High IRT test results warrant further testing through the sweat chloride test, the industry standard diagnostic test. X-ray and CT scan show tubular, air-filled pockets, normally in the upper lobes of the lungs. Lung, pancreas, and intestinal function tests and a fecal fat test may also be ordered and monitored.

HOLTER MONITOR

A Holter monitor is worn continuously for 24 to 48 hours. This is helpful when a regular, brief electrocardiogram (ECG) has not shown any abnormalities, but the patient is presenting with symptoms such as pain, dizziness, palpitations, or a change of consciousness that could still be cardiac health related. While a Holter monitor does allow for an extended view and perspective on heart health, it is also partially dependent on accurate reporting/journaling on the part of the patient while wearing the monitor. It may also be a little bothersome to the patient, and they will not be able to shower or bathe until the monitor is removed at the end of testing.

CLOSTRIDIOIDES DIFFICILE INFECTION

Clostridioides difficile (*C. diff*) is a gram-positive, anaerobic, spore-forming bacillus that causes diarrhea and colitis. The proliferation of *C. diff* is usually the result of antibiotic therapy and is seen most often in the elderly patient. There can be an extended period of time (weeks to even months) before the patient shows signs and symptoms of the infection. The bacteria release toxins that increase mucosal inflammation and damage to the colon. The patient presents with frequent diarrhea and abdominal discomfort. In advanced cases, fever, nausea, dehydration, weight loss, and blood or pus in the stool will also be present. If symptoms are severe or persistent, they may need to be treated with metronidazole (first choice) or vancomycin.

IMAGING FINDINGS IN RHEUMATIC HEART DISEASE

Rheumatic heart disease, caused by a streptococcal infection (generally in children), most frequently affects the mitral valve, causing stenosis and regurgitation. **Stenosis** is created by inflammation of the valve leaflets, fibrin deposits on the cusps, fusion of leaflet adhesions (commissures), and formation of the classic "fish-mouth deformity" to the valve. X-ray, computed tomography (CT), and magnetic resonance imaging (MRI) will show edema or inflammation in the acute phase, calcifications, cardiomegaly, specific chamber enlargements in established disease, and in severe cases pericardial effusion and alveolar hemorrhage.

FRACTURE TYPES AND SALTER-HARRIS CLASSIFICATION

Types of fractures include:

- **Avulsion**: bone fragment pulled away by a ligament or tendon
- **Torus (buckle)**: compression of two bones
- **Comminuted**: bone in many pieces
- **Complete**: fracture continues all the way across the bone
- **Incomplete**: fracture does not go all the way across the bone
- **Compound (open)**: bone breaks through skin
- **Simple (closed)**: a non-displaced fracture; it's aligned
- **Displaced**: fracture ends are not lined up
- **Greenstick**: bone is bent/partially fractured
- **Stress**: hairline fracture from repetitive force

Salter-Harris classification for epiphyseal fractures (growth plate):

- **Type I**: a fracture that follows along the epiphyseal plate (growth plate)
- **Type II**: an epiphyseal plate fracture that continues into the metaphysis, causing a metaphyseal fragment
- **Type III**: an epiphyseal plate fracture that extends through the epiphysis (articular surface)
- **Type IV**: an epiphyseal plate fracture that extends through the epiphysis and metaphysis
- **Type V**: a compression fracture of the epiphyseal plate

CT SCAN

A **computed tomography** (CT) scan is a more detailed and intricate series of x-rays that allow for examination of bones and soft tissues. While there are often more cost-effective screening methods, CT scan is the first choice in the presence of a head injury. Other uses might include diagnosing muscle and bone disorders, internal injuries, and bleeding. It can also detect and monitor tumors, infection, blood clots, and heart and lung disease. A CT scan is not recommended in the pregnant patient. CT creates radiation exposure and creates a risk of an allergic reaction to any contrast used.

ELECTROCARDIOGRAM

Electrocardiography, or the electrocardiogram (**ECG**), is the study of electrical impulses through the heart. Correct placement of the 12 monitor leads must be executed in order to receive accurate results. Leads are divided into three divisions:

- **Limb leads**: leads I, II, and III.
- **Augmented leads**: aVR, aVL, and aVF.
- **Precordial leads**: V1 to V6.
  - V1 is placed at the fourth intercostal space, to the right of the sternum.
  - V2 is also in the fourth intercostal space, to the left of the sternum.
  - V3 is located directly between V2 and V4.
  - V4 is placed in the fifth intercostal space at the midclavicular line.

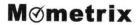

- o   V5 is also in the fifth intercostal space at the anterior axillary line directly between V4 and V6.
- o   V6 is also in the fifth intercostal space at the midaxillary line.

Additional leads are placed on each limb.

> **Review Video: EKG Rhythms - Reading the Graph**
> Visit mometrix.com/academy and enter code: 872282
>
> **Review Video: EKG Interpretation: Atrial Fibrillation and Atrial Flutter**
> Visit mometrix.com/academy and enter code: 263842

CBC

Normal diagnostic ranges of a **complete blood count** (CBC) are as follows:

- **White blood cells**: $4,500 - 11,000/mm^3$
- **Red blood cells**:
  - o   Males: $4.3 - 5.9$ million/mm^3
  - o   Females: $3.5 - 5.5$ million/mm^3
- **Hemoglobin**: Carries oxygen and is decreased in anemia and increased in polycythemia. Normal values:
  - o   Males >18 years: $14.0 - 17.46$ g/dL
  - o   Females >18 years: $12.0 - 16.0$ g/dL
- **Hematocrit**: Indicates the proportion of red blood cells (RBCs) in a liter of blood (usually about 3 times the hemoglobin number). Normal values:
  - o   Males >18 years: $45 - 52\%$
  - o   Females >18 years: $36 - 48\%$
- **Mean corpuscular volume (MCV)**: Indicates the size of RBCs. Normal values:
  - o   Males >18 years: $84 - 96 \ \mu m^3$
  - o   Females >18 years: $76 - 96 \ \mu m^3$
- **Mean corpuscular hemoglobin (MCH)**: $25.4 - 34.6$ pg/cell
- **Mean corpuscular hemoglobin concentration (MCHC)**: $31 - 36\%$ Hb/cell
- **Platelets**: $150,000 - 400,000/mm^3$

RISKS ASSOCIATED WITH ENDOSCOPY

A patient consenting to endoscopy needs to be aware of the **risks** of an adverse reaction to the sedation used, arrhythmia, infection, pain, bleeding, or perforation. **Upper endoscopy**—also called esophagogastroduodenoscopy (EGD)—can also lead to aspiration or respiratory depression. **Lower endoscopy** (colonoscopy, sigmoidoscopy, and enteroscopy) can cause dehydration and an uncomfortable bloating from the gases used during exploration and polyp removal. These risks are greater in those with preexisting conditions such as lung, liver, or cardiac disease. A thorough history and screening for potential problems should be completed, and prophylactic intravenous fluids and antibiotics should be considered.

CLEAN-CATCH URINE SPECIMEN

The following are the instructions that should be given to a patient on how to gather a **clean-catch urine specimen**:

- Begin with clean hands.
- For females, instruct them to sit on the toilet and spread apart the labia with two fingers. They should then gently cleanse the inner labia, from front to back, twice. Continue to hold open the labia, then begin urinating. Stop the urine flow and hold the collection container a few inches away from the urethra before beginning the stream of urine again. Only a few inches of urine need to be collected in the specimen cup. Cover and label the specimen clearly.
- For males, instruct them to clean the head of the penis. Retract the foreskin as needed and begin cleaning at the urethral opening, and continue down and away from the head of the penis. Begin urinating. Stop the urine flow, and hold the collection container a few inches away from the penis before beginning the stream of urine again. Only a few inches of urine need to be collected in the specimen cup. Cover and label the specimen clearly.

PATHOPHYSIOLOGICAL MECHANISMS OF DYSPNEA

The **vascular bed** begins to decrease from thromboemboli, tumor emboli, vascular obstruction, radiation, chemotherapy toxicity, or concomitant emphysema. As the vascular bed decreases, the physiological dead space causes **increased ventilation demands**. This results in hypoxemia and severe deconditioning with metabolic acidosis, alterations in carbon dioxide output (VCO_2), and arterial partial pressure of carbon dioxide (PCO_2). This also increases neural reflex activity, anxiety, and depression. Inspiratory muscle weakness from cachexia, electrolyte imbalances, neuromuscular abnormalities and steroid use, pleural or parenchymal disease, reduced chest wall compliance, and airway obstruction (such as asthma, tumor growth, and COPD) can produce impaired mechanical responses and ventilatory pump impairment.

CK RESULTS FOLLOWING MI

The expected pattern of **creatine kinase** (CK) results in the hours and days following a **myocardial infarction** (MI) are as follows:

- CK and CK-MB levels are evaluated every 6 to 8 hours in a suspected myocardial injury. Total CK and CK-MB (specific to cardiac cells) initially rise within the first 4 to 6 hours of an MI. A normal range would be 30 IU/L to 180 IU/L for CK, and CK-MB totaling 0% to 5% of the CK level.
- Assuming no further damage is sustained, peak levels (in excess of six times the normal range) are reached between 12 to 24 hours after the injury.
- CK levels will return to normal within 3 to 4 days of the event.
- Small spikes in CK level might also occur following invasive cardiac procedures.

HYPERKALEMIA

A normal **potassium level** is between 3.5 and 5 mEq/L. Elevated potassium, or **hyperkalemia**, is normally classified as a level greater than 6 mEq/L. It is possible to see a false-high potassium level if the blood cells rupture during or after the lab draw. Hyperkalemia is caused by renal disease, adrenal insufficiency, metabolic acidosis, severe dehydration, burns, hemolysis, and trauma. It rarely occurs in the absence of renal disease but may be induced by drugs such as NSAIDs and potassium-sparing diuretics. Untreated renal failure results in reduced excretion of potassium. Patients with Addison's disease and deficient adrenal hormone levels experience a sodium loss that results in potassium retention. Along with elevated blood potassium levels, the electrocardiogram will show peaked T waves, flattened P waves, prolonged PR interval, and wide QRS complexes. The patient may also complain of muscle fatigue, weakness, partial paralysis, or nausea.

SLEEP STUDIES

Sleep study options include the polysomnogram (PSG), multiple sleep latency test (MSLT), maintenance of wakefulness test (MWT), actigraphy, and home-based portable monitoring devices. The **PSG test** requires an overnight sleep center visit. It monitors bodily functions (electroencephalogram, heart rate, respirations, oxygen level) during sleep in order to identify and properly diagnose sleep-related disorders such as sleep apnea, restless leg syndrome (RLS), and related conditions such as sleep-triggered seizures. **Home-based monitoring** may be an abbreviated option for extensive PSG studies. The **MSLT** and **MWT** are daytime measurements of wakefulness. **Actigraphy** is a portable, continuous monitoring system of activity levels and sleep patterns. Sleep studies may be considered if a patient mentions having trouble falling asleep or staying asleep, snores, or complains of extreme tiredness and fatigue during most waking hours.

INITIAL TESTING FOR SHOCK

Shock can be classified into several causative categories: hypovolemic, hemorrhagic, cardiogenic, neurogenic, glycemic (hypo- or hyper-), and anaphylactic. **Shock** is treated as an emergency situation, with the highest priority going toward assessing and maintaining the ABCs (airway, breathing, circulation). While some necessary additional information may vary depending on whether or not the type of shock is known, other information is universally gathered. This testing includes vital signs, electrolytes, glucose, ABGs (arterial blood gases), urinalysis, serum creatinine, CBC, blood type and match, coagulation studies, pulse oximetry, and blood gases. Blood lactate, BUN (blood urea nitrogen) and creatinine, ionized calcium, C-reactive protein, cultures (when indicated), total bilirubin, and alanine aminotransferase may also be useful to assess **septic shock**. Chest x-ray may be useful in patients with **hypovolemic shock** who do not show improvement after being given fluids. In **hypovolemic shock with possible hemorrhage**, PT/INR and focused assessment with sonography for trauma are useful as well. In patients with **cardiogenic shock**, ECG and possible echo are useful in diagnosis.

WBC COUNT AND DIFFERENTIAL

White blood cell (leukocyte) count is used as an indicator of bacterial and viral infection. WBC is reported as the total number of all white blood cells.

- Normal WBC for adults: 4,800–10,000
- Acute infection: 10,000+, with 30,000 indicating a severe infection
- Viral infection: 4,000 and below

The **differential** provides the percentage of each different type of leukocyte. An increase in the white blood cell count is usually related to an increase in one type, and often an increase in immature neutrophils, known as bands. This is referred to as a "shift to the left," an indication of an infectious process.

- Immature neutrophils (bands):
  - Normal: 1–3%
  - Changes: Increase with infection
- Segmented neutrophils (segs):
  - Normal: 50–62%
  - Changes: Increase with acute, localized, or systemic bacterial infections
- Eosinophils:
  - Normal: 0–3%
  - Changes: Decrease with stress and acute infection
- Basophils:
  - Normal: 0–1%
  - Changes: Decrease during acute stage of infection
- Lymphocytes:

- o Normal: 25–40%
- o Changes: Increase in some viral and bacterial infections
- Monocytes:
  - o Normal: 3–7%
  - o Changes: Increase during recovery stage of acute infection

Formulating Most Likely Diagnosis

RIGHT- AND LEFT-SIDED HEART FAILURE

Right-sided heart failure (**cor pulmonale**) generally results from long-term high blood pressure or chronic lung disease, such as chronic obstructive pulmonary disease (COPD). It is a failure of the right side of the heart to efficiently retrieve blood from the body, and it causes fluid retention. Symptoms can include an activity-dependent altered level of consciousness, complaints of chest pain or discomfort, dependent edema, and altered breathing state (wheezing or cough). Patients may also present with ascites, gastrointestinal complaints, cyanosis, swollen liver, abnormal heart sounds, and neck vein distension. Right-sided heart failure can also result from preexisting left-sided heart failure.

Left-sided heart failure is a result of a dysfunction in the heart's ability to pump blood to the rest of the body correctly (the responsibility of the left ventricle). This causes fluid retention in the lungs (pulmonary edema). The patient may present with cardiomegaly and marked dyspnea.

Cor Pumonale

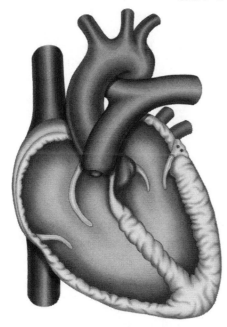 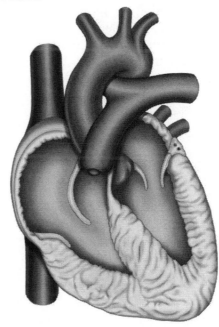

Normal   Right Ventricular Hypertrophy

PARONYCHIA AND HERPETIC WHITLOW

Herpetic whitlow can form tiny pustules resembling blisters (clear fluid), and their location is further away from the nail bed than paronychia lesions (deeper yellow-green abscess). **Herpetic whitlow** often affects more than one finger at a time; **paronychia** is generally focused on one nail bed. Paronychia is caused by fungus or bacteria, with complete resolution with treatment. Herpetic whitlow is a herpes simplex viral infection, which

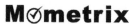

will remain dormant in the body. Herpetic whitlow is not treated by draining the infected area as paronychia often is; herpetic whitlow will often resolve itself.

APHTHOUS ULCERS AND ORAL HERPES

Aphthous ulcers (also known as **canker sores**) are small, shallow, round or oval lesions occurring inside the mouth. Canker sores are not contagious and are more likely to be the result of injury to the area, malnutrition, or stress. **Cold sores (oral herpes)** most often occur on the lips, have a more blister-like appearance, and are highly contagious. Only oral herpes is caused by the herpes virus, which lies dormant within the body and manifests during times of illness or high stress levels. Both conditions can be painful and create difficulties eating, drinking, and talking. Both types of lesions will heal on their own within two weeks.

TYPES OF TRANSPLANT REJECTION

Hyperacute rejection occurs within minutes to hours of the transplant. This type of reaction occurs when the donated tissue (or blood cells) has not been properly matched to the new host. **Acute rejection** happens within days and up to three months after transplant. Acute rejection is the most common form. Most patients will experience at least some degree of acute rejection, and this is the primary focus of immunosuppressive medication regimes. **Chronic rejection** occurs after four months and up to years after the transplant, after a slow and constant fight by the body against the tissue that is foreign to the system.

VIRAL AND BACTERIAL MENINGITIS

Viral meningitis: There are approximately 10,000 cases of viral meningitis in the US each year, and this is the most common form of meningitis. It is most common in those younger than five years old or those with compromised immune systems. This most commonly results from infection with enteroviruses, arboviruses, and type 2 herpes simplex virus. The virus is transmitted through contact with an infected person through saliva, sputum, mucus, or fecal matter; however, only a small percentage of those infected actually contract meningitis. Patients may present with fever, nausea/vomiting, light sensitivity, head and neck pain, and a change in mental status. LP (lumbar puncture) shows normal opening pressure, elevated WBC, normal or slightly reduced glucose, normal or slightly elevated protein. Viral meningitis will often run its course without medical intervention other than monitoring fluids and using universal precautions. Complications include seizures, hearing loss, brain damage, kidney failure, and death.

Bacterial meningitis: Approximately 4,000 cases of bacterial meningitis occur yearly within the United States, resulting in 500 deaths each year. Even in the presence of recovery, there are often lasting consequences of the disease, including brain damage, hearing damage, and learning disabilities. Leading causes include *Streptococcus* strains, *Neisseria meningitidis* (meningococcal; most common in 16- to 23-year-olds), *Haemophilus influenzae*, and *Listeria monocytogenes*. Contamination results from contact with bacterial-infected saliva, sputum, and mucus. The patient may present with fever, nausea, vomiting, light sensitivity, head and neck pain, and a change in mental status. LP shows a high opening pressure, elevated WBC, decreased glucose, elevated protein. Immediate treatment with antibiotics is needed. Prevention through vaccination is key.

ANGINA PECTORIS AND MYOCARDIAL INFARCTION

Angina pectoris often serves as a warning sign for myocardial infarction. **Angina** is chest pain occurring from reduced blood flow to the myocardium. **Stable angina** is described as squeezing, pressure, or burning, and is focused on the chest cavity. It is intermittent, often correlating with increased activity and dissipating with rest and/or the use of nitroglycerin. **Unstable angina** will present with the above symptoms, but the symptoms do not abate with rest or medication. **Myocardial infarction** occurs when the lack of oxygen perfusion to the heart causes myocardial tissue death. This pain is more extreme, often referred to as crushing, and it extends beyond the chest to radiate out toward the back, shoulder, neck, and jaw. Rest and nitroglycerin will have no effect on this type of pain. Initial treatments will include oxygen, reperfusion, and medications (nitrates, β-blockers, antiplatelets, anticoagulants). Morphine can be given for extreme pain control. In an ST-elevated myocardial infarction (STEMI), an electrocardiogram will show ST changes and laboratory results will show elevated troponin and creatinine levels. Unstable angina and a non-ST elevated MI (NSTEMI) may present very similarly in pain and other factors, but can primarily be differentiated by the elevation of cardiac biomarkers that will be present in an MI.

IRRITABLE BOWEL SYNDROME AND INFLAMMATORY BOWEL DISEASE

Irritable bowel syndrome (**IBS**) is the most common intestinal disorder in America. It does not affect the actual tissue of the bowel, although there may occasionally be an infection present. The cause is unknown, and it occurs in women more than men. The patient may present with complaints of abdominal pain, cramping, bloating, and changes in bowel habits. **Inflammatory bowel disease (IBD)** is an actual inflammation or abnormality of the bowel caused by an immune response, such as Crohn's disease or ulcerative colitis. The initial cause is also unknown. Symptoms may include fever, stomach cramps, and bloody diarrhea. Joints, eyes, skin, and liver may also show signs of the disease, and it increases the patient's risk for colon cancer.

GONORRHEA AND CHLAMYDIA

Gonorrhea is a bacterial infection (gram-negative diplococci) caused by *Neisseria gonorrhoeae* and is spread through oral, vaginal, penile, or anal contact. Symptoms may appear within 1 day of exposure or can be delayed up to a month in men. Females are usually asymptomatic, but may have vaginal discharge, dysuria, dyspareunia, infertility, and symptoms of pelvic inflammatory disease (PID). Males may be asymptomatic but usually seek help for penile discharge and may also have pain and epididymitis. Gonorrhea and chlamydia coexist in up to 50% of cases. Diagnosis is made by cervical or urethral culture or NAAT (nucleic acid amplification test). Treatment consists of ceftriaxone 250 mg IM in 1 dose AND azithromycin 1 g PO in 1 dose; **OR**, if ceftriaxone is not available: cefixime 400 mg PO in 1 dose AND azithromycin 1 g PO in 1 dose. Diagnose and treat sexual partners. Report STDs to the CDC through the local health department.

Chlamydia is an STD caused by the bacteria *Chlamydia trachomatis* and is the most common STD in the United States. It is very common to be asymptomatic and incubation is usually 1–3 weeks. Signs and symptoms in males are urethritis, epididymitis, or proctitis. Females may experience mild cervicitis with vaginal discharge and dysuria, but it can lead to pelvic inflammatory disease and infertility. Reactive arthritis (also called Reiter syndrome: urethritis, conjunctivitis, arthritis) has been associated with chlamydia infection. Diagnosis is by cervical, vaginal, or penile swab or first-catch urine using NAAT. Treatment includes azithromycin 1 g PO in 1 dose **OR** doxycycline 100 mg PO bid for 7 days. Avoid sexual contact for 1 week after symptoms resolve. Treatment of the patient's sexual partner is critical to avoid reinfection. Report to the health department.

MIGRAINE AND CLUSTER HEADACHES

A **migraine** is classified as a throbbing headache accompanied by nausea, vomiting, photophobia, and sensitivity to sound that can last for hours or days. The headache may be preceded by a sensory warning, an aura, a smell, a change in vision, or a sensation on the skin. Each patient's sensory warning is unique. There may also be other subtle changes in bowel habits, mental outlook, appetite, and mood in the day or two prior to each episode. Migraines are more common in women.

Cluster headaches are so named because of their tendency to occur in "clusters." Attacks will happen frequently over a few weeks or months and then go into a remission period. There is no defining aura or warning sign of pending attacks. The patient is often awakened in the night to pain on one side of their head. Cluster headaches are more common in men.

ADL ASSESSMENT TOOLS

All of these assessment tools are used to help determine a patient's overall ability to function in general **activities of daily living (ADLs)** and review the patient's ease in meeting their own needs.

- The **Karnofsky Performance Scale (KPS)** is a 0 to 100 scale rating the patient's success in completing their own ADLs. Higher scores indicate higher levels of competence, with 100 representing full ability without patient complaint. As the numbers decrease, the patient's need for outside help with ADLs increases.
- **Eastern Cooperative Oncology Group (ECOG) Performance Status** uses a 0 to 5 scale as a correlation between the patient's disease process and its effects on their own ADL competencies. Lower numbers indicate a lower level of restriction related to the disease process.
- The **Palliative Performance Scale (PPSv2)** rates the patient's abilities in five areas: ambulation, activity and current disease manifestations, self-care, nutritional intake, and level of consciousness. These are rated as a percentage that correlates to their success in these functions.

CIRRHOSIS OF THE LIVER

When toxins, inflammation, or metabolic changes within the liver create nodules and fibrosis, **cirrhosis** is the resulting condition. Cirrhosis of the liver is incurable, although in some cases a liver transplant might be considered as an option. The nodules and fibroids interfere with blood flow through the liver, which can cause blood to back up in the spleen. When blood pools within the spleen, it becomes enlarged and blood platelet counts fall. Cirrhosis can also cause gastric and esophageal varices. If not treated, these varices can rupture and bleed, which can result in death. Abdominal ascites and peripheral edema often result from the blood flow restrictions as well. The patient begins to exhibit jaundice in the eyes and then in the skin. Rectal hemorrhoids are also common. Hormonal, metabolic, and kidney disturbances can also result from cirrhosis.

Treatment varies according to the symptoms, and is supportive rather than curative, as the fibrotic changes in the liver cannot be reversed. Options include abstaining from alcohol use or hepatotoxic drugs. Medications such as prednisone, ursodiol (Actigall), lactulose, and azathioprine (Imuran) can be administered. Diet alterations include low-sodium and low-protein diets with increased vitamin K intake, dietary supplements and vitamins. Other treatments include diuretics (potassium-sparing) such as Aldactone and Dyrenium to decrease ascites, colchicine to reduce fibrotic changes, and liver transplant (the definitive treatment).

DEPRESSION

The depressed patient may present with any number of the following: depressed mood; insomnia or hypersomnia; an absence of pleasure in previously enjoyed activities; psychomotor retardation; fatigue; feelings of worthlessness and guilt; and an inability to concentrate, make decisions, or remember important information. The patient may experience significant and unexplained weight loss or weight gain. In severe cases, they may also disclose recurrent thoughts of death or suicide. Severity is assigned by the presence of an expressed intent with a plan and means to carry out a suicide attempt, as well as previous attempts. The hallmark symptoms of depression are appetite and sleep changes and decreased energy and concentration. However, in the presence of physical illness, these symptoms can be masked or created by the disease process or corresponding treatments. With preexisting illness, the following symptoms may be more reliable indicators of depression: fearfulness, depressed or changed appearance, social withdrawal, brooding, self-pity and pessimism, and a depressed mood or affect that cannot be changed or lifted.

MEDICAL CONDITIONS ASSOCIATED WITH DEPRESSION

Patients experiencing depression have a greater tendency toward **medical illnesses** and vice versa. Underlying causes and links may be found in multiple areas of the assessment. Patients with cardiovascular disease, congestive heart failure, arrhythmias, and heart attacks are prone to a higher incidence of depression. Patients with the following central nervous system conditions are at increased risk: cerebrovascular anoxia or accident, Huntington disease, subdural hematoma, Alzheimer disease and dementia, human immunodeficiency virus (HIV) infection, carotid stenosis, temporal lobe epilepsy, multiple sclerosis, post-concussion syndrome,

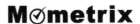

myasthenia gravis, narcolepsy, and subarachnoid hemorrhage. Other causes can include rheumatoid arthritis, thyroid disease, diabetes, Cushing disease, Addison's disease, anemia, lupus, liver disease, syphilis, encephalitis, alcoholism, and general malnutrition.

ANXIETY

Anxiety is marked by feelings of excessive worry, irritability, restlessness, intense feelings of danger, and agitation. The source of the disquiet is unknown or very vague. The patient may have trouble falling or staying asleep and experience interference with other normal activities in their daily life. **Physically**, the patient may be identified as having frequent crying spells, headaches, muscle tension, stomach and intestinal distress, palpitations, shortness of breath, anorexia, or overeating. **Psychologically**, the patient is vulnerable to unrealistic fears, obsessions with harmful ideas, and compulsions. Patients may also try to self-medicate with multiple chemicals or substances in attempts to alleviate any of these symptoms. An **anxiety disorder** is identified by the persistence of these symptoms over a period of six months or more.

Health Maintenance, Patient Education, and Preventive Measures

MANAGEMENT OF HYPERTRIGLYCERIDEMIA

Hypertriglyceridemia is a major health concern in the US. The main goal of any dietary changes should focus on weight loss because, in the absence of other causative diseases, weight is often directly connected to the **triglyceride level**. A recommendation to **limit total fat intake** to 10% of the daily calorie consumption, and to introduce exercise, can often be made. Careful examination of the total LDL and HDL cholesterol levels will help with fine-tuning dietary and exercise recommendations. Testing should also be done to rule out metabolic syndrome. Medication supplements such as statins, fibrates, niacin, and fish oil can also assist in the preventative and recovery process. A referral to a lipidologist or endocrinologist may be needed.

DIET FOR PHENYLKETONURIA

Phenylketonuria (**PKU**) causes a buildup of the amino acid phenylalanine (found in protein-based foods) in the blood. Therefore, the main focus of diet recommendations for PKU is on **restricting protein intake**. General diet restrictions include avoiding milk, eggs, cheese, nuts, beans, soy, chicken, beef, pork, fish, peas, beer, chocolate, and foods containing aspartame. Limits on fruits, vegetables, and simple carbohydrates (starches) are also common. Diet, growth, and blood levels of phenylalanine will need to be frequently monitored in order to make adjustments in the individual patient's dietary needs. Pegvaliase is a new option for adults and is the first enzyme substitute to be released by the FDA (in 2018).

FECAL IMPACTION

Fecal impaction happens when it becomes impossible for a hard, dry portion of stool to pass through the rectum. This most often occurs in a patient experiencing chronic constipation who has been using laxatives for extended periods of time, then stops suddenly. The muscles of the intestines and colon have atrophied and can no longer move stool without assistance. Other risk factors include immobility and side effects from medications such as anticholinergics, antidiarrheal agents, and pain medications with methadone or codeine. Treatment options may include manual extraction, suppositories, or surgery. Preventative maintenance includes diet and activity modifications and setting specific parameters for laxatives and stool softeners.

COMMON HEALTH SCREENINGS FOR ADULT FEMALES

Although clinical judgment should be used to decide how many, and which, screenings should be focused on for the individual patient, there are common **health screenings** that should be almost universally provided. Interview questions should include tobacco, alcohol, and recreational drug use; personal safety and abuse; mental health; and personal health beliefs and practices, including any alternative health treatments the patient is pursuing. Physical and laboratory assessments should cover hypertension; vision; skin, colon, rectal, cervical, and breast cancer screenings; cholesterol; and chlamydia and other sexually transmitted diseases.

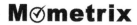

DIETARY CONSIDERATIONS FOR GOUT

Treatment for acute episodes includes monitoring water and food intake and medications (pain reliever and anti-inflammatory agents). **Gout** can be exacerbated by obesity, high blood pressure, impaired kidney function, alcohol, fructose and corn syrup, dehydration, illness, and fever or injury. Long-term control depends on adequate hydration, weight loss, dietary restrictions (avoidance of grain alcohol, shellfish, organs, and sweets), aerobic exercise, and medications (probenecid, sulfinpyrazone, allopurinol, and febuxostat) to help lower uric acid levels. When medication is being given to control uric acid, monitoring levels through blood testing is essential to find and maintain optimal treatment levels. Reducing purine ingestion can reduce uric acid levels by up to 1 mg/mL. This may help decrease the number of flare-ups. **Purines** are amino acid and are therefore found in protein-containing food. Since proteins are necessary for metabolism, patients should not avoid all proteins, but should try decreasing those foods highest in purines, including: sweetbreads (highest), organ meats, sardines, mackerel, anchovies, mussels, shrimp, and lobster.

SOMOGYI EFFECT

In the diabetic, the **Somogyi effect** is the body's tendency to overreact to low blood sugar levels. This overcompensation—in which glucagon and epinephrine communicate to the liver to convert glycogen stores into readily available glucose—creates a new spike in the blood sugar. This phenomenon most often occurs as a result of nighttime hypoglycemia that goes untreated. If a patient is consistently awakening with elevated blood glucose levels, they may need to wake up in the middle of the night in order to perform another blood sugar reading. Their evening intake and insulin dose can then be adjusted to prevent further episodes.

MODIFIABLE AND NON-MODIFIABLE RISK FACTORS FOR CARDIOVASCULAR DISEASE

Risk factors that the patient (and their healthcare provider) can exercise some control over are identified as **modifiable**. These can include smoking, excess weight, alcohol use, cholesterol levels, and blood pressure; risk may be reduced by active management of diabetes and stress, and the amount of exercise the patient engages in. Risk factors **beyond the patient's control** include age, male sex, and genetic tendencies including race (Caucasian, black, or Native American) and family history. The greatest risk is to those who have already experienced a cardiovascular event or have been previously diagnosed with a cardiac vascular disease such as peripheral vascular disease, aortic aneurysm, or carotid artery disease. Others with high risk include those who have at least two of the modifiable or non-modifiable risk factors or type 2 diabetes.

MANAGEMENT AND MAINTENANCE OF MAJOR DEPRESSION

Medication and therapy are normally needed in order to begin resolving **major depression**. However, it is important to note the differences in the amount of time it may take for these approaches to work. The patient, especially, needs to understand that their progress may seem slow. **Selective serotonin reuptake inhibitors (SSRIs)** take between 2 and 6 weeks to reach a therapeutic level and should not be adjusted until after that time. **Tricyclic antidepressants (TCAs)** can also take several weeks and carry an increased risk of adverse effects. **Monoamine oxidase inhibitors (MAOIs)** should not be combined with SSRIs. There should be a cleansing period of 4 to 5 weeks between administration of SSRIs and MAOIs. Other treatments that may be considered include light therapy, transcranial magnetic stimulation (TMS), and electroconvulsive therapy (ECT). The patient should also be advised that alcohol and recreational drug use can feed the problem rather than provide the relief they are seeking.

AIDS DEMENTIA COMPLEX (ADC)

The exact cause of AIDS dementia complex (ADC) is unknown, but it is a primary result of the disease process itself. Current theories suggest that the HIV infection stimulates an invasion of **macrophages** in the brain (microglia). These release cytokines that directly damage the nervous tissue by disrupting the neurotransmitter functions and causing encephalopathy. This condition affects as many as 15% of all AIDS patients. Prognosis is poor, and the disease is not reversible. However, retroviral drugs can delay its onset. Central nervous system HIV infections in children tend to have a more dramatic and pronounced effect than those occurring in adults. ADC is characterized by gradual memory loss, decreased concentration and

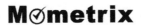

cognition, and mood disorders. The patient may also experience physical symptoms of ataxia, incontinence, and seizures.

OSTEOPOROSIS

Osteoporosis describes bones that have become weak, brittle, and prone to fractures from even mild stress. Early signs and symptoms may include complaints of back pain, diminished height, hunched or stooped posture, and eventual fracture that occurs from what otherwise would have been considered a minor injury. Postmenopausal Caucasian and Asian women carry the greatest risk for developing osteoporosis. Other risk factors include immobilization/sedentary lifestyle, low BMI, reduced dietary intake (calcium, phosphorus, magnesium, vitamin D), a positive family history, previous fragility fracture, and smoking/alcohol use. Diagnosis is made through measuring bone density with dual-energy x-ray absorptiometry (DXA). **DXA screening** for osteoporosis should be performed in all women ≥65 years old, and in those between menopause and 65 years old if risk factors are present. Therapy often includes the prescription of bisphosphonates (alendronate, risedronate, ibandronate, or zoledronic acid). **Hormone replacement therapy (HRT)** after menopause can help prevent osteoporosis. Prevention counseling might also include weight-bearing exercise, smoking cessation, minimal alcohol consumption, and guidance in safe environments and practices to avoid falls.

EDUCATION FOR PATIENTS WITH ACUTE OR CHRONIC ILLNESSES

Education for patients with acute or chronic illnesses should include the following:

- **Diagnosis**: Establish a basic understanding of the disease process, including areas of the body affected, causes, prognosis, and whether or not it is contagious.
- **Complications**: Clarify possible signs and symptoms, early warning signs, and signals of disease progression and healing.
- **Management**: Define what the patient can expect from their care and recovery, including treatments, diet, activity levels, and medications.
- **Aggravating factors**: Help the patient understand what behaviors or triggers may increase their symptoms and what can be done to avoid or control them.
- **Prognosis**: Patients need both an immediate idea of what to expect and a long-term picture of what to expect.
- **Prevention**: Establish self-care habits that can help prevent recurrence of the problem.
- **Resources**: Make sure the patient is informed of all available resources to help them on their healthcare journey.

COMMON HEALTH SCREENINGS FOR ADULT MALES

Though clinical judgment should be used to decide how many, and which, screenings should be focused on for the individual patient, there are **common health screenings** that should be almost universally provided. Interview questions should include tobacco, alcohol, and recreational drug use; personal safety; mental health; and personal health beliefs and practices, including any alternative health treatments the patient is pursuing. Physical and laboratory assessments should cover hypertension; vision; skin, colon, rectal, prostate, and testicular cancer screenings; cholesterol; and chlamydia and other sexually transmitted diseases. **Testicular cancer** usually affects males 15–35 years old and presents as a painless testicular mass that does not transilluminate. Therefore, it is important to encourage monthly self-exams, especially in young men.

CHILDHOOD IMMUNIZATIONS

Childhood immunizations should be administered at the following ages:

Immunization	Birth	1–2 mo.	4 mo.	6 mo.	12–15 mo.	15–18 mo.	2 y.	4–6 y.	11–12 y.	16 y.
Hepatitis B (**Hep B**)	1	2		3						
Rotavirus vaccine (**RV**)		1	2							
RV if RotaTeq		1	2	3						
DTaP		1	2	3		4		5		
Haemophilus influenzae type B (**Hib**) if ActHIB, Hiberix, Pentacel		1	2	3	4					
Hib if PedvaxHIB		1	2		3					
Pneumococcal conjugate vaccine (**PCV**)		1	2	3	4					
Inactivated polio vaccine (**IPV**)		1	2	3				4		
Measles, mumps, rubella (**MMR**)					1			2		
Varicella					1			2		
Hepatitis A (**Hep A**)					1		2*			
Tetanus, diphtheria, acellular pertussis (**Tdap**)									1	
Human papillomavirus (**HPV**)									1**	
Meningococcal A, C, W, Y									1	2

*Give 6–18 months after first dose.   **Give second dose 6–12 months after first dose.

ADULT IMMUNIZATIONS

Adult immunizations should be administered at the following times:

- **Influenza**: Annually
- **Tdap** (one time), then **Td**: Every 10 years
- **Pneumococcal**: ≥65 years old—one dose of Prevnar 13 (PCV13, conjugate vaccine), then Pneumovax 23 (PPSV23, polysaccharide vaccine) 1 year following the PCV13 if immunocompetent; if immunocompromised, may give the PPSV23 8 weeks after the PCV13

32

- **Zoster:** RZV—2 doses, 2–6 months apart if ≥50 years old (give even if previous shingles or previous Zostavax, ZVL). This is preferred, but may give 1 dose of ZVL if ≥60 years old.
- **Check to make sure these are up to date:** MMR, varicella, HPV, Hep A, Hep B, Hib, and meningococcal. (The necessity of these may depend on underlying medical conditions of patients.)

ENVIRONMENTAL FACTORS THAT CAN AFFECT THE SEVERITY OF ASTHMA

Common environmental triggers for **asthma exacerbation** include seasonal allergies created by pollen, weather patterns, mold spores, animal dander, smoke, smog, other odors such as perfumes, and household and cleaning chemicals. Exposure to things such as dust mites during infancy can even be a key factor in the initial development of asthma. Other factors to consider include hormone fluctuations, exercise, foods, and medications used for other conditions (NSAIDs and β-blockers). Any effort made to control or remove known triggers creates positive results for overall lung heath as well as the number of acute asthma attacks.

IMPACTS OF STRESS ON HEALTH

Excessive stress occurs when the body's natural "fight-or-flight" instinct becomes overstimulated. This creates an overload of adrenaline, cortisol, and glucose in the system and reduces the function of body systems not needed for immediate response to a crisis. Stress alters the immune, cardiac, digestive, and reproductive systems. It increases the patient's risk for heart disease, sleep disorders, skin disorders, digestive problems, altered thought processes (including memory and emotion), tobacco, alcohol and drug abuse, obesity, and autoimmune disorders, as well as exacerbating these conditions once they exist.

SIGNS OF ABUSE

Regular **screening for domestic violence** in a healthcare setting is a helpful and inoffensive method of identifying victims. **Abuse** may occur with any gender and at any age and situation, including children, elderly people, women, and even pregnant women. Watch for injuries that do not seem to match the story given; overbearing or overprotective partners who answer for or dominate your interview with the patient; frequent nonspecific complaints, such as headache and stomach, neck, and back pain; insecurity, stammering, or avoidance in giving responses to simple questions; intestinal complaints; and sexually transmitted disease. In the abused adolescent female, the following are more common: tobacco, alcohol, and drug use; decreased school attendance; isolation; and bulimia. History and physical findings must be carefully documented, and it is required that confirmed cases are reported to the appropriate agency (e.g., child protective services, adult protective services, police). Some states also require reporting suspected abuse cases. Rape kits should be collected within 72 hours of the assault for legal purposes. Refer patients to the appropriate community and counseling services.

NATIONAL ENVIRONMENTAL PUBLIC HEALTH TRACKING PROGRAM

The National Environmental Public Health Tracking (**EPHT**) program was designed by the Centers for Disease Control (CDC) in response to a need for a way to accurately record and analyze the correlations between **environmental factors** and **health trends**. The goal is to help find ways to prevent diseases such as poisoning, birth defects, developmental disabilities, cancer, and neurologic and respiratory diseases. Information is gathered through **biomonitoring** (measurements of how much of various chemicals are actually absorbed into the body) from local, state, and federal agencies as well as academic institutions and other nongovernment organizations. The collected data can be accessed through the CDC.

Clinical Intervention

HEALTH BELIEF MODEL

The health belief model is a theory framework that helps define how likely an individual is to make or maintain **positive health choices**. Adherence to any treatment regime is based on the patient's belief that their disease is serious and threatening to their well-being. Action is determined by cues to action, perceived benefits of action, and reduced barriers to action. In order to promote change, the individual's (or group's) core

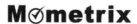

motivations and beliefs must be identified and promoted. It is not a system of negative reinforcement or scare tactics, but a way to promote positive internal attitude changes toward positive health outcomes.

> **Review Video: Diabetes Education: Health Belief Model**
> Visit mometrix.com/academy and enter code: 954833

TREATMENT OPTIONS AND GOALS FOR HYPERTENSION IN DIABETIC PATIENTS

Because of the higher risk for nephropathy, myocardial infarction, and stroke associated with diabetes, it is highly important to adequately treat **hypertension**. The contributors to hypertension in **diabetes** are believed to be diabetic neuropathy, hyperinsulinemia, arterial stiffness, and expansion of extracellular fluid. Antihypertensives in the diabetic patient prevent the progression of kidney disease; lower the risk of MI, stroke, and heart failure; and lower the risk for mortality. The first line of defense is angiotensin-converting enzyme (ACE) inhibitors; the next choice would be angiotensin II receptor blockers (ARBs), although multiple antihypertensives may be needed. Diuretics are often needed as well. The Eighth Joint National Committee suggests that blood pressure in diabetics be kept less than 140/90. Outside of medication, the diabetic patient should be encouraged to keep their blood sugar levels under tight control, lose weight as needed, exercise, and quit smoking. All of these will help mitigate the patient's increased risk for atherosclerosis and high blood pressure.

TREATMENT OPTIONS FOR SEIZURES

The treatment of **epilepsy** attempts to find a balance for the patient between controlling seizures, maintaining a high quality of life, and managing side effects. Because of this, antiepileptic medications are usually not necessary after a single seizure, and will only be used for patients who have risk for recurrent seizures. Selecting the antiepileptic drug should take into account the type of seizures, possible adverse effects of medication, other medical conditions, whether the patient wishes to have children, and other lifestyle and patient factors. **Broad-spectrum seizure medications** control all seizure types: valproate, zonisamide, clobazam, lamotrigine, levetiracetam, and topiramate. **Narrow-spectrum seizure medications** usually work on specific types of seizures: carbamazepine, vigabatrin, ezogabine, gabapentin, phenobarbital, phenytoin, pregabalin, and primidone. A ketogenic diet—a strict diet intended to induce a long-term starvation effect in order to burn ketones—may be tried in the child whose seizures aren't easily controlled by medication. This diet is high in fat and low in carbohydrates, and requires careful monitoring. Alternative medicine includes biofeedback, melatonin (may worsen seizures), and folic acid supplements. Surgery is effective for some medication-refractory focal seizures. Complications include a high risk of mortality due to injury and motor vehicle accidents (MVAs), with seizures and the risk of seizures recurring when medications are tapered or stopped.

SMOKING CESSATION OPTIONS

Nicotine dependence is the most common addiction in the United States. The first intervention is simply to begin a conversation with the patient and assess their interest in quitting and history of quitting attempts. Counseling, behavioral modification therapy, and one-on-one support can be offered from various sources, but medication may be needed. **Nicotine replacement therapy** is safe for most patients. Over-the-counter options include nicotine patches, gum, and candy. Prescription options include nicotine inhalers and nasal spray. Non-nicotine medications that may also be helpful include bupropion SR and varenicline. Bupropion is contraindicated in patients with a history of seizures. Counseling must include the possibility of weight gain and advice about diet and exercise. Clonidine and nortriptyline may be considered, but they are not currently FDA approved and carry many more side effects. The Public Health Service recommends the "5 A's" approach to aid patients with smoking cessation:

- **Asking** about smoking.
- **Advising** on how to approach quitting and setting a date to quit.
- **Assessing** the patient's willingness and readiness to consider quitting.

34

- **Assisting** with counseling as well as pharmacologic aids.
- **Arranging** a follow-up appointment 2 to 4 weeks after the date set for quitting.

The combination of counseling and support groups with drug therapy has a smoking cessation success rate of about 50%.

HDL, LDL, AND TRIGLYCERIDE LEVELS

Hyperlipidemia is defined as an elevation of serum lipid levels. Diagnosis is made by performing a screening lipid profile. A fasting lipid profile is most accurate and should be routinely performed in all adults ≥20 years old every 4–6 years regardless of risk factors, according to the AHA (American Heart Association). Patients should be routinely checked for risk factors throughout their lives. A 10-year risk for heart disease should be calculated. Levels at which to begin treatment depend on individual patient characteristics, including age, sex, and presence of other risk factors for coronary artery disease. In general, **optimal levels** are considered to be:

- LDL <100 mg/dL
- HDL >60 mg/dL
- Triglycerides <150 mg/dL
- Total cholesterol <200 mg/dL
- Cholesterol/HDL ratio <3.5

Low-density lipoprotein (LDL) represents the "bad" cholesterol that is responsible for atherosclerosis. LDL increases heart disease risk. **High-density lipoprotein (HDL)** represents "good" cholesterol that helps to remove buildup from the vessel walls. Higher levels of HDL can help reduce the risk of heart disease. Triglyceride level correlation is still unclear, but elevated levels are linked with an increased risk of heart disease, especially in conjunction with elevated LDL levels.

UNIVERSAL PRECAUTIONS

Universal precautions are designed to promote a reasonable degree of safety for the patient and provider in any caregiving situation. They emphasize acting as if every patient is a carrier of an infectious agent such as hepatitis B or HIV. **Universal precautions** require protective barriers (gloves, gown, mask, and/or goggles) when there is any chance of coming in contact with blood; semen; or vaginal, synovial, spinal, pleural, peritoneal, amniotic, or pericardial fluids.

AIRBORNE, CONTACT, AND DROPLET PRECAUTIONS

Airborne precautions apply to tuberculosis, chicken pox, shingles, and measles. Doors must remain closed, respirators must be worn at all times within the room, and strict hand-washing procedure is observed. **Contact and enteric precautions** apply to cases of antibiotic-resistant infections [methicillin-resistant *Staphylococcus aureus* (MRSA) and vancomycin-resistant enterococci (VRE)], respiratory syncytial virus (RSV), diphtheria, herpes, impetigo, abscesses and skin ulcerations, pediculosis, scabies, staphylococcal furunculosis, zoster, *Clostridioides difficile,* and *Escherichia coli.* Gown and gloves are required within the room, as well as strict hand-washing procedure. **Droplet precautions** apply to meningitis, pneumonia, epiglottitis, pneumonia, bacteremia, group A streptococcal pharyngitis, influenza, scarlet fever, adenovirus, mumps, rubella, and parvovirus B19. These precautions require a simple mask and strict hand-washing procedure.

COMPROMISED STERILE FIELD

A sterile field does not extend below the table or platform it is set up on. **Contamination** can occur if anything below this level comes in contact with the field (such as if the sterile gown below the waist level, or a portion of the sterile drape folding over the edge of the table, touches the field). Hands dropped below the level of the table, arms 3 inches above the wrist, and the back of the sterile gown are also considered contaminated. Sneezing or coughing over the field is contaminating, as is replacing an implement in the field that has been transported out of the field or dropped. Fields that are established on a moist surface are considered

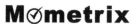

contaminated. So is a field that is left unattended or uncovered, or that one has completely turned away from during a procedure.

DISCHARGE PLANNING

Discharge planning is a formal process that allows care providers to coordinate the individual needs of the patient extending beyond their time in a hospital or long-term-care setting. This assessment process examines how to provide the appropriate care once they no longer meet criteria for hospitalization. Also considered is an understanding of the patient's insurance and benefit coverage to ensure that needed services will be available without unreasonable financial burden. The patient must receive clear and accurate teaching about their condition and about self-care, as well as community resources that will be available to them.

CANCER TREATMENT

There are three main types of cancer treatment available: surgery, radiation, and chemotherapy. These may be used alone or in combination. **Surgery** attempts to remove the entire tumor, as well as surrounding tissues that may have been affected, in order to produce a curative/cancer-free state in the patient. When this is not possible, surgery can be used as a palliative effort to remove as much of the tumor as possible in order to lessen the associated pain and symptoms for the patient. **Radiation therapy** provides localized cancer treatment focusing on the removal of cancer cells before they produce clinical symptoms. Radiation can also be palliative, or used in the treatment of medical emergencies such as spinal cord compression or superior vena cava syndrome. **Chemotherapy** uses medications to target and help destroy cancer cells. This therapy can be used alone, but it is often combined with other treatments for either a curative objective or a palliative focus on symptom and pain control.

COMPLEMENTARY AND ALTERNATIVE MEDICINE

The following are the five main types of complementary and alternative medicine, as defined by the National Center for Complementary and Integrative Health (NCCIH):

- **Biologically based practice**: A focus on the use of naturally occurring substances and diet for health promotion.
- **Energy medicine**: Asian-based energy, magnetic, and biofield beliefs such as Reiki and qigong.
- **Manipulative and body-based practice**: The practice of manipulating body parts or systems as a way to improve or manipulate their performance, such as chiropractic, massage, and reflexology.
- **Mind–body medicine**: A focus on the way mental outlook and belief systems affect health, promoting relaxation and meditation techniques.
- **Whole medical systems**: More conventional medicine working in conjunction and harmony with a specific cultural belief system, such as traditional Chinese medicine.

INTERPERSONAL AND COMMUNICATION SKILLS

The interpersonal and communication skills that are important for quality patient care are:

- The ability to establish a **therapeutic relationship** with appropriate boundaries.
- Effective and tolerant **listening skills**, as well as the ability to correctly interpret nonverbal cues.
- An understanding of open-ended and guided **questions and interview skills**.
- Clear and concise writing and documentation skills.
- Comfort and confidence in **communicating** with individuals from all walks of life.
- Appropriately accommodating messages to optimize **understanding** in the recipient.
- Remaining **level-headed and emotionally stable**, even in disruptive or contentious situations.
- Ability to maintain strict **patient confidentiality**.

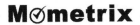

Pulmonary Embolism

Pulmonary embolism is a leading cause of sudden death. Immediate recognition and treatment for **pulmonary embolism** is crucial to the patient's chances of survival. Symptoms can be vague and nonspecific but might include chest pain, dyspnea, tachypnea, cough, abnormal lung sounds, low blood pressure, or even a sense of impending doom or nonspecific agitation. Computed tomography pulmonary angiography is used to make a positive diagnosis. However, using pulmonary embolus risk assessments like the **Wells score** can help the clinician make decisions, especially if the patient is not stable. Bedside echo is sometimes used in an unstable patient to justify giving certain medications. Priority care is given to basic life functions, including monitoring oxygen saturation levels and administering oxygen as needed. Anticoagulants and thrombolytics may be used to dissolve the clot, or it may need to be surgically removed. A vena cava filter may also be inserted to prevent further clots from reaching the lungs. Complications include recurrent thromboembolism, pulmonary hypertension, and death.

Status Epilepticus

Status epilepticus is a seizure lasting longer than 5 minutes, or the state of repeated seizures without a subsequent return to consciousness, or return of normal brain function, between each separate episode. Most common etiologies include noncompliance with antiepileptic drug therapy, drug withdrawal, metabolic dysfunction, and acute brain injury. Each type of seizure has characteristic movements, but general signs are jerking movements, decreased level of consciousness, and tonic posturing. Diagnosis is made by clinical assessment. An EEG should be assessed later to check for less obvious forms of status epilepticus.

Treatment for status epilepticus focuses on maintaining a clear airway, protecting the patient from imminent harm, and administering medication in an attempt to resolve the episode. Assess for adequate patient perfusion, give a glucose solution, evaluate the electrolytes, and administer IV benzodiazepines followed by IV fosphenytoin. Lorazepam is generally the first line of defense; however, if the seizure does not respond to treatment within the first 5 to 7 minutes, phenytoin or fosphenytoin should be added. In extreme cases, barbiturates, anesthesia, neuromuscular blocks, and propofol may be needed to control seizure activity. Complications include death, cerebral anoxia, neurologic damage, possible long-term injuries as a result of syncope/convulsions, cardiac arrhythmias, aspiration pneumonitis, respiratory failure, and cardiac injury.

Successful Lifestyle and Health Changes

Change begins with the patient making a firm, concrete commitment to a goal or positive outcome. No change can be achieved without a decision to pursue that change. **Goals** that are measurable, gradual, and within the realistic reach for the patient must be established. A clear path needs to be visualized. A realistic view of negative life events and relapses must be established—one that allows the patient to be forgiving of their perceived failures and maintain long-term resolve toward the change. The patient must receive **support and encouragement** from outside sources that they trust and value.

Facilitating Better Collaboration and Coordination

Tools for facilitating better collaboration and coordination include **practice guidelines** to help define each participant's role in care, as well as clinical protocols or pathways to focus care and to clarify procedure and strategies to be followed. The goal is to create a **team** in which the members understand their own, and each other's, role within the group; understand the goals of the team; share responsibility; reach collective decisions; and actively include the patient and their family in the care process. An effective **collaboration effort** includes all stages of care, including assessment of needs, action, communication, and evaluation of goals upon completion. A primary key is streamlined **communication** and respect for each individual's unique contribution.

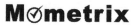

SUBACUTE CARE FACILITIES

For the patient who faces hospital discharge but is still too ill for home or nursing home care, the four types of subacute care facilities that might be available are as follows:

- **General**—Patients discharged to this level of care are stable and healing well but still require skilled care for such things as long-term intravenous treatments.
- **Chronic**—Chronic care facilities are for terminal and end-of-life patients that cannot be cared for in an at-home setting because of choice or complexity of care, as with ventilator dependency.
- **Transitional**—At this level, the patient still needs complex medical and nursing care, such as deep-wound management.
- **Long-term transitional**—This level identifies a need for continued complex medical care that is expected to have an extended treatment time.

COMMON NON-PAIN COMPLAINTS WITH TERMINAL ILLNESSES

Patients with cancer often express **fatigue** and **anorexia** as the top two reasons for emotional and physical distress. Nausea, constipation, states of delirium or other alterations of mental status, and dyspnea are also frequent. Fatigue encompasses symptoms of tiredness, a lack of energy not related to the amount of rest the patient is getting, diminished mental capacity, and weakness. These symptoms interfere with the ability to perform activities of daily living and are often underdiagnosed or downplayed by the patient as inevitable. Anorexia and cachexia are associated with the general wasting of many terminal illnesses, and they require careful nutritional management. Nausea and constipation are often related to medications and other treatments but are easily treated if assessed and planned for. **Palliative treatments** are helpful for altered mental states and dyspnea as well if they are assessed and planned for.

Pharmaceutical Therapeutics

NYSTATIN

Nystatin (Mycostatin, Nadostine, Nilstat, Nystex) can be used to treat **oral candidiasis** (thrush) in children and adults as an oral suspension at a dose of 400,000 to 600,000 units (200,000 units for infants) four times a day for up to 2 weeks. For treatment of **intestinal candidiasis** in adults and children, oral tablets of 500,000 to 1,000,000 units of nystatin are given three times a day. For treatment of **vaginal candidiasis**, nystatin in the form of vaginal tablets of 100,000 units is given once a day for 2 weeks. Adverse reactions might include nausea, vomiting, stomach discomfort, diarrhea, rash, or vaginal irritation.

COLCHICINE

Colchicine (Colcrys) is sometimes prescribed for **gout**. It used to be a primary treatment for acute gout, but now NSAIDs are favored over colchicine. This is because there is a narrow therapeutic window for colchicine to be effective (it should be given within 36 hours of the onset of the attack), and there is a risk of toxicity. The function of colchicine is to counteract the swelling and pain from uric acid buildup, but this is now better achieved with NSAIDs. For acute attacks, an initial dose of up to 1.2 mg of colchicine can be given, followed by 0.6 mg 1 hour later. The IV form of colchicine is no longer approved or used in the US. Nausea, vomiting, stomach discomfort, and diarrhea are common reactions. It is contraindicated in those with renal or hepatic impairment. Grapefruit juice, and many medications, can interfere with the action of colchicine.

COMBANTRIN

Combantrin (pyrantel pamoate) is an anthelmintic used for treatment of infections caused by **parasitic worms** such as roundworm and pinworm. Normal dosage for pinworms is 11 mg/kg (maximum of 1 g) orally, followed by a second dose after 2 weeks (dosage recommended by the CDC). It is important to treat all family members and others who have close contact with the infected individual and to emphasize fastidious personal hygiene habits. Piperazine salts should not be used during the time of treatment, and caution should be used when treatment is needed in patients with severe malnutrition, anemia, or liver impairment.

38

MINOXIDIL

Oral minoxidil (Loniten) is an **antihypertensive** used in adult patients with severe high blood pressure. Therapeutic dosages must be built up to, and usually range from 10 to 40 mg a day. It may cause edema, tachycardia, or other cardiac side effects. Loniten should not be used with NSAIDs or the herb ma huang because they interfere with its action.

Topical minoxidil (Rogaine) is a **hair growth stimulant** available in 2% and 5% topical solutions. These solutions can be applied to areas of thinning hair up to twice a day. Patients should be educated about the possibility of skin irritation and what to expect for results. About 40% of patients will begin to see moderate hair growth after 4 months of use.

OPIATE ABUSE AND WITHDRAWAL SYMPTOMS

Opioid analgesic therapy is a widely used method of chronic pain control. The severity of symptoms is dependent on the amount and duration of use. Common side effects of **abuse** may mimic the flu and include increased respirations, diarrhea, runny nose, sweating, coughing, lacrimation, muscle twitching, and increased temperature and blood pressure. Withdrawal symptoms will overlap with abuse symptoms and become worse. Agitation, anxiety, nausea and vomiting, chronic goose bumps, and dilated pupils are also present. Overdose is treated with naloxone, and withdrawal symptoms can be eased with methadone.

ACETAMINOPHEN

Acetaminophen is a non-narcotic analgesic for mild to moderate **pain and fever**. This pain relief effect can be enhanced when combined with caffeine. Likewise, when acetaminophen is combined with narcotics, it can enhance the pain relief quality of the narcotic. Acetaminophen has no effect on inflammation. It can be safely used in children. It also does not affect blood clotting time. Those with a history of heavy alcohol use should use it cautiously because the combination of the two has a greater chance of creating damage to the liver. Overdose is treated with N-acetylcysteine (NAC).

ASPIRIN

Aspirin is an NSAID (nonsteroidal anti-inflammatory), salicylate analgesic for mild to moderate **pain and fever reduction**. Use in children is not recommended because of an increased risk of Reye syndrome. Aspirin is also often used as a prophylactic to reduce the risk of myocardial infarction, stroke, and transient ischemic attacks (TIAs) because of its blood thinning quality. It is beneficial in treating inflammation. However, aspirin can also decrease the reabsorption of uric acid, increase gastric irritation, and increase risk of occult blood loss. Signs of **aspirin poisoning** include tinnitus (ringing in ears), hearing impairment, hyperventilation, vomiting, and confusion. Treatments for aspirin poisoning include gastric lavage, activated charcoal, and IV fluids.

METHYLDOPA

Methyldopa (Aldomet, Dopamet) is an **antihypertensive** that can be administered orally or by IV. IV dosing is usually 250–1,000 mg infused over 30–60 minutes every 6–8 hours. Oral maintenance is a daily dose of 250–1,000 mg PO divided every 6–12 hours. In long-term use, it is often recommended that this medication be taken at bedtime because of its tendency to cause sedation. Other common side effects are headache, orthostatic hypotension, nasal congestion, and dry mouth. Use cautiously with amphetamines, β-blockers, norepinephrine, phenothiazines, tricyclic antidepressants, anesthesia, barbiturates, haloperidol, levodopa, lithium, MAO inhibitors, and tolbutamide. Monitor blood pressure and liver function closely.

POTASSIUM-SPARING DIURETICS

Potassium-sparing diuretics include amiloride, triamterene, spironolactone, and eplerenone. They are used to prevent **sodium reabsorption and potassium secretion** in the collection tubules while still promoting **urinary excretion of excess fluid**. Potassium-sparing diuretics are often used in conjunction with antihypertensive medications to manage high blood pressure or congestive heart failure. Although this class of

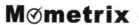

medications can help prevent hypokalemia, they should not be used at the same time as potassium supplements, and potassium levels still need to be monitored.

OCCUPATIONAL HEALTH HAZARDS

The most common **accidents** to occur in the workplace involve system and mechanical failures. Musculoskeletal complaints such as back pain accompany heavy lifting and repetitive activities. Injuries can be to large muscles (such as the back) or smaller muscle groups (wrists, neck, ankles). Hearing loss is common in construction and manufacturing industries. Chemical and biological agents that can cause liver damage, reproductive disorders, and cancer are most common in professions that have constant exposure to pesticides, heavy metal, and corrosive substances. Healthcare workers are particularly vulnerable to HIV, tuberculosis, and hepatitis B and C.

PHARMACEUTICAL TREATMENTS FOR MILD TO MODERATE ACNE

Over-the-counter options include lotions containing benzoyl peroxide, sulfur, resorcinol, or salicylic acid. These products are best for mild cases of **acne**. For more severe cases, the strength of the lotions can be increased through the prescription of tretinoin, adapalene, or tazarotene. Beyond topical agents, antibiotics (tetracycline or clindamycin) can be considered, as well as oral contraceptives. Chemical peels, microdermabrasion, and laser and light therapy can also be useful. Isotretinoin (Amnesteem, Claravis, Sotret) is an extremely powerful medication, which, while highly effective for scarring cystic acne, carries many risks and side effects and should be considered as a last resort.

PHARMACEUTICAL TREATMENTS FOR HEARTBURN (GERD)

Occasional heartburn may be normal, but sometimes heartburn is a symptom of **GERD (gastroesophageal reflux disease)**. The diagnosis of GERD can be made on clinical assessment information alone, or in combination with endoscopy. In some patients, endoscopy will be needed to rule out other conditions. Symptoms include a burning feeling in the chest that seems worse after eating or when lying down, and is exacerbated by bending over. Nausea, vomiting, and difficulty swallowing are also common symptoms. Medication options include antacids (Maalox, Mylanta, Rolaids, and Tums) to neutralize stomach acid; however, long-term use can result in changes in bowel habits. H2-receptor blockers (Tagamet HB, Pepcid AC, Zantac, and Axid AR) are meant to reduce the stomach's production of acid. Relief isn't as instant as with antacids, but it will last longer. Proton pump inhibitors (Prevacid 24HR and Prilosec) can both reduce acid production and heal the trauma caused to the esophagus. Patient counseling should include weight loss, if needed; avoidance of tight clothing; specific trigger foods; eating smaller, more frequent meals; smoking cessation; and remaining upright after eating. Complications include erosive esophagitis, esophageal bleeding, esophageal cancer, ulcers, and Barrett esophagus.

TETRACYCLINE ANTIBIOTICS

It is important to remember that children should not be given **tetracycline antibiotics** (e.g., doxycycline) due to alterations that can occur in tooth or bone development, causing a permanent discoloration of the teeth. This drug should only be used in pediatrics if the benefits outweigh the risks. To indicate the use of this drug, the patient should be >8 years old or have a severe/life-threatening infection such as Rocky Mountain spotted fever or anthrax.

TREATMENT OPTIONS FOR COPD

Chronic obstructive pulmonary disease (COPD) cannot be cured, but it can be controlled with medication. Inhalers can be coupled with anti-inflammatory medications. The first line of defense is usually recommended as ipratropium and albuterol (β-2 adrenergics and anticholinergics). The second-line option is albuterol, and the third choice would be methylprednisolone sodium succinate, followed by theophylline. Acute flare-ups may also require assistance from steroids, nebulizers with bronchodilators, oxygen therapy, and breathing assistance through aids such as a BiPAP portable ventilator. Other recommendations for the patient might include weight management, pulmonary rehabilitation, and reducing triggers in their environment such as smoke or perfumes. Surgery to remove severely damaged lung tissue may also be considered.

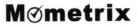

INITIAL DOSING OF LEVOTHYROXINE SODIUM

Considerations for dosing must include patient age, duration and severity of hypothyroidism, and presence of any preexisting cardiac disease, such as angina. There is a high level of sensitivity to thyroid medications, so the initial dose should begin at a very low level, generally 25 mcg a day, increasing as needed every 1 to 2 months in order to reach therapeutic levels. Adults older than age 60 will require less medication than younger adults. **Levothyroxine** increases cardiac workload and elevates heart rate—the patient should inform you of any chest pain, palpitations, sweating, anxiety, or shortness of breath.

CHRONIC, STABLE ANGINA

Initial medication choices include **β-blockers** such as metoprolol in order to lower the heart rate, blood pressure, and oxygen requirements of the heart. Long-acting **nitrates**, including isosorbide dinitrate, may be considered if β-blockers prove ineffective, but there is a tendency to develop a tolerance to these medications. Ranolazine is also a good choice. Angiotensin-converting enzyme (ACE) inhibitors lower blood pressure. Calcium-channel blockers help the heart relax to reduce workload and blood pressure. Preventive measures against myocardial infarction may also be considered using aspirin, clopidogrel, or prasugrel.

CYSTITIS

Cystitis is most often caused by *Escherichia coli* (*E. coli*). The patient presents with urinary frequency, urgency, and pain, and there may also be a pain response to light pressure on the suprapubic area. Urinalysis will show white and red blood cells. Because of the increase in strains of *E. coli* that are resistant, current recommendations/drugs of choice for uncomplicated cystitis include nitrofurantoin, TMP-SMX, or fosfomycin, but local susceptibility patterns should be considered. These recommendations change frequently according to the mutations of the bacterial strains and should be frequently revalidated in a dependable resource such as *The Sanford Guide to Antimicrobial Therapy*.

HEPARIN AND WARFARIN

Heparin is an **anticoagulant** that works on the intrinsic pathway of the clotting cascade, and its activity is checked with a partial thromboplastin time (PTT) or an anti-Xa assay. **Heparin** comes in several forms: low molecular weight heparin (LMWH) and unfractionated heparin (UFH). Heparin sodium has a short half-life, is injectable, and can be given intravenously or subcutaneously for more acute illnesses such as deep vein thrombosis, MI, and pulmonary embolism. PTT, prothrombin time (PT), and international normalized ratio (INR) will be monitored frequently. Protamine reverses the effects of heparin. Heparin sodium is used cautiously in the patient who has had or will be undergoing surgery.

Warfarin (Coumadin) is an **anticoagulant** that works on the extrinsic pathway of the clotting cascade by inhibiting vitamin K-dependent clotting factors (factors 10, 9, 7, 2); its activity is checked with a PT. It is normally given in oral form (2 to 10 mg a day) as long-term therapy for those patients needing blood thinners (e.g., those with atrial fibrillation, mechanical heart valves, or thromboembolism). It can be given concurrently with heparin the first 4–5 days of treatment. Warfarin requires both baseline and frequent PT and INR levels to maintain a therapeutic level. The patient should also be monitored for unusual bruising and bleeding, and should be cautioned against aspirin, NSAIDs, and other over-the-counter supplements (e.g., ginkgo biloba, St. John's wort) that affect bleeding times. Vitamin K can be administered to reverse the effects of warfarin.

> **Review Video: Heparin—An Injectable Anticoagulant**
> Visit mometrix.com/academy and enter code: 127426
>
> **Review Video: Warfarin - Uses and Side Effects**
> Visit mometrix.com/academy and enter code: 844117

HYPERTENSIVE PATIENTS WITH HEART FAILURE AND REDUCED CARDIAC OUTPUT

The optimal treatment goal for the hypertensive patient with heart failure is to reach a stable blood pressure of less than 130/80 mmHg. This usually requires more than one medication. An angiotensin-converting enzyme

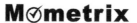

(ACE) inhibitor with thiazide diuretic therapy slows cardiac remodeling, improves cardiac function, and reduces further cardiovascular events after a myocardial infarction. β-blockers are also commonly added. Other medications that might be considered are dihydropyridine calcium antagonists, angiotensin receptor blockers (ARBs), aldosterone inhibitors, and isosorbide dinitrate/hydralazine.

OPIOID ROTATION

Opioid rotation is a process of systematically switching a patient's prescribed opioid when they no longer seem to be receiving effective pain relief on their current medication, rather than increasing the dosage. Changing from one opioid to another, or altering the delivery method, may become necessary under the assumption that incomplete cross-tolerance among opioids occurs. Changing analgesics or the method of delivery may result in a decreased drug requirement. When altering opioid delivery regimes, use morphine equivalents as the common factor for all dose conversions. This method will help reduce medication errors.

SPASMOLYTICS

Spasmolytics for the bladder include flavoxate hydrochloride (Urispas), oxybutynin chloride (Ditropan, Oxytrol), phenazopyridine hydrochloride (AZO Standard, Geridium, Pyridium, Urodine), and tolterodine tartrate (Detrol). These are used to offer relief to patients with urinary disorders such as urinary frequency, urgency, nocturia, incontinence, pain, and bladder spasms. Carisoprodol, cyclobenzaprine, metaxalone, and methocarbamol are used in conjunction with rest and physical therapy to treat acute/painful musculoskeletal conditions causing muscle spasms. These conditions frequently include fibromyalgia, tension headaches, and myofascial pain syndrome. These are contraindicated in neurologic conditions such as cerebral palsy and multiple sclerosis.

ANTIARRHYTHMIC DRUGS

Antiarrhythmic drugs include sodium-channel blockers, β-blockers, potassium-channel blockers, calcium-channel blockers, adenosine, digitalis, atropine, and even electrolyte supplements when given for the express purpose of helping to correct a cardiac rhythm anomaly. It is important to understand the action of each medication and match it carefully to the individual patient's needs. **Antiarrhythmics** are always given with caution because not only do they stabilize cardiac excitability or depression, but they could also cause a secondary arrhythmia or other unwanted cardiac complication, such as hypotension.

ANTIBIOTIC CHOICE FOR OTITIS MEDIA

The current recommendation by the American Academy of Pediatrics is a 10-day course of **amoxicillin**. Secondary choices are erythromycin or sulfonamide. It is important to note that some cases of **otitis media** are viral in origin and require no antibiotic. These ear infections will resolve on their own. Treatment with antibiotics may be delayed by 48 to 72 hours in the child between the ages of 6 months and 2 years to avoid overuse of antibiotics if the cause may be viral.

ACE INHIBITORS

Angiotensin-converting enzyme (ACE) inhibitors are used to lower **blood pressure** by promoting vasodilation as well as acting as a diuretic. This is a recommended treatment option for heart failure patients and those recovering from myocardial infarction. ACE inhibitors are identified by the ending "**pril**": benazepril, captopril, enalapril, fosinopril, lisinopril, moexipril, quinapril, and ramipril. Side effects are rare, but the patient may experience some dizziness or lightheadedness when therapy begins. ACE inhibitors should not be taken during pregnancy or when breastfeeding.

BETA-BLOCKERS

Beta-blockers (β-blockers) block norepinephrine and epinephrine from binding with their receptors to **slow the heartbeat and lower blood pressure**. β-blockers include acebutolol, bisoprolol, esmolol, propranolol, atenolol, labetalol, carvedilol, and metoprolol. Note the identifying ending of "**lol**." β-blockers are recommended for patients who have diabetes, cardiac arrhythmias, heart failure, myocardial infarction recovery, and angina pectoris. β-blockers are generally not used in combination with calcium-channel blockers. Side effects are rare, but β-blockers are able to cross the blood–brain barrier, and this may result in central nervous system (CNS) symptoms such as headache or dizziness. β-blockers may also mask symptoms of hypoglycemia and exacerbate asthma. Gradual tapering over 1 to 2 weeks is advisable. Abrupt cessation can lead to rebound hypertension, tachycardia, sweating, unstable angina, myocardial infarction, and possibly death.

CALCIUM-CHANNEL BLOCKERS

Calcium-channel blockers (amlodipine, felodipine, diltiazem, verapamil, nifedipine, nicardipine, nisoldipine, and bepridil) **relax blood vessels and reduce cardiac workload** by preventing calcium from entering the cardiac tissue. This lowers pulse and blood pressure. They may be prescribed for cardiac disease, coronary spasms or angina, arrhythmias, hypertrophic cardiomyopathy, or right-sided heart failure. Patients should be instructed not to consume grapefruit, grapefruit juice, or alcohol while on this medication. Dosages may need to be lowered in older adults because they are more prone to side effects.

> **Review Video: Calcium Channel Blockers and Antiarrhythmics**
> Visit mometrix.com/academy and enter code: 942825

PARKINSON'S DISEASE

A combination of levodopa and carbidopa (Sinemet, Parcopa) is the treatment of choice for **Parkinson's disease**. **Levodopa** acts to reduce tremor, rigidity, bradykinesia, and postural inability, but it cannot slow or halt disease progression. **Carbidopa** facilitates the ability of levodopa to reach the brain in optimal amounts. When it is working well, mobility is improved; however, the patient can experience dyskinesia. There is also a varied cycle of effectiveness with prolonged use. When the medication is less effective, motor symptoms become more spasmodic and unpredictable. Possible interactions may be experienced when the patient is also taking antacids, antiseizure medications, antihypertensives, or antidepressants or is on a high-protein diet.

CONSTIPATION

Before medication is considered, review the patient's fiber and fluid intake, as well as their activity level. Encourage dietary modifications, exercise, and bowel training activities before a prescription is issued. Medication choices fall into four categories, listed by order of choice: bulk laxatives, stool softeners, osmotic laxatives, and stimulant laxatives. **Bulk laxatives** (methylcellulose, polycarbophil, and psyllium) are dietary fiber supplements taken when the patient's normal consumption is still inadequate. **Stool softeners**, also called emollient laxatives (docusate calcium, docusate sodium), encourage water to enter into the bowel. **Osmotic laxatives** (lactulose, magnesium citrate, magnesium hydroxide, polyethylene glycol, sodium biphosphate, and sorbitol) stimulate osmosis and create more available water in the intestine. **Stimulant laxatives** (bisacodyl, cascara sagrada, castor oil, and senna) encourage greater intestinal motility and increase water in the bowel.

ORAL CONTRACEPTIVES

Hormone-based oral contraceptives (**OCs**) are the most common choice among women for birth control. OCs inhibit the release of **gonadotropin-releasing hormone (GnRH)** and increase the viscosity of cervical mucus. The most common type of OCs are a combination of both estrogen and progestin. These are most effective when used accurately; options include either a 28-day or 91-day cycle. Combined estrogen/progestin OCs are contraindicated in women older than age 35 who smoke or have migraines; in those with unexplained uterine bleeding, untreated high blood pressure, cerebrovascular accident (CVA), congestive heart failure (CHF), cardiovascular/vascular disease, thrombosis/embolism, or active liver disease; in breast cancer/other neoplasms that are estrogen- or progestin-sensitive; and in women who are pregnant. Also, effectiveness may be altered by rifampin and antiepileptics, phenytoin, and carbamazepine. The patient must also be aware that oral contraceptives do not prevent the spread of HIV or STDs. Oral contraceptives may be prescribed to stabilize symptoms of premenstrual syndrome (PMS) or help treat acne. Progesterone-only contraceptives are recommended for those breastfeeding or those with a contraindication to estrogen use, but they must be taken

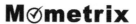

at the same time every day to be effective, and breakthrough bleeding is a common side effect. Other forms of **contraception** include contraceptive rings, patches, or injections, female or male sterilization, condoms, female barrier methods, abstinence/periodic abstinence, coitus interruptus, and intrauterine devices.

EMERGENCY CONTRACEPTION

Emergency contraception can be provided to women who have a fear that they may have been unintentionally impregnated. This may occur because of sexual assault or rape, protective device failure (condom breakage or dislodged diaphragm), or when no birth control was used at all (including forgetting to regularly take prescribed birth control pills). **Emergency contraceptive pills** that are available without a prescription contain levonorgestrel (e.g., Plan B One-Step, Next Choice One Dose) and are most effective if taken within 72 hours after unprotected sex. Both ulipristal acetate and copper-bearing IUDs require a prescription, and can be taken or inserted up to 5 days after unprotected sex.

ANTIPSYCHOTICS

First-generation antipsychotics include haloperidol, chlorpromazine, perphenazine, and fluphenazine. They are used to treat schizophrenia and related disorders. These antipsychotics can produce Parkinson-like symptoms such as akinesia, bradykinesia, stoic facial expression, tremor, cogwheel rigidity, postural abnormalities, and tardive dyskinesia.

Second-generation (atypical) antipsychotics include clozapine, risperidone, olanzapine, quetiapine, ziprasidone, aripiprazole, and paliperidone. When prescribing clozapine, special care must be taken to monitor the patient's white blood cell count. Other medications should be considered before clozapine. Atypical antipsychotics often cause weight gain.

NSAIDS FOR RHEUMATOID ARTHRITIS

NSAIDs (e.g., naproxen) can be used to treat symptoms and pain related to diseases such as **rheumatoid arthritis**, but they cannot slow or halt disease progression. Patients may benefit from NSAID use through its anti-inflammatory, analgesic, and antipyretic properties. NSAIDs tend to be the first line of defense against pain caused by inflammatory conditions. They may also be used in conjunction with opioid therapy to reduce the amount of opioid needed. Adversely, gastrointestinal bleeding or ulceration, decreased renal function, and impaired platelet aggregation may occur. Studies have also indicated that the therapeutic effects of NSAIDs may not extend beyond 6 to 12 months of use. Short-term memory loss may occur in older patients. There may be an increased cardiovascular risk with prolonged use. Patients allergic to sulfa drugs can also experience a cross-sensitivity to some types of NSAIDs.

TRIPTANS

Triptans (sumatriptan, eletriptan, almotriptan, frovatriptan, rizatriptan, zolmitriptan) are **serotonin receptor agonists** that help relieve pain from **acute migraine attacks** by causing vasoconstriction of the intracranial blood vessels and relieving swelling. Sensitivity to light and noise, nausea, and vomiting also associated with migraines will be quickly resolved as well. Combining triptans with acetaminophen or naproxen can boost their effectiveness even further. They can cause irritation at the point of administration (injection or nasal spray) and may cause some dizziness, drowsiness, or lightheadedness. Triptans cannot be used in patients with cerebrovascular disease. Patients should also be educated about rebound headaches.

METRONIDAZOLE

Oral metronidazole (**Flagyl**) is an antibiotic used to treat **infections of the reproductive system or gastrointestinal tract** such as pelvic inflammatory disease (PID), trichomoniasis, and *Clostridioides difficile* (*C. diff*). Nausea and headache are common side effects. Flagyl may also be given intravenously. Topical cream metronidazole is applied to the skin once a day for the treatment of rosacea. It does not, however, cure the disease process. It may also be used as vaginal treatment for bacterial infections (500 mg PO bid for 7 days). Either application has the potential to cause skin irritation.

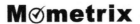

ADVERSE SIDE EFFECTS AND ALLERGIC REACTIONS TO MEDICATION

Adverse side effects to a medication can be, at times, very severe; however, with adverse side effects, the body does not form antibodies against the medication. A true **allergic reaction** means that the body's immune system has created antibodies against the foreign substance it perceives as a threat. These antibodies cause an anaphylaxis reaction with hives, facial and throat swelling, wheezing, light-headedness, vomiting, and even shock. These reactions are usually almost immediate, occurring in under an hour, although there may be a delay of several hours.

PERMETHRIN CREAM

Over-the-counter permethrin 1% cream can be used to treat **lice** (leave on for 10 minutes and rinse; may be repeated in 7 days). Permethrin 5% (Elimite) cream can be prescribed as treatment for **scabies**. The patient should be instructed to wash and dry their entire body, then apply the cream to every exposed surface, paying particular attention to the creases and folds. Permethrin 5% cream needs to remain on the skin for at least 8 to 14 hours. Then the patient should again wash and dry thoroughly and put on clean clothing. Patients should be aware that the itching will ease somewhat within the first 24 hours, but may not be completely relieved for up to 4 weeks after treatment. The treatment may also cause temporary redness of the skin. Permethrin is safe for use in infants after 2 months of age, and for patients of all other ages, including the elderly.

PANIC ATTACKS

Antidepressants can often be used for long-term treatment and prevention of **panic attacks**. Selective serotonin reuptake inhibitors (SSRIs) such as fluoxetine (Prozac), paroxetine (Paxil), citalopram (Celexa), escitalopram (Lexapro), and sertraline (Zoloft) are the initial choices. The next choice is selective serotonin and norepinephrine reuptake inhibitors (SSNRIs). Treatment of an **acute attack** may require a sedative such as Xanax, Klonopin, Valium, or Ativan. In addition to medication, psychotherapy, cognitive behavior therapy, relaxation, and meditation training should also be considered.

UPPER RESPIRATORY INFECTIONS

Upper respiratory infections are the most common cause of doctor visits. An **upper respiratory infection** involves the sinuses, nasal passages, pharynx, and larynx. There is typically inflammation of these areas that causes pain, congestion, and cough. The patient may also complain of difficulty breathing and fatigue. These types of illnesses are most common during the fall and winter months. The virus is contagious through respiratory droplets that are inhaled or transferred by touch. The risk of contracting an upper respiratory infection is highest among those who spend long hours in close quarters with many other people, those with poor hand-washing habits, smokers, immunocompromised individuals, and those working in healthcare settings. These illnesses are not caused by a bacterial infection and cannot be relieved through the use of antibiotics.

GENTAMICIN

Gentamicin is an antibiotic used to treat **bacterial infections**. In its injectable form, it is often used to treat serious infections such as *Pseudomonas*, *Escherichia coli*, and *Staphylococcus*. Standard dosing is 1 mg/kg every 8 hours. Common side effects include nausea, vomiting, and loss of appetite. When it is given as an intramuscular injection, patients often complain of pain and irritation at the injection site. Gentamicin in this form also carries a high risk of renal toxicity and ototoxicity. Gentamicin can also be prescribed in a solution for use as eye drops to treat infections such as **conjunctivitis**.

BACK PAIN MANAGEMENT OPTIONS

Depending on the source, amount, and consistency of the pain, **treatment options** can vary greatly. Treatment options include: physical therapy, mild anti-inflammatory medications, chiropractic referrals, transcutaneous electrical nerve stimulation (TENS) or intradiscal electrothermal therapy (IDET) units, injections, and surgical interventions. Any intervention is aimed at reducing pain and recovering movement. For an acute episode, an ice pack and anti-inflammatory agent may be sufficient. Long-term bed rest is not recommended. For more

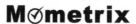

chronic needs, treatment options should progress from the most noninvasive that is needed for the patient to receive relief.

DOXORUBICIN

Doxorubicin is an antineoplastic drug common in the treatment of **breast, bladder, ovarian, and endometrial cancers**. It may also be used in certain types of lymphoma and leukemia, thyroid, and skin cancers. Injections are provided every 21 to 28 days. Common side effects include nausea, vomiting, mouth and throat lesions, changes in appetite, fatigue, and weight loss. Long-term monitoring of the heart should also be planned for because doxorubicin can have a damaging effect on cardiac health.

SALICYLIC ACID

Salicylic acid is a popular medication used for treatment of various **skin disorders** such as psoriasis, ichthyosis, dandruff, corns, calluses, and warts. It works by reducing swelling, redness, and irritation while unclogging pores in the treatment of acne. For other conditions, it loosens and softens areas of thickened or calloused skin until it falls off naturally or can be easily removed. Mild concentrations are used for most conditions. Solutions of 2% to 10% concentration are used for treatment of corns, and up to 17% for warts. However, salicylic acid should not be used to treat warts on the face, mouth, or nose; any wart with a hair follicle; genital warts; moles; or birthmarks.

ANTIHISTAMINES

There are two types of antihistamines: H1 (allergies) and H2 (reduced gastric acid secretion). They affect either the H1 or H2 receptors in the body.

H1 antihistamines block histamines that are triggered by allergies in order to calm the body's reaction to the allergen. There are two generations of H1 antihistamine medications. The most marked side effect of first-generation antihistamines (diphenhydramine, clemastine, brompheniramine) is sedation and anticholinergic effects (dry mouth/eyes, dizziness, urinary retention), as compared to second-generation antihistamines (fexofenadine, loratadine, desloratadine, cetirizine). Also, the sedative effects of first-generation antihistamines may have the opposite effect and cause excitability in children. There are precautions to H1 antihistamine use in both angle-closure glaucoma and benign prostatic hyperplasia (BPH).

H2 antihistamines include cimetidine and famotidine. These are usually used along with PPIs or as a second-line medication for GERD and gastric ulcers. Side effects include headache, confusion, and dizziness. Most of the above medications should not be used in pregnant women or nursing mothers; most H1s are not recommended for children <2 years old, with some not recommended for children younger than 6 years old.

INSULIN

Rapid-acting insulin (Humalog, NovoLog, Apidra) is designed to act on the body's needs for insulin during meal consumption. Onset is in 12–30 minutes, with peak action within 30 minutes to 3 hours, with its full duration of action between 3 and 5 hours. **Short-acting insulin** (regular Humulin, regular insulin) is used when a meal is anticipated within 30 minutes to an hour. Onset is 30 minutes, peak action is 2.5 to 5 hours, and the duration is 12 to 18 hours. **Intermediate-acting insulin** (NPH insulin) covers an extended period when the patient's need will be steady, such as the time when the patient is asleep. Onset is 1 to 1.5 hours, peak action is anywhere from 6 to 10 hours, and the full duration is 14 to 24 hours. **Long-acting insulin** (Lantus, Levemir) gives coverage for a full 24 hours. Peaks are very gentle or nonexistent, and the duration is typically >24 hours with a range of 11 to 32 hours. **Combinations of insulin (premixed)** with different durations can be premixed to provide a more complex level of coverage. Premixed insulins include Humulin 70/30, Novolin 70/30, NovoLog 50/50 and 70/30, and Humalog mix 75/25.

ADDICTION AND PSEUDOADDICTION

Addiction is a primary and constant neurobiological disease with genetic, psychosocial, and environmental factors that create an obsessive and irrational need or preoccupation with a substance. **Addictive behaviors**

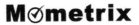

include unrestricted, continued cravings and compulsive, persistent use of a drug despite harmful experiences and side effects. **Pseudoaddiction** is an assumption that the patient is addicted to a substance, when in actuality the patient is not experiencing relief from the medication. It is prolonged, unrelieved pain that may be the result of undertreatment. This situation may lead the patient to become more aggressive in seeking medicated relief, thus resulting in the inappropriate "drug-seeker" label.

PHYSICAL DEPENDENCE, TOLERANCE, AND PSEUDOTOLERANCE

Physical dependence is a condition of bodily adaptation to the presence of a specific drug or chemical. Abrupt removal or a rapid reduction of dosage will result in **withdrawal symptoms**. The patient does not present with the psychological and environmental dependence that are evident in addictions, such as an obsessive and irrational need for or preoccupation with a substance; unrestricted, continued cravings; and compulsive, persistent use of a drug despite harmful experiences and side effects. **Tolerance** is the adaptation of the body to continued exposure to a drug or chemical. The effects of the drug at the same level of exposure are minimized over time. Additional dosing is required to maintain the same outcomes. **Pseudotolerance** is the misguided perception by the caregiver that a patient's need for increasing doses of a drug is due to the development of tolerance, when in reality disease progression or other factors are responsible for the increase in dosing needs.

Applying Basic Scientific Concepts

NORMAL HEART SOUNDS

Heart sounds are created by the noise of the blood pushing through the heart valves. **S1**, or the "lub" sound, is created by the mitral and tricuspid valves. **S2**, or the "dub" sound, is created by the aortic and pulmonary valves. During youth, a third benign heart sound, **S3**, or gallop, may also be present after S2. In the adult, this is usually an indication of cardiac disease. Abnormal sounds that might be observed occur when these valves do not close at the proper times or do not close completely.

ABNORMAL BREATHING PATTERNS

The following are abnormal breathing patterns:

- **Cheyne-Stokes**: respiratory depression caused by heart failure and uremia.
- **Kussmaul**: deep, rapid, labored breathing related to acidosis.
- **Obstructive**: obstructive lung disease, or COPD, causing prolonged expiration due to narrowed airways and increased resistance.
- **Ataxic**: unpredictable irregularity, both shallow and deep breaths, apnea, from brain damage and respiratory depression.
- **Tachypnea**: rapid shallow breathing, with multiple causes.

HYPOVOLEMIA

Hypovolemia is a state of decreased blood plasma volume. Common causes of **hypovolemia** are dehydration, bleeding, vomiting, and burns. Dehydration can be a cause, but is not interchangeable with the term *hypovolemia*. Dehydration is a decrease in the available water within the body. A specific loss of blood plasma (hypovolemia) also includes a marked depletion in sodium levels. If the loss is greater than 10% to 20% of the body's total volume, the patient can begin to exhibit symptoms such as tachycardia, hypotension, pale skin, dizziness, change in mental status, nausea, and excessive thirst. **Hypovolemic shock** (tachycardia, tachypnea, clammy skin, reduced pulse pressure, blood pressure changes, reduced capillary refill, oliguria, hypoperfusion of organs) can also result. If needed, treatment involves both fluid and blood replacement.

FRANK-STARLING LAW OF THE HEART

The Frank-Starling law (also known as Starling's law or Maestrini's heart law) describes the correlation between **cardiac blood volume** and **stroke volume**. End diastolic volume is directly proportional to stroke volume (increased end diastolic pressure equals increased ventricular output). The greater the amount of fluid within the ventricles during diastole, the greater the amount of force that will be exerted during the systolic contraction. This process is independent from any neural or hormonal influences. When the heart's ability to contract is compromised, heart failure may be suspected. The heart will resort to the **Law of Laplace** to try and compensate, and S3 may be detected.

LAW OF LAPLACE

The Law of Laplace states the relationship between **pressure** and **volume** in elastic spheres like the heart and alveoli. If a sphere has radius r, wall thickness w, and wall tension t, then the pressure inside the sphere P would be:

$$P = \frac{2wt}{r}$$

So, the pressure within a tube is inversely proportional to the radius and the tension within the sphere's wall can be decreased by increasing the thickness of the wall. This helps us understand left ventricular hypertrophy within the **heart**. Another way to apply this is that, as pressure increases within a sphere, it is less likely the sphere will rupture if the diameter also increases. In **alveoli**, the pressure that is needed to expand the alveoli is directly proportional to the surface tension and inversely proportional to the radius. Surfactant allows alveoli to remain open and not collapse into larger alveoli by decreasing the surface tension. Smaller alveoli have proportionally more surfactant, which helps them remain easier to expand even though the radius is smaller.

POISEUILLE'S LAW/EQUATION

Poiseuille's law explains the relationship between **pressure** and **resistance**, which affects blood or air flow. The longer and smaller a lumen is, the greater the resistance, causing a need for increased pressure that raises blood pressure and decreases oxygenation. For a tube of length l and radius r carrying a fluid of viscosity (thickness) v, with a pressure difference Δp between the ends of the tube, the equation for flow rate R is:

$$R = \frac{\pi r^4 \Delta p}{8vl}$$

SODIUM-GLUCOSE TRANSPORT PROTEINS

Sodium-glucose linked transporters (**SGLTs**) are found in the mucous membranes of the small intestine. Their role is to help with **renal glucose reabsorption** because sodium and glucose transport across membranes in the same direction. In cases where blood glucose levels have become too high, SGLT allows glucose to be excreted in the urine by creating a sodium gradient for the glucose to follow. This knowledge is currently being explored for its usefulness in treating type 2 diabetes mellitus.

PURINE METABOLISM

Purine and xanthine are **nucleotides** involved in both DNA and RNA formation, as well as **energy transference** and **nitrogen disposal**. The **purine** family includes adenine, guanine, caffeine, xanthine, uric acid, and others. Purine is metabolized by hypoxanthine-guanine phosphoribosyltransferase (HGPRT). Disruptions in this process can cause DNA genetic disorders that are hereditary. Health problems such as Lesch–Nyhan syndrome, gout, anemia, epilepsy, developmental delays, deafness, kidney disease, and immune disorders, as well as many others, can be caused by the resulting disruptions in the purine metabolism, that in turn cause DNA disruptions. The action of allopurinol inhibits the conversion of **xanthine** into uric acid, making it an effective treatment for gout.

SA NODE AND AV NODE

The cells of the **sinoatrial (SA) node**, which are located in the upper wall of the right atrium near the superior vena cava, are specialized to act automatically, regardless of the electrical impulses in the surrounding cardiac tissue. This allows it to act as the "pacemaker for the heart." The impulses travel from the SA node to the **atrioventricular (AV) node**, located near the base of the right atrium, through it to the bundle of His and Purkinje fibers to the rest of the cardiac tissues, causing coordinated ventricular contractions. The SA node's natural rhythm under normal conditions is a steady 60 to 100 beats per minute. If there is a greater oxygen demand by the cells of the body, this message is relayed to the SA node through the sympathetic or parasympathetic autonomic nervous system, which responds by sending out more rapid impulses to increase blood circulation through the heart and lungs to the body. If there is a malfunction of the SA node, the AV node will act as a fail-safe and take over the regulation of the heart at a slower rhythm (25–55 bpm).

Professional Practice

INFLUENCE OF CULTURAL AND RELIGIOUS BELIEFS

Cultural and religious beliefs can have a large influence on how medical care is provided, including formulating a treatment plan that is acceptable to the patient. Many cultures are skeptical of traditional medical care, and some people prefer to adhere to specific beliefs and to traditions that follow their beliefs. For example, some cultures may have one person in the family who makes most of the decisions, such as the oldest male or female, and communication regarding the diagnosis and treatment plan should be discussed with that person.

Some religions have very strict guidelines regarding which medical treatments are acceptable and which are not. There are also cultural and religious groups that believe in certain home remedies or treatments. These should be inquired about to ensure they are not harmful to the patient or counteractive against the treatment that will be prescribed. It is important for the PA to respect the patient's cultural and religious beliefs while communicating to them the importance of the recommended medical treatment.

INFORMED CONSENT

The laws that govern the required information to be included in an **informed consent** vary from state to state. It is important that the PA knows the informed consent requirements for the state in which they practice. In general terms, the informed consent is the legal document that identifies the specific procedure to be performed, along with any potential risks present as a result of the procedure. This should also include the risks present if the patient should opt to not undergo a recommended procedure. It is the PA's responsibility to provide this information and disclose these risks.

Once the patient has received the information within the informed consent, they usually have the right to refuse the treatment. Exceptions exist if the patient has an altered mental status, if the condition affecting the patient is a threat to community safety, or if the patient is a minor. The parents or guardians of a minor may refuse treatment for their child, but they are not legally allowed to refuse life-sustaining treatment for the child.

ASPECTS OF LEGAL AND MEDICAL ETHICS

The following are aspects of legal/medical ethics:

- **Living will:** A written legal document that specifies the medical treatments a person does or does not wish to have performed. For example, a person may not wish to be intubated and placed on a ventilator if they are in respiratory arrest.
- **Advance directive:** Oral or written instructions regarding treatment preferences a person has if they should become seriously ill. A living will is an example of an advance directive.

- **Organ donation:** Ideally, the decision of whether to donate organs following death is discussed with family members so they are aware of the person's wishes. Many people opt to designate their position as an organ donor, and in most states, this is indicated on the driver's license. If a person has not designated themselves as an organ donor, or if they have not discussed this with family members, the decision of whether to donate any body tissues is made by the family members, or by the person making medical decisions for someone at the end of life when they cannot make the decision themselves.
- **Code status:** This is indicated on a patient's chart, and it clarifies what measures a person wishes to be taken if they are in a situation of cardiac or respiratory arrest.
- **DNR:** Stands for "Do Not Resuscitate." It means that, in the event a person enters a state of cardiac arrest, efforts will not be made to perform CPR or provide artificial breathing to a person.
- **DNI:** Stands for "Do Not Intubate." It means that, while medical interventions can be performed to save a person's life, the person does not wish to be intubated and placed on a ventilator.
- **Medical power of attorney:** A person designated, through legal documentation, to make medical decisions in the event that a person cannot make these decisions on their own. Ideally, the wishes of the person regarding end-of-life treatment will be communicated beforehand to the person who is designated as the medical power of attorney.

ETHICAL PRINCIPLES OF PATIENT RIGHTS

There are **four main principles** that serve as a foundation for patients' rights:

- **Justice**: There should be fairness in all medical decision-making. This means that the risks and benefits of a medical treatment should be considered, and all available resources should be made available equally to all patients.
- **Autonomy**: Patients have the right to make their own decisions regarding medical treatment. The patient should be fully informed so that an educated decision can be made, but the patient should not be persuaded to make a certain decision, even if it is in their best interest to do so. Autonomy is closely related to the right to self-determination.
- **Nonmaleficence**: This refers to the principle of "do no harm." Medical providers must decide whether the patient may be harmed by a medical treatment, even if it is in the best interest of the patient.
- **Beneficence**: Medical providers must make decisions regarding treatment of a patient with the patient's best interest in mind. This may vary from patient to patient depending upon the particular situation.

HIPAA PRIVACY AND SECURITY

HIPAA is the **Health Insurance Portability and Accountability Act**, established in 1996 to instill rules regarding the protection and transmittal of patient health information.

- The **HIPAA Privacy Rule** was enacted in 2003 to protect patient information. For patients, this protects their health information and outlines who is allowed, and not allowed, access to the information. For those who have access to patient information, it outlines specific rules that must be followed when sharing patient information. HIPAA protects a patient's medical record by outlining what entities are allowed information obtained from the patient's record. HIPAA works at many levels to ensure a patient's rights are not violated by preventing the sharing of personal health information with those who are not involved in their healthcare.
- The **HIPAA Security Rule**, also established in 2003, pertains to the electronic health record and requirements to ensure that the medical record system is secure. This rule outlines the guidelines to be followed at the administrative and technological level of healthcare recordkeeping.

MEDICAL INFORMATICS

Medical informatics is the combination of medicine and technology to improve documentation and medical care for the patient. This has improved communication by allowing the patient access to their health record so they can be involved in their care. Most healthcare record systems also allow the patient to communicate electronically with their provider so they can be more involved with their care. Medical informatics has also improved communication between healthcare entities, as access to a patient's medical record may be shared between different providers to improve the coordination of care.

Medical informatics also allows healthcare providers to be more efficient in treating patients by having all of their information available in one location. Review of medical history, easier charting methods, and easier communication with other members of the healthcare team through the patient's electronic health record can improve the overall delivery of care. There is also increased safety with an electronic healthcare system because of built-in functions alerting providers to repeat procedures, medication interactions, and other actions that may be harmful to the patient.

BILLING AND CODING SYSTEMS

The billing and coding systems utilized in the American healthcare system are:

- **ICD-10**: Created by the World Health Organization to assign a code to specific diseases and health states, the International Statistical Classification of Diseases and Related Health Problems is now in its 10th revision. Work on the 10th version started in 1983 and was finished in 1992. The United States started to use this version in 2015. The ICD-10 contains over 14,000 disease states and symptoms for which there is a diagnosis code. Every disease diagnosed during a medical visit will have a corresponding ICD-10 code.
- **CPT**: The Current Procedural Terminology code is established by the American Medical Association. A CPT code is designated for a specific medical, surgical, or diagnostic procedure. New editions of the standard CPT codes are released every October. It is similar to the ICD-10 code, except it identifies the services that were performed rather than the medical diagnosis. The CPT simplifies medical record charting for clarity between medical providers and for billing purposes.

CHARACTERISTICS OF THERAPEUTIC COMMUNICATION

Communication can be verbal or nonverbal. The PA can practice **therapeutic communication** with a patient in a nonverbal way by remaining silent, nodding the head, and actively listening to their concerns. Facial expressions should remain relaxed and eye contact should be non-judgmental. A hand on a shoulder if a patient is upset can also be effective.

Verbal communication that is therapeutic includes using close-ended or open-ended questions at appropriate times.

- Close-ended questions will generally elicit a yes or no or another simple answer.
- Open-ended questions allow a patient to expand on their symptoms or concerns.

Restating what the patient has stated lets them know that their concerns were heard and that the PA is clarifying to understand how they are feeling. At the end of a visit, the main points can be summarized to the patient in order to explain the plan or what is to happen next. The patient should always be asked if they have any questions, to ensure communication was clear and understood.

BARRIERS TO THERAPEUTIC COMMUNICATION

When communicating with a patient and their family, the PA should be aware of their **level of understanding**. While some people are more visual learners, others are more audible learners. Some may understand an explanation by hearing it, while others need to read written material or see diagrams and pictures to understand. The teaching style should be based on the patient's most preferred method of learning.

Language barriers can compromise communication with a patient and their family. If English is not their first language, they may have difficulty understanding some medical terms. This can also affect compliance with the treatment plan if instructions are not understood.

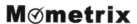

Hearing and vision loss can affect communication with a patient and their family. Of course, if the patient is hearing impaired, they may not clearly hear or understand spoken information that is given to them. It may be helpful to provide educational materials that can be read. If there is vision loss, printed materials may not be helpful.

SCOPE OF PRACTICE OF THE PHYSICIAN ASSISTANT

The scope of practice of the PA varies depending upon the practice setting. Depending upon the practice and the collaborative agreement established with the supervising physician, the responsibilities of the PA may vary. In general, the following duties are within the scope of practice for the PA:

- Taking a medical history from a patient
- Performing a physical exam on a patient
- Ordering and interpreting laboratory and diagnostic tests
- Formulating a diagnosis
- Prescribing appropriate medication for a patient, depending upon state prescribing laws
- Performing in-office procedures and assisting in surgery

LIMITATIONS

Limitations to the scope of practice of the PA vary depending upon state law. These can further vary depending upon the responsibilities delegated to the PA within a specific practice. These limitations include:

- Performing surgery independently
- Administering general anesthetic
- Prescribing outside of the parameters established by the state in which they practice
- Performing any duties that are prohibited as outlined in the collaborative agreement established with the supervising physician

SUPERVISION PARAMETERS

The supervision parameters in the PA's scope are as follows:

- **Malpractice:** PAs need to have malpractice insurance to protect them if they are sued for malpractice or negligence. This is usually provided by the employer, but it may be necessary for the PA to purchase this at their own expense. A PA can be sued independently, without their supervising physician being implicated, if the PA was given advice and guidance from the physician and opted to not follow that medical advice. Often, the supervising physician is also named in a lawsuit if the PA is sued, as well as any healthcare professionals who were involved in the care of the patient. The healthcare facility may also be named in a lawsuit.
- **Mandated reporting:** PAs are legally obligated to be mandated reporters of any cases of suspected abuse or neglect of children, the elderly, and the disabled. If the PA suspects that this is the case with a patient, the local social services department should be contacted if the patient is a minor. In the event of suspected elder abuse, the local branch of adult protective services should be contacted.
- **Conflict of interest:** A conflict of interest can arise if the PA has a vested, financial interest in a specific pharmaceutical product, procedure, or treatment. The PA would then be in a position to financially benefit from promoting these services to the patient. A conflict of interest can also occur if the provider's judgment is influenced. This can occur in caring for family members or close friends because of the difficulty in remaining objective. Most states have policies against providers caring for family members due to a potential for conflict of interest.

- **Impaired provider:** If a provider is under the influence of a medication or drug that interferes with their ability to perform their job duties, or if a medical condition has caused the provider to be unable to safely and effectively treat patients, then the provider is impaired. Most states have an impaired provider program that offers a means by which an impaired provider can receive treatment in order to safely return to practice. The impaired provider may be subject to disciplinary measures at the state level.

PROFESSIONAL DEVELOPMENT REQUIREMENTS

In order to work as a physician assistant, several professional development requirements must be met and maintained:

- **State level**: State licensure must be current; requirements vary depending on the state in which the PA practices. Licensure usually renews on an annual basis.
- **National level**: Certification by the National Commission on Certification of Physician Assistants (NCCPA) must be renewed every 2 years. This is also dependent upon CME obligations for the PA being met. The PA must retake their certification exam every 10 years in order to remain active.
- **Continuing medical education (CME)**: The PA is on a 2-year cycle with CME requirements. They must obtain a total of at last 100 continuing education credits within that 2-year cycle, with at least 50 being considered Category 1 and 50 classified as Category 2. (Category 2 is any medical education activity or patient care that has not been classified as Category 1.) Educational articles with CME credits, conferences, and specific activities are outlined by the NCCPA.

IMPORTANCE OF EVIDENCE-BASED MEDICINE IN HEALTHCARE

Evidence-based medicine involves utilizing research-proven protocols for treating specific health conditions in order to provide the highest-quality care possible. The results of practicing evidence-based medicine include:

- Treating and monitoring specific chronic health conditions by using methods that are proven to provide high-quality results
- Minimizing healthcare costs by avoiding duplicate or unnecessary tests
- Providing consistent treatment for specific conditions

There are several ways the PA can put evidence-based medicine into practice:

- Stay current on recommended protocols and treatment for specific conditions. This provides better outcomes for the patient and minimizes wasted time and resources on trying multiple treatments that may not be as effective.
- Communicate the treatment protocol to the patient and explain the research-based results that have been proven in the past. This can help to increase patient compliance as they see an improvement in their health.
- Use the technological resources available in practice. This can also help the PA to put evidence-based medicine into practice.

ELEMENTS OF DISASTER PREPAREDNESS

The main elements of disaster preparedness are:

- **Communication**: This includes communication between those responding to the disaster and the community at large. Open communication between everyone involved provides more effective resolution of the disaster.
- **Training**: Training should be up to date and comprehensive before a disaster strikes. Keeping everyone involved current on their training will increase the effectiveness of managing a disaster situation.

- **Asset preparedness**: Before a disaster occurs, the assets available should be inventoried. Know beforehand what assets and resources will be necessary to provide food, water, medical care, and other services to those affected by a disaster.
- **Technological needs**: A plan should be in place before a disaster occurs to accommodate the computer or other technological resources that must be made available, including software and hardware needs, as well as the space required.
- **Leadership**: At the healthcare level, there must be people assigned to the role of providing leadership during a disaster. Teams with specific responsibilities should be established beforehand to avoid confusion and chaos when a disaster occurs.

INFECTION CONTROL MEASURES TO IMPLEMENT IN RESPONSE TO OUTBREAKS

The World Health Organization (WHO) has established an **event management system** to be implemented in the event of a disease outbreak. Elements of this system include:

- **Monitoring information on epidemics and outbreaks to investigate trends**. Reviewing past outbreaks of specific diseases can also help to forecast situations that may occur in the future. This includes monitoring the trends of the disease, reviewing the epidemiological information from past outbreaks, and tracking current confirmed outbreaks of a specific disease.
- **Evaluating the logistics of managing a disease outbreak, to include resource management and personnel management.** This includes continually educating and informing response teams on areas of concern that may require activation of the personnel needed to manage an outbreak. It is important to ensure that the resources necessary to manage and treat a disease outbreak are available.
- **Regularly reviewing past successes and failures**, and identifying areas of improvement, based on past performance of managing disease outbreaks. This evaluation of response should be an ongoing process before, during, and after implementation of the response system.

OCCUPATIONAL HEALTH ISSUES AND RISKS

There are several different types of **occupational health risks** to the PA:

- **Infectious agents**: Caring for patients with infectious diseases, even illnesses as benign as a cold or stomach virus, places the PA at risk for contracting these conditions. Depending upon the field of medicine in which the PA is practicing, some of these exposures can be life-threatening.
- **Chemical and radiation hazards**: Depending upon the practice setting, the PA may be exposed to various chemical hazards, such as hazardous gases, or sources of radiation, such as x-rays.
- **Physical hazards**: Musculoskeletal injuries can occur on the job from lifting or moving patients, or from excessive strain on the legs or back from standing all day. There is also the possibility of being exposed to physical harm from patients in certain healthcare settings, or in the event of workplace violence.
- **Psychological stress**: The PA can be under a tremendous amount of stress at work, which can have long-term psychological effects. Identifying those stressors and taking steps to decrease work stress can be helpful in preventing the effects of stress.

EPIDEMIOLOGY

Epidemiology is the field of medicine that focuses on the occurrence and trends of specific diseases within a population. The specialization of epidemiology is very important to public health for several reasons:

- **Studying the course of a disease**: For example, examining the onset and symptoms of influenza in the US, and the course that influenza follows.
- **Identifying frequency of disease**: For example, examining the incidence of influenza cases in the US, or in elderly patients in the US.
- **Identifying pattern of disease**: For example, identifying specific populations or regions in which influenza is identified in the US and the pattern followed as the disease spreads.

- **Identifying risk factors and causes of disease**: For example, identifying those with pre-existing medical conditions, the very young, and the elderly as being at greater risk for contracting influenza, especially with exposure to those with influenza.
- **Evaluating disease prevention and treatment methods**: For example, evaluating the effectiveness of the annual flu vaccine in preventing a population from contracting the disease, and evaluating the antiviral medications available for treatment of influenza.

QUALITY AND RISK MANAGEMENT IN HEALTHCARE

Quality management: Evaluating and improving services offered to ensure they are free of error and completed in an efficient manner. In healthcare, providing high-quality services and care should be done in an economically efficient way in order to minimize unnecessary costs. Evaluating a healthcare organization's quality level is an ongoing process that is constantly evolving and improving to meet its goals.

Risk management: The constant evaluation of the processes within a healthcare system to identify areas in which an error could occur. The purpose of risk management is to correct the problems that contributed to an error so that it does not occur again. Risk management also strives to identify any potential problems so that changes can occur to prevent them from becoming an issue. The goal of effective risk management in healthcare is to provide high-quality care while minimizing cost and any potential dangers to the patient.

Organic Areas

Cardiovascular System

CARDIOMYOPATHIES

Cardiomyopathies are chronic conditions involving a diseased heart muscle. There are three main types: dilated, hypertrophic, and restrictive. **Dilated cardiomyopathy** is the most common type of cardiomyopathy. It results in a reduction in strength of the ventricular contraction, which causes dilation of the left ventricle and a decreased ejection fraction. The most common causes are genetics, alcohol abuse, toxins and drugs, coronary heart disease (CHD), infections, and endocrinopathies (diabetes, thyroid disease), but it can also be due to an autoimmune or an idiopathic process. Infective myocarditis due to the coxsackievirus and other viruses can lead to dilated cardiomyopathy. **Hypertrophic cardiomyopathy** causes a significant hypertrophy of the left ventricle, especially the septum, which results in obstruction of the left ventricle. This is most often genetic in etiology (autosomal dominant) and may be first seen in young athletes as a sudden cardiac arrest. Hypertension may also contribute to development of this type of cardiomyopathy. **Restrictive cardiomyopathy** is rare and occurs due to some type of infiltrative process that results in decreased elasticity of the ventricles, which causes diastolic dysfunction and heart failure. It can be idiopathic or due to conditions that result in endomyocardial fibrosis, such as sarcoidosis or amyloidosis.

DILATED CARDIOMYOPATHY

Dilated cardiomyopathy will cause patients to feel short of breath, especially on exertion, and orthopnea and paroxysmal nocturnal dyspnea (PND) may be present, resulting in complaints of **fatigue**. Patients may also report edema and weight gain, especially around the abdomen. As the ejection fraction decreases, symptoms of congestive heart failure may present, such as rales, edema, S3 gallop, and an increase in jugular venous distension (JVD).

An echocardiogram will assess valvular function, flow, and chamber sizes, and estimate the ejection fraction (EF). A cardiac catheterization can be done to determine the extent of coronary artery disease (CAD) present, and also ejection fraction. A myocardial biopsy may be done during a cardiac catheterization if an autoimmune or infiltrative process is suspected. Cardiac MRIs are increasingly being used in diagnosis. An ECG may show nonspecific ST-T wave changes with left ventricular hypertrophy and possible conduction abnormalities. A chest x-ray may show cardiomegaly, pulmonary venous congestion, interstitial pulmonary edema (Kerley B lines), and pleural effusions. Lab work includes CBC, comprehensive metabolic panel, B-type natriuretic peptide assay (indicates fluid overload), cardiac biomarkers, and thyroid function tests. Finally, a urine or serum drug screen can identify the presence of alcohol/illicit drug use.

Treatment is aimed at reducing preload and afterload, diuresis, and airway support. ACE inhibitors are primarily used, but other treatments include β-blockers, angiotensin II receptor blockers (ARBs), and aldosterone antagonists, to slow left ventricular enlargement. Idiopathic dilated cardiomyopathy is highly familial, so when a new diagnosis is made, genetic screening should be done.

HYPERTROPHIC CARDIOMYOPATHY

Hypertrophic cardiomyopathy may not give any warning signs to patients and is frequently the cause of **sudden cardiac arrest** in the young athlete. If symptomatic, patients commonly complain of dyspnea on exertion (most common), episodes of syncope, angina, palpitations, or fatigue. A systolic crescendo-decrescendo murmur and S4 can be heard with hypertrophic cardiomyopathy, but unlike the other types of cardiomyopathies, the intensity of the murmur will increase when patients are standing or performing the Valsalva maneuver, especially noted if it is obstructive. Also, a double carotid pulse and a jugular venous pulse with a prominent 'a' wave may be noted. A 2-D echocardiogram is diagnostic and assesses diastolic function, valvular function, and EF. ECG changes seen with hypertrophic cardiomyopathy include ST-T wave changes, left ventricular hypertrophy, and deep Q waves.

Treatment focuses on improving diastolic dysfunction by slowing the heart rate and decreasing the contractility of the heart, maintaining euvolemia, and controlling any arrhythmias. β-blockers and calcium channel blockers (e.g., verapamil) are used. Drugs that decrease preload (e.g., ACE inhibitors, angiotensin II receptor blockers, nitrates) should be avoided. Also, because hypertrophic cardiomyopathy is primarily a genetic condition, patients' families should undergo a thorough cardiac evaluation. Complications include left ventricular outflow tract obstruction, CHF, endocarditis, thrombus, and sudden death.

RESTRICTIVE CARDIOMYOPATHY

Restrictive cardiomyopathy is the rarest **cardiomyopathy**. It is marked by **diastolic dysfunction** due to noncompliant ventricular walls that resist diastolic filling, which leads to pulmonary venous hypertension. It must be distinguished from constrictive pericarditis, which has a similar clinical presentation. It may cause dyspnea on exertion, fatigue, orthopnea, and paroxysmal nocturnal dyspnea, as well as peripheral edema and an increase in jugular venous distension. A heart murmur (AV valve regurgitation) may be auscultated, and patients may have chronic atrial fibrillation. This is a diagnosis of exclusion, as this physiology can be seen in many other disorders. Echo may show bilateral atrial enlargement and a restrictive pattern of filling. Though this can be idiopathic in etiology, a myocardial biopsy can be done to determine if an infiltrative process (sarcoidosis or amyloidosis) is present. Cardiac MRI is helpful in detecting pericardial thickening. Treatment is aimed at treating the underlying cause and symptoms, decreasing end-diastolic pressure, and correcting any arrhythmias. Complications include systemic emboli and a progressive decrease in cardiac function. Symptomatic restrictive cardiomyopathy has a poor prognosis.

CONDUCTION DISORDERS
ATRIAL FIBRILLATION

Atrial fibrillation (**AFib**), also known as "holiday heart," is the most common **tachyarrhythmia** and results in an **irregularly irregular rhythm with no visible P waves on ECG**. The QRS complex is usually narrow, ≤0.12 seconds. The AHA classifies AFib as paroxysmal (terminates spontaneously or with intervention within 7 days of onset), persistent (does not terminate within 7 days), long-standing persistent (occurring for >12 months), or permanent. AFib can also be classified as valvular (with moderate to severe mitral stenosis) or nonvalvular (without rheumatic mitral stenosis, heart valve, or mitral valve repair). Common complaints include weakness, dizziness, dyspnea, and palpitations. However, some patients are asymptomatic.

Diagnosis is confirmed through ECG. Assess causes (e.g., alcohol use or withdrawal) and associated diseases, and perform a complete cardiovascular evaluation. Check TSH and T4. Treatment focuses on rate control, anticoagulation, and rhythm control (if AFib symptoms limit the patient). For rate control, diltiazem, verapamil, or β-blockers can be used. Digoxin may be used in patients with AFib due to heart failure, but is contraindicated in patients with preexcitation syndrome. Anticoagulation is based on stroke risk and includes aspirin, warfarin, heparin, and newer anticoagulants (dabigatran, rivaroxaban, etc.). Rhythm control options include cardioversion and ablation. Cardioversion is most effective when started within 48 hours of the onset of AFib. Cardioversion can be performed either chemically (ibutilide, dofetilide, flecainide, propafenone, or amiodarone) or electrically. For new-onset AFib, effectively anticoagulate (>3 weeks with warfarin [INR of 2–3] or a new agent, or use a heparin bridge for a TEE [transesophageal echocardiography] cardioversion) and perform a TEE to assess for atrial thrombus before electrical cardioversion is performed. Continue anticoagulation for 4 weeks post-procedure. If >150 bpm and patient is unstable, immediate synchronized cardioversion should be done to normalize the rate. Complications include reduced cardiac output, thrombus formation, CVA, and heart failure.

ATRIAL FLUTTER

Atrial flutter, the second most common **tachyarrhythmia**, results in a **regular rhythm on ECG** with an atrial rate of **240–360 bpm**. The P waves will follow a "sawtooth" pattern (most obvious in leads II, III, and aVF) two or more times followed by a narrow QRS. This is a macro reentrant arrhythmia with the reentry point just above the AV node. Atrial flutter commonly occurs when the atrial focus is irritated (e.g., atrial enlargement), resulting in multiple firings. The AV node will block some of these impulses from being sent to the ventricles, which can cause an abnormal ventricular rhythm. Signs and symptoms include palpitations, fatigue, and presyncope. The heart rate is typically about 150 bpm due to the AV node block.

Diagnose with ECG, and vagal maneuvers or adenosine may help unmask atrial flutter waves if not visualized clearly on ECG. Evaluate with a transthoracic echocardiogram (TTE). If the patient is unstable, the initial treatment of choice is immediate synchronized cardioversion. IV amiodarone is another option. If stable, the acute patient should undergo synchronized cardioversion or use oral dofetilide, IV ibutilide, and/or rapid atrial pacing for rhythm control, or use IV β-blockers, IV diltiazem, or IV verapamil for rate control. Amiodarone may also be considered. In patients with ongoing atrial flutter, radiofrequency catheter ablation is the treatment of choice for rhythm control, or β-blockers, diltiazem, or verapamil may be used for rate control. For patients with >48 hours (or unknown length) of atrial flutter, check TEE for thrombus, and give anticoagulation before and for a minimum of 4 weeks after cardioversion. If there is recurrent or chronic atrial flutter, continued use of anticoagulants is necessary and based on current stroke risk guidelines. Complications include syncope, CHF, and embolism.

PREMATURE ATRIAL CONTRACTIONS

With a premature atrial contraction (**PAC**), also known as an **atrial premature beat (APB)**, there is an area within the atria that is irritated and is triggering delivery of sporadic impulses. This results in the atria contracting at a time out of sync with the regular rhythm of the atria. PACs are typically benign and found in both the young and elderly, and in those with and without heart disease. There are some known PAC precipitants: smoking, caffeine, stress, and alcohol. PACs are generally asymptomatic and not considered dangerous. Some patients may feel a palpitation or "skipped" beat. Diagnosis is made by ECG with an abnormally shaped P wave (but extra P waves may be hidden within the QRS complex or T waves) with a normal or narrow QRS. A Holter monitor may be worn to assess the frequency of PACs. Treatment is not required unless there is an underlying problem that needs to be managed (usually found in patients with frequent PACs). Avoid or minimize precipitants. If the patient has ongoing, symptomatic PACs, β-blockers can be used. Typically, there are no complications. However, PACs may trigger other dysrhythmias, especially AFib or atrial flutter.

PAROXYSMAL SUPRAVENTRICULAR TACHYCARDIA (PSVT)

Paroxysmal supraventricular tachycardia (PSVT) is an **elevated heart rate** that begins and ends abruptly, originating within the **atria** due to a reentry mechanism. The rate (usually >150 bpm and regular) is so fast that the underlying rhythm cannot be diagnosed. PSVTs can be seen in healthy patients or those with underlying heart or lung disease, as well as in digoxin toxicity and alcohol intoxication. Signs and symptoms vary depending on rate, but can include dizziness, syncope, shortness of breath, diaphoresis, chest pain, and palpitations.

Diagnose clinically and on ECG. P waves are usually not present, or they are buried behind the QRS complex. The PR interval cannot be determined because of the absence of P waves, and the QRS complex is usually very narrow. Screen for Wolff-Parkinson-White syndrome (due to increased risk of sudden death). If patients have a heart rate >150 bpm and are clinically stable, vagal maneuvers may help convert the rate to a sinus rhythm. If this does not work, the next step for acute cases with a narrow QRS complex should be to give IV adenosine, or alternatively, IV verapamil or IV diltiazem. Avoid these AV node blockers if QRS is wide. Instead use synchronized cardioversion, procainamide, or amiodarone. If a patient has a heart rate of >150 bpm and is unstable, immediate electrical synchronized cardioversion is necessary to attempt to return to sinus rhythm. Long-term care options include radiofrequency ablation (first line) or calcium channel blockers, β-blockers, or digoxin. Complications are rare, but may include MI, CHF, and cardiac arrest.

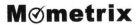

SICK SINUS SYNDROME (SINUS NODE DYSFUNCTION)

Sick sinus syndrome, or sinus node dysfunction, is a group of arrhythmias where the **sinoatrial (SA) node** doesn't function properly, causing **bradycardia**; this is most common in patients >50 years old and tends to be progressive. It is represented by a pattern of irregular sinus bradycardia with possible long pauses (sinus pause; temporary disappearance of P waves) in conduction. There can even be sinus arrest (failure to generate an electrical impulse). There may also be an accelerated atrial rate or a pattern of bradycardia–tachycardia as the heart tries to correct its rhythm. Patients are often asymptomatic early on, and there are often no clear symptoms, but vague complaints that could mimic other disorders. Signs and symptoms include a feeling of fluttering or "wrongness" in the chest, dizziness, fatigue, presyncope, syncope, dyspnea on exertion, a change in mental status, and altered consciousness.

Diagnosis is made by ECG (possibly with a Holter monitor). If the patient is asymptomatic, no treatment is necessary. If possible, stop medications causing bradycardia. Permanent treatment is provided by an internal pacemaker, and the associated surgical risks should be discussed with the patient. Complications of sinus node dysfunction include syncope, CHF, AFib or flutter, AV block, tachycardia-bradycardia syndrome, thrombi, emboli, stroke, and sudden death.

ECG CHANGES PRESENT WITH FIRST-DEGREE AV BLOCK

First-degree AV block occurs when there is a delay in the transmission of the electrical impulse in the heart somewhere along the path from the SA node and through the AV node/His-Purkinje system. The most likely cause is a problem in the AV node itself, and incidence increases with age. This condition can also be caused by drugs (e.g., β-blockers, amiodarone, calcium channel blockers, digoxin) or can be found in well-trained athletes or those with increased vagal tone. First-degree AV block typically does not cause symptoms in patients. Diagnosis is made by ECG. There is usually no change in the heart rate, but the ECG will exhibit a lengthened **PR interval** of >0.2 seconds. There are regular P waves followed by a QRS complex (all P waves conduct to the ventricles, therefore there are no missed beats). The rest of the ECG should be normal. No treatment is necessary. If patients have an underlying condition that could be contributing to the first-degree AV block, such as hypoxia, MI, Lyme disease, collagen vascular disease, or dehydration, then treat those conditions appropriately. There are usually no complications from first-degree AV block, but a few patients will progress to second-degree AV block.

SECOND-DEGREE AV BLOCK (MOBITZ TYPE I AND MOBITZ TYPE II)

In second-degree AV block, not all atrial beats are conducted to the ventricles. This condition can be categorized as **Mobitz type I** or **Mobitz type II**. It may occur after a MI and can be transient and asymptomatic, or it can be due to digoxin, β-blockers, or calcium channel blockers. It must be determined whether a 2:1 AV block is type I or type II, as treatment varies.

Type I second-degree AV block occurs when the time it takes for the electrical impulse to travel from the SA node to the AV node increases until a **ventricular beat** is finally skipped. On the ECG, this will look like a gradually increasing PR interval until a QRS is dropped. If it results in symptomatic bradycardia, it can be treated with atropine, and transcutaneous pacing can help normalize the rate. Further workup will determine if additional intervention is necessary.

Type II second-degree AV block occurs when the electrical impulse signal travels from the SA node to the AV node, but the signal does not always continue on to the ventricles to cause a **contraction**. On ECG, this results in a normal PR interval and a QRS that is usually dropped in the 3rd (3:1) or 4th (4:1) cycle. These patients are more likely to experience symptoms of dizziness, light-headedness, or syncope. This is treated with pacing, and transcutaneous pacing is necessary even in asymptomatic patients. Reversible causes should be investigated, and if none are found, patients should get a permanent pacemaker, as they have a high likelihood of progressing to complete heart block.

THIRD-DEGREE AV BLOCK

Third-degree AV block is considered **complete heart block**. The SA node continues to send its electrical impulse to the AV node, but the AV node is not transmitting this signal on to the ventricles. The ventricles are contracting, but this contraction is due to stimulation of the ventricular fibers, so the heart rate is usually decreased to <40 bpm. Some causes include idiopathic conduction disease, drugs that depress AV conduction, increased vagal tone, and myocardial infarction. Myocardial infarction, resulting in cardiac hypoxia, can cause a disruption in the electrical system of the heart by damaging the AV node so the impulse cannot be transmitted from the SA node to the ventricles.

Signs and symptoms include dizziness, angina, syncope, and exacerbation of heart failure symptoms. Diagnosed by ECG; this condition results in regularly occurring P waves and regularly occurring QRS complexes that are completely independent of each other. The atrial rate is normal at 60–100 bpm, but the ventricular rate will be bradycardic. The QRS complexes may appear wide, indicating an infranodal block with escape rhythms coming from the His or both bundle branches, usually resulting in a hemodynamically unstable patient who doesn't respond to atropine. Treatment of this condition requires transcutaneous pacing until permanent pacing can be established. Patients should be closely monitored for a change in symptoms. Complications include asystole, ventricular fibrillation/ventricular tachycardia, and death.

BUNDLE BRANCH BLOCK

A bundle branch block (**BBB**) can occur within the left or right ventricle. It is usually due to an area of **muscle damage**. As the electrical impulse travels from the atria to the ventricles, the undamaged ventricle will transmit the signal normally. The damaged ventricle, however, will be delayed in transmitting the signal, and this will result in **two QRS complexes** on ECG. Patients are most often asymptomatic and will have a normal heart rate and rhythm. The patient presenting with new-onset BBB should have a complete cardiac workup.

A quick way to diagnose a patient with a BBB is to look at the V1, V2, V5, and V6 leads. With an RBBB (right BBB), the V1 and V2 leads will exhibit an abnormal, wide QRS complex with a "rabbit ears" appearance, with an upward deflection of the QRS complex in V1. With an LBBB (left BBB), leads V5 and V6 will exhibit a widened QRS complex with a notched appearance, with a downwardly deflected QRS in V1. Ventricular rhythms, Brugada syndrome (a genetic disease with increased risk of sudden cardiac death), and ventricular pacing should be ruled out. It is important to remember that a patient with clinical symptoms representing an acute MI cannot be diagnosed with an MI by ECG alone if an LBBB is present. Sgarbossa criteria, as well as other diagnostic labs, will be helpful in this situation. Typically, a BBB does not require treatment. However, a pacemaker would be indicated with syncope (more often seen in LBBB). Prognosis of BBB is tied to underlying heart disease (e.g., an RBBB associated with an MI is associated with increased mortality).

PREMATURE VENTRICULAR CONTRACTIONS (PVCs)

Premature ventricular contractions (**PVCs**) occur when there is an area of irritability within a ventricle, causing it to **contract early**. The cause of PVCs is often unknown, but can be due to electrolyte imbalance, medications (e.g., digitalis), alcohol/drugs, adrenaline (caffeine, anxiety, etc.), or myocardial injury (ischemia, acute MI). Most patients are asymptomatic, but some experience palpitations. The heart rate can vary and will depend upon the underlying rhythm. PVCs generally cause an irregular heart rate, but there can be regularity if bigeminy is present (occurs when a PVC is present after every regular ventricular beat). Trigeminy is present when a PVC occurs during every third ventricular beat. On ECG, P waves are not present before a widened and unusually long QRS, usually followed by a fully compensatory pause. A pattern of bigeminy or trigeminy may be present. Check electrolytes and perform a cardiac workup if indicated.

Treat the underlying cause, if it can be identified (e.g., oxygen if hypoxia is present). Often no treatment is necessary. β-blockers suppress PVCs in patients with ischemia and excess catecholamines. Antiarrhythmic medications (lidocaine, amiodarone, etc.) may be necessary if the PVCs are complex and the patient is symptomatic, especially in the setting of an MI. It is important to consider amiodarone in the peri-MI period to reduce the risk of ventricular tachycardia or ventricular fibrillation. Complications include increased risk of other arrhythmias and cardiomyopathy.

VENTRICULAR TACHYCARDIA

Ventricular tachycardia is a fast (>100 bpm) but regular rhythm with ≥3 **irregular beats** in a row that occurs when the ventricles repeatedly contract without coordinated atrial contractions. It can be **sustained** (>30 seconds) or **non-sustained** (<30 seconds). This can be a deadly arrhythmia and is considered a cardiac emergency. Signs and symptoms include syncope, palpitations, chest pain, shortness of breath (SOB), anxiety, and dizziness. The rate is usually regular at around 150 up to 250 bpm. Diagnosis is on ECG, with widened QRS complexes and typically no P waves present. If the patient is unconscious or unstable, diagnosis is only made by physical findings and rhythm strip. If the patient does not have a pulse, advanced cardiac life support (ACLS) protocol should be started, making sure to defibrillate the patient as quickly as possible. If the patient does have a pulse, assess whether the patient is otherwise hemodynamically stable or unstable. If stable, antiarrhythmics—such as amiodarone, sotalol, or procainamide—should be given to convert to sinus rhythm. If the patient is unstable, cardioversion is indicated (sedate if able). If the patient loses their pulse, defibrillation is indicated. In patients with monomorphic V-tach, with structurally normal hearts, catheter ablation or medication is the usual management. In patients with more complicated issues, an implantable cardioverter-defibrillator should be placed, especially if there is a history of heart disease, to decrease risk of sudden cardiac death. Correct electrolyte disturbances. Complications include sudden death.

VENTRICULAR FLUTTER, TORSADES DE POINTES, AND RMVT

Three types of ventricular tachycardia are ventricular flutter, torsades de pointes, and repetitive monomorphic ventricular tachycardia.

Ventricular flutter is a type of **rapid monomorphic ventricular tachycardia** that can degenerate into ventricular fibrillation. The rate is often about 300 bpm. The ventricles will spasm without any discernible pattern of organized activity. On ECG, there will be a monomorphic sine wave that looks the same even when the ECG is turned upside down. Ventricular flutter can resemble artifact, so the leads must be placed correctly on patients, and patient pulse checked.

A magnesium or potassium deficiency can cause a form of polymorphic ventricular tachycardia called **torsades de pointes**. It is associated with a congenital or acquired (medication/electrolyte disturbance) prolonged QT interval. The name means "twisting of points" because of the changing axis of this rhythm. This rhythm will appear as a series of **widened QRS complexes** that vary in height in a wave pattern. This can also degenerate into ventricular fibrillation. Magnesium sulfate (usually 1–2 gm over 1–2 mins.) should be given.

Repetitive monomorphic ventricular tachycardia (RMVT) is a recurring, monomorphic tachycardia. It is the most common type of idiopathic V tach. It occurs in those without cardiac structural disease. On ECG, it may appear as prolific ventricular ectopy or alternating nonsustained V tach with sinus rhythm.

VENTRICULAR FIBRILLATION

Ventricular fibrillation (**VF**) occurs when the ventricles are in a state of uncontrolled **spasm** (quivering) without being able to complete a forceful contraction. This causes cardiac arrest and is a true emergency, with death occurring within minutes of the arrhythmia. On ECG, the heart rate cannot be determined because of the irregularity. There are no discernible P waves, QRS complexes, or T waves. The rhythm can appear to be coarse or fine. VF can resemble artifact, so the leads must be placed correctly on patients, and pulse checked. For treatment of VF, ACLS protocol should be followed, including high-quality CPR, immediate defibrillation, epinephrine 1 mg every 3–5 minutes, and amiodarone 300 mg bolus (and possible 150 mg second dose). Patients should be well oxygenated and intubated if necessary. Look for causes, such as the 5 Hs & 5 Ts. The 5 Hs are hypovolemia, hypoxia, hydrogen ions (acidosis), hypo/hyperkalemia, and hypothermia. The 5 Ts are tension pneumothorax, tamponade, toxins, thrombosis (cardiac), and thrombosis (pulmonary). Prognosis is often related to time of onset of VF and medical treatment. Anoxic encephalopathy and death may follow, even after initial successful resuscitation.

CONGENITAL HEART DISEASE

COARCTATION OF THE AORTA

Coarctation of the aorta is a non-cyanotic, congenital heart defect (which may present later in life) in which there is **narrowing of the aorta**, usually distal to the left subclavian artery. This results in the development of **collateral circulation** through the intercostal arteries and the branches of the subclavian artery. It is most common in male children and is often associated with Turner syndrome in females. Clinically, the patient may exhibit hypertension with blood pressure and pulse discrepancies between the upper and lower extremities. Symptoms of congestive heart failure may be present, along with weak or absent femoral pulses. A systolic murmur will be heard predominantly over the back.

Coarctation of the aorta is diagnosed using a chest x-ray and ECG. X-ray shows a "figure 3" sign in the left upper mediastinal shadow, and rib notching will be evident due to the development of collateral vessels trying to pass over the coarctation. An ECG usually shows right ventricular hypertrophy in infants and left ventricular hypertrophy in adults. Echocardiogram may also be done; this helps measure peak pressure gradients. Diagnosis can be confirmed using a cardiac catheterization/angiogram. Treat symptomatic neonates with prostaglandin E1 to open the ductus arteriosus. Treatments include balloon angioplasty and possible stent placement to widen the aorta, resection, left subclavian flap aortoplasty, or patch aortoplasty. Post-op endocarditis prophylaxis treatment is required 6 months after the repair. Lifelong follow-up is necessary. Complications include hypertension, CHF, stroke, aortic dissection/rupture, cerebral aneurysm, coronary artery disease, and organ failure.

> **Review Video: Pediatric Cardiology & Cardiac Defects**
> Visit mometrix.com/academy and enter code: 674392

ATRIAL SEPTAL DEFECT (ASD)

An atrial septal defect (**ASD**) is a non-cyanotic, congenital heart defect in which there is an **opening between the left and right atrium** causing a left-to-right shunt. This can result in failure to thrive in the infant, but it is often not diagnosed until adulthood because minimal symptoms may be present in the first few decades of life. Although ASD is typically asymptomatic, the infant may exhibit dyspnea and excessive fatigue. On exam, a systolic murmur and a widely split and fixed S2 will be heard. An ASD is diagnosed initially through a combination of exam findings, ECG changes, and chest x-ray. ECG findings may include right- or left-axis deviation (depending on the position of the defect), an rSR′ pattern in V1, or a right bundle branch block. An echocardiogram and an angiogram can be done to confirm the diagnosis. ASD is not diagnosed in utero because of the presence of the patent foramen ovale. It is usually detected within a couple of days of birth if the defect is large, or in the second or third decade of life. Treatment includes observation, or closure if the defect is significant. Repair is accomplished using cardiac catheterization techniques to patch the defect (preferred when possible) or through surgical repair. Post-op endocarditis prophylaxis treatment is required 6 months after the repair. A small ASD, especially if central, may close during childhood and never cause an issue. Complications are often related to the size and can include heart failure, arrhythmias, stroke, and pulmonary hypertension.

VENTRICULAR SEPTAL DEFECT

A ventricular septal defect (**VSD**) is a non-cyanotic, congenital heart defect in which there is an **opening between the left and right ventricles**. This condition can be associated with Eisenmenger syndrome (a VSD with cyanosis and pulmonary hypertension). Clinically, the infant may exhibit signs of pulmonary hypertension and congestive heart failure. Very rapid respirations may be present with sweating and pallor. The infant may have great difficulty eating because of the difficulty breathing, resulting in failure to thrive. On exam, a harsh, holosystolic murmur (with or without a thrill) can be heard at the lower left sternal border (LLSB). A VSD is suggested with exam findings and chest x-ray, but diagnosed with an echocardiogram. An ECG usually shows

62

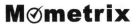

left ventricular hypertrophy, but if the defect is large, the ECG may show combined ventricular hypertrophy or right ventricular hypertrophy. Small VSDs may not need treatment. Treat heart failure with diuretics, digoxin, and ACE inhibitors. Closure of the VSD can be attempted using cardiac catheterization techniques, but open surgery may be necessary or preferred. Post-op endocarditis prophylaxis treatment is required 6 months after the repair. Complications include arrhythmias, endocarditis, and pulmonary hypertension.

PATENT DUCTUS ARTERIOSUS

Patent ductus arteriosus (**PDA**) is a non-cyanotic, congenital heart defect in which the **ductus arteriosus** fails to close after birth, causing a left-to-right shunt. The ductus arteriosus is an opening, present in utero, that serves as a shunt between the left pulmonary artery and the aorta. After birth, it normally closes within 10–18 hours of life. However, this opening can fail to close due to a rubella infection while in utero, or due to other causes (e.g., prematurity, maternal use of phenytoin or amphetamines). If the PDA closes spontaneously after this time, it typically occurs by 3 months of age. Clinically, the infant may be asymptomatic, or may exhibit pulmonary hypertension, difficulty feeding, and a failure to thrive. On exam, there will be a continuous machinery murmur heard at the left upper sternal border (LUSB). The apical impulse is displaced laterally, a thrill may be palpated, and a widened pulse pressure may also be present. PDA is diagnosed through a combination of exam findings, ECG, and chest x-ray, but is confirmed by echocardiogram. Closure of the PDA may be achieved using IV COX inhibitors (e.g., indomethacin) or IV ibuprofen. Other options include less invasive cardiac catheterization techniques; or surgery may be necessary. Complications include pulmonary hypertension, heart failure, and endocarditis.

TETRALOGY OF FALLOT

Tetralogy of Fallot (**TOF**) is a cyanotic, congenital heart defect that comprises four conditions: a ventricular septal defect, right ventricular hypertrophy, right ventricular outflow obstruction (pulmonary stenosis), and overriding of the aorta. This is the most common **cyanotic infant heart disease**. Genetic factors, maternal rubella/other viruses, and some medications are associated with the development of this condition. Clinically, the infant will be cyanotic with dyspnea, and will exhibit poor feeding/poor weight gain, and eventually clubbing. "Tet" spells, or severe cyanotic spells, may occur when feeding or crying. A holosystolic murmur can be heard on exam, as well as a prominent right ventricular impulse and thrill noted at the left sternal border (LSB). TOF can be diagnosed using physical exam (PE) findings, chest x-ray, ECG, and echocardiogram. A CBC will show polycythemia (elevated RBCs, elevated Hgb/Hct). Surgery is necessary, and is usually performed in the first year of life. Patients will always require endocarditis prophylaxis before all dental procedures and other invasive procedures throughout their lifetimes. Complications include endocarditis, emboli, and CHF. If untreated, this defect leads to disability and death by adulthood.

HYPERTENSION AND HYPOTENSION

PRIMARY, SECONDARY, AND MALIGNANT HYPERTENSION

Primary (essential) hypertension is the most common form of hypertension, accounting for 90–95% of cases. The cause of this type of hypertension is unknown, but genetic and environmental factors play a role. Most patients are unaware that they are suffering from this type of hypertension. It is diagnosed after patients have three separate episodes of blood pressure 140/90 or higher that are not found to be due to some type of medical condition.

Secondary hypertension only affects about 2–10% of the population of patients who have been diagnosed with hypertension. It is due to another medical condition, such as renal disease (most common), renal artery stenosis, primary aldosteronism, or pheochromocytoma.

Malignant hypertension (hypertensive emergency) is uncontrolled severe hypertension that causes end-organ damage and can be life-threatening. It can be due to secondary causes (e.g., renal artery stenosis, abrupt clonidine withdrawal), or the cause may be unknown. The goal is to provide immediate treatment by decreasing the mean arterial blood pressure slowly, no more than 15–25% over the first minutes to 1–2 hours, with further titration based on symptoms. After the patient is stabilized, gradually reduce blood pressure over

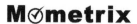

24–48 hours. Nitroprusside, clevidipine, nicardipine, labetalol, and fenoldopam are the most common IV medications used to initially treat this condition.

HYPERTENSION
CLASSIFICATIONS*

Standard classifications of hypertension in adults (from JNC 7; based on two or more readings):

Classification	Systolic BP mmHg		Diastolic BP mmHg
Normal	<120	*and*	<80
Pre-hypertension	120–139	*or*	80–89
Stage 1 hypertension	140–159	*or*	90–99
Stage 2 hypertension	≥160	*or*	≥100

* Guidelines from American College of Cardiology and American Heart Association in 2017 lower these: **Normal** as <120/80; **Elevated** as 120–129 *and* <80; **Stage 1** as 130–139 *or* 80–89; **Stage 2** as ≥140 *or* ≥90.

Hypertensive crises (blood pressure >180/120) can be classified as follows:

- **Hypertensive urgency**: severe hypertension without target-organ damage found.
- **Hypertensive emergency**: severe hypertension with acute target-organ damage.

Severe hypertensive retinopathy (malignant hypertension) is severe hypertension with papilledema and flame-shaped retinal hemorrhages and exudates. Hypertensive encephalopathy may be present as well.

TREATMENT

β-blockers help to lower blood pressure by decreasing the heart rate and the force that is exerted by the ventricles with each heartbeat. β-blockers work on **β-receptors**, though not all β-blockers are created to work just on cardiac β-receptors. Some of these medications, especially the older medications, work on all the β-receptors in the body. β-blockers are now thought to be helpful in patients with known CAD, those who have had an MI, and those patients with known CHF. Although β-blockers are a routine part of therapy for those with heart failure, in patients with acute decompensated heart failure, they may exacerbate acute heart failure symptoms. Because β-blockers reduce the heart rate, there is a risk that they can cause bradycardia and hypotension. This can result in dizziness, confusion, and possibly even syncope. The most commonly reported side effects of β-blockers are sexual dysfunction, depression, and fatigue. β-blockers are associated with increased airway resistance in patients that already have lung disease. β-blockers are contraindicated in those with second- and third-degree AV block, symptomatic bradycardia associated with sick sinus syndrome, asthma, and severe COPD. Sudden withdrawal from β-blockers can cause ischemic symptoms, especially for those with coronary artery disease. Therefore, slowly reduce over several weeks. Some examples of β-blockers include metoprolol (Lopressor), atenolol (Tenormin), carvedilol (Coreg), and acebutolol (Sectral).

ACE inhibitors work on the **arteries** to cause dilation, which decreases the total peripheral vascular resistance (resistance of blood flow thorough the systemic blood vessels) and leads to a decrease in blood pressure. They work through inhibiting the **renin-angiotensin-aldosterone system**. Their effects help decrease morbidity and mortality in patients with heart failure, recent MI, renal disease, and proteinuria. Their antihypertensive effects are additive when used with thiazide diuretics. ACE inhibitors are not used as first-line treatment in African American patients due to a possible increased risk of stroke. Because ACE inhibitors cause arterial dilation, they can—in rare cases—cause angioedema, resulting in excessive dilation in the arteries of the lips, face, and larynx. Though rare, this type of allergic reaction is a medical emergency. A common potential side effect of ACE inhibitors is a chronic, nonproductive cough (5–20% of patients), which can be a reason for noncompliance in patients. Hypotension, pruritus, and rash are other related side effects. ACE inhibitors may cause the kidneys to decrease excretion of potassium, so patients should be monitored for hyperkalemia (especially patients taking potassium supplements or potassium-sparing diuretics). ACE

64

inhibitors are contraindicated in pregnancy and in patients with bilateral renal artery stenosis. Some examples of ACE inhibitors include captopril (Capoten), enalapril (Vasotec), and quinapril (Accupril).

Diuretics classes include thiazide, potassium-sparing, and loop diuretics. **Thiazide diuretics** are used as first-line therapy in most patients and can be used alone or in combination (e.g., with a β-blocker or ACE inhibitor). Thiazides are particularly helpful in African American patients with or without diabetes mellitus (DM). **Potassium-sparing diuretics** work better in combination with other antihypertensive drugs. **Loop diuretics** can be used in patients with a decreased glomerular filtration rate or CHF.

Diuretics work on the kidneys to increase the amount of water and sodium that is excreted from the body through the urine. This helps to reduce the actual fluid volume in the body, thus decreasing the amount of pressure within the arteries and resulting in a lowered blood pressure. Because diuretics work on the kidneys, they may not be appropriate for all patients, especially those with renal disease. Along with the water and sodium that is increasingly excreted from the body, potassium is also depleted with some of the diuretics. This can result in hypokalemia, so a potassium supplement is often prescribed along with the diuretic. Eating foods high in K^+ may also help patients prevent a decrease in potassium levels. An increase in urinary frequency is often seen, so patients should take diuretics in the morning to prevent having to get up frequently during the night. Examples of some diuretics are as follows. Thiazide diuretics: hydrochlorothiazide (HCTZ) and chlorthalidone (Thalitone). Potassium-sparing diuretics: spironolactone (Aldactone) and triamterene (Dyrenium). Loop diuretics: furosemide (Lasix) and torsemide (Demadex).

Calcium channel blockers are particularly helpful in African American patients with or without DM. There are two categories of Ca^{++} channel blockers (CCBs): dihydropyridines and non-dihydropyridines. The **dihydropyridines** bind Ca^{++} channels in vascular smooth muscle to dilate the arteries, resulting in a decrease in blood pressure. The **non-dihydropyridines** bind Ca^{++} channels in the SA and AV nodes and also have cardiac and some vascular effects, thereby decreasing the heart rate and the force of ventricular contractions. The newer CCBs, the dihydropyridines, only work to cause peripheral arterial dilation and may sometimes cause reflex tachycardia. They should be used cautiously in patients with CHF. The non-dihydropyridines, which cause a decrease in ventricular force, may worsen CHF and are contraindicated in severe left ventricular dysfunction, in moderate to severe CHF, and in patients with second- and third-degree heart block. Nifedipine is associated with an increase in mortality in the acute period after MI. Possible side effects while taking CCBs: headaches, flushing, dizziness, and edema. Constipation and gingival hyperplasia are specific adverse effects of the CCB verapamil. Dihydropyridines ("-pines") include amlodipine (Norvasc), nifedipine (Procardia), and felodipine (Plendil). The non-dihydropyridines are diltiazem (Cardizem) and verapamil (Calan).

Angiotensin-receptor blockers (**ARBs**) work similarly to ACE inhibitors by working on the **renin-angiotensin system**. However, they block the effects of angiotensin II by binding to angiotensin type I receptors, causing the arteries to dilate, which decreases the pressure within the arteries and leads to a decrease in blood pressure. Their effects also help patients with CHF by decreasing the risk of stroke and decreasing the risk of a future MI. ARBs are usually used when ACE inhibitors are not well tolerated. Both ARBs and ACE inhibitors are helpful in patients with DM (especially white, non-African American patients), chronic kidney disease, and stroke. However, ACE inhibitors and ARBs should not be used in combination with each other. An ARB may be prescribed instead of an ACE inhibitor due to a lower incidence of chronic cough and angioedema. Shared side effects between the two drugs include hyperkalemia, renal dysfunction, and syncope due to hypotension. ARBs do have a higher rate of hypotensive symptoms than ACE inhibitors. They are contraindicated in pregnancy and in diabetic patients on aliskiren. Examples of ARBs include losartan (Cozaar), telmisartan (Micardis), and valsartan (Diovan).

ORTHOSTATIC HYPOTENSION

Orthostatic hypotension is a sudden drop in **blood pressure** that is symptomatic and affects approximately 20% of the elderly. It usually occurs when a patient stands up quickly or is rising from a lying to sitting or standing position. It is typically caused by autonomic dysfunction or hypovolemia. Another common cause of orthostatic hypotension is medication, including antihypertensives, antidepressants (especially tricyclic), vasodilators (e.g., nitrates), and diuretics. Excessive alcohol use, prolonged bed rest, and adrenal insufficiency are other causes. Patients will describe a sudden dizziness or light-headed sensation, syncope, or near syncope when getting up too quickly. Other symptoms are leg buckling, blurry vision, confusion, and weakness/fatigue. Some patients may also experience these symptoms after eating.

Diagnosis is based on a sustained >20 mmHg decrease in systolic pressure, a 10 mmHg decrease in diastolic pressure, or both, that is noted within 3 minutes of standing after a 5-minute time of resting in the supine position. If there is not a corresponding increase in the heart rate, consider autonomic dysfunction, whereas a corresponding increase in heart rate by >30 bpm suggests hypovolemia or postural orthostatic tachycardia syndrome (POTS). Treatment includes discontinuing medications that could be responsible (if able), correcting hypovolemia, increasing sodium intake, using elastic stockings, and exercising. Advise patients to rise slowly from a seated or lying position. If severe symptoms remain after nonpharmacologic intervention, consider fludrocortisone or midodrine. Complications include falls, strokes, and cardiovascular disease.

CARDIOGENIC SHOCK

Cardiogenic shock is a condition of **decreased cardiac output**, but with adequate intravascular volume. The heart is not able to supply the body with the necessary blood, oxygen, and nutrients that are necessary for proper functioning. It is most often secondary to MI damage that reduces the contractibility of the ventricles, interfering with the pumping mechanism of the heart and decreasing oxygen perfusion. Cardiogenic shock has three characteristics: increased preload, increased afterload, and decreased contractibility. Together, these result in a decreased cardiac output and an increase in systemic vascular resistance (SVR) to compensate and protect vital organs. This results in an increase of afterload in the left ventricle with increased need for oxygen. As the cardiac output continues to decrease, tissue perfusion decreases, coronary artery perfusion decreases, fluid backs up, and the left ventricle fails to adequately pump the blood, resulting in pulmonary edema and left ventricular failure. Decreasing oxygen consumption is a major initial goal of treating cardiogenic shock.

Symptoms include:

- Hypotension with systolic blood pressure <90 mmHg
- Tachycardia >100 bpm with weak, thready pulse and dysrhythmias
- Decreased heart sounds, chest pain
- Tachypnea and basilar rales
- Oliguria
- Cyanotic, cool, clammy skin, pallor, and mottled extremities

Treatment includes:

- IV fluids
- Inotropic agents
- Anti-dysrhythmics
- Intra-aortic balloon pump (IABP) or left ventricular assist device

CORONARY HEART DISEASE

ANGINA (STABLE, UNSTABLE, PRINZMETAL VARIANT)

Angina is chest pain due to myocardial ischemia that is usually brought on by stress or exertion and relieved by rest and/or nitrate medications. Angina can be classified as stable, unstable, or Prinzmetal variant type.

Stable angina usually lasts <5 minutes. It is increased with activity and decreased with rest and/or nitrates. It is described as a clenching sensation over the chest, and the physical exam is usually normal.

Unstable angina (also known as preinfarction or crescendo angina) is a progression of coronary artery disease and occurs when there is a change in the pattern of stable angina. The pain may increase, last longer (>5–20 minutes), fail to respond to a single nitroglycerin, become more frequent, occur at rest, and be accompanied by pallor, diaphoresis, and ST-segment depression, but without elevated biomarkers. Unstable angina may indicate an upcoming myocardial infarction.

Prinzmetal variant angina results from spasms of the coronary arteries, and is often related to stress, cold weather, smoking, or illicit stimulants. Variant angina frequently occurs cyclically, usually at night or the early morning, and at rest. Elevation of ST segments usually occurs with variant angina. Nitroglycerin or calcium channel blockers are used for treatment. Patients presenting with chest pain should be treated with SL nitroglycerin (0.3–0.6 mg every 5 minutes up to 3 times), daily aspirin and β-blockers, and an appropriate stress test. It is extremely important to determine the presence of **acute coronary syndrome (ACS)**, which includes unstable angina, NSTEMI, and STEMI, so directed treatment can begin as soon as possible.

ACUTE MYOCARDIAL INFARCTION (MI)

Acute myocardial infarction (MI) may be classified as **NSTEMI** (non-ST-segment elevation MI) or **STEMI** (ST-segment elevation MI). Clinical manifestations of MI may vary considerably, with males having the more "classic" symptom of sudden-onset crushing chest pain, and females and those under 55 often presenting with atypical symptoms. Elderly patients and diabetics may have reduced pain sensation, may not have any of the classic symptoms of an acute MI due to neuropathy or dementia (elderly), and may complain primarily of weakness. About two-thirds of patients have prodromal symptoms (chest discomfort, fatigue, SOB) weeks to days preceding the MI, and most MIs occur in the early morning hours. Patients may complain of crushing pressure or pain throughout the chest, radiating into the neck, jaw, or left arm. They may also have epigastric pain or a feeling of weakness or anxiety. Patients may be nauseated, pale, diaphoretic, and short of breath, and may appear restless or lethargic.

On exam, an S4 gallop is usually present, blood pressure may be high or low, and acute symptoms of CHF may also be seen. Serial ECGs may show ST elevation, though depression can also be seen. Serial cardiac enzymes (troponin) should be drawn at presentation and 3 hours later. Troponin I and T are contractile proteins that appear in the serum after cardiac necrosis, and are the new standard of measuring cardiac injury. Troponin levels increase within 3–12 hours of cardiac injury, peak at 24–48 hours, and return to normal after 5–14 days. An echocardiogram may show a decreased EF, and cardiac wall stiffness may be seen.

ACUTE MYOCARDIAL INFARCTION TREATMENT

Remember the mnemonic: MONA. This stands for immediate acute MI treatment with **morphine**, **oxygen**, **nitrates**, and **aspirin**. Also start β-blockers and heparin (or another anticoagulant). Determine as soon as possible if chest pain is due to unstable angina, NSTEMI, or STEMI, as the treatment course is different (obtain a 12-lead ECG within 10 minutes of arriving to ER). Early reperfusion is key.

STEMI (ST-segment elevation MI) corresponds to an ECG with ST elevation not easily reversed with nitroglycerin, and elevated troponin I or T. STEMI treatment is:

- Immediate percutaneous coronary intervention (PCI) within 90 minutes **or** thrombolytics
- Coronary artery bypass graft (CABG) if unable to perform PCI

NSTEMI (non-ST-segment elevation MI) corresponds to an ECG with no ST elevation, but with ST depression and/or T wave inversion, and elevated cardiac markers. NSTEMI treatment is:

- If **unstable**: immediate angiography with PCI or CABG
- If **stable**: PCI or CABG within 24–48 hours

Thrombolytic therapy works best when begun within 12 hours of the onset of chest pain, with the goal of starting within 30 minutes of ER arrival, if that course of reperfusion is chosen. These medications can have serious side effects, so a careful assessment of the patient's medical history should be done. Thrombolytics/fibrinolytics are contraindicated with any known intracranial hemorrhage, tumor, or stroke. In the case of STEMI or unstable NSTEMI, ideally, patients should be stabilized and taken for angiography and PCI or CABG within 90 minutes of presenting to the ER. PCI involves percutaneous transluminal coronary angioplasty (PTCA), usually with stent placement. The decision of whether to use PCI or CABG is based on multiple factors, including availability of PCI, symptoms, comorbidities (e.g., DM), the number and location of blocked arteries, and the degree of narrowing of arteries. At discharge, start lifestyle changes and continue antiplatelets, β-blockers, ACE inhibitors, and statins.

VASCULAR DISEASE
AORTIC ANEURYSM

An aortic aneurysm is a dilation of the aorta ≥50% of normal arterial size. It is usually seen as an **abdominal aortic aneurysm** (AAA) >3 cm at a level below the renal arteries, but it can be common in the **thoracic aorta** in patients who have connective tissue disorders (e.g., Marfan syndrome). High-risk patients for developing an aortic aneurysm are men age >65 who smoke, have hypertension, and have atherosclerosis. Many aortic aneurysms are found incidentally during an imaging study. Most are asymptomatic, but patients may have complaints of vague back pain before dissection or rupture occurs. An abdominal pulsatile mass may be felt, or a bruit may be heard, and if dissection or rupture occurs, there will be hypotension and decreased pulses below the level of the aneurysm. A dissected AAA classically presents with abdominal pain, a pulsatile abdominal mass, and hypotension, and requires immediate emergency surgery without imaging studies.

If diagnosis is unclear, ultrasound or CT will visualize the aneurysm. CT angiography or magnetic resonance angiography (MRA) can confirm the diagnosis in patients who have not ruptured. If a patient has a known but asymptomatic aneurysm, an annual ultrasound should be done to monitor its growth. The risk of surgical repair typically outweighs the risk of aneurysm rupture until the ascending aorta reaches >5–6 cm, the descending aorta is >6–7 cm, and the abdominal aneurysm is >5–5.5 cm. Patients with Marfan syndrome require surgery when it reaches ≥4.5–5 cm in any location. Repair is with endovascular stent grafting, or open surgery for more complicated cases. In the asymptomatic patient, medical management includes aggressive control of blood pressure with β-blockers, serial imaging, smoking cessation, and patient education on signs of complications (sudden intense back or abdominal pain). Complications include thrombus/embolus, dissection, rupture, or death.

DISSECTING AORTIC ANEURYSM

A dissecting aortic aneurysm occurs when the wall of the aorta is torn and blood flows in the channel created between the intima and media, dilating and weakening it until it risks rupture (which has 90% mortality). This most often occurs in the proximal ascending aorta.

DeBakey classification uses anatomic location as the focal point:

- **Type I** begins in the ascending aorta, but may spread to include the aortic arch and the descending aorta (50%). (i.e., Stanford type A)
- **Type II** is restricted to the ascending aorta (35%). (i.e., Stanford type A)
- **Type III** is restricted to the descending aorta (15%). (i.e., Stanford type B)

Patients will describe a fairly sudden onset of mid-abdominal pain or back pain that is ripping or tearing in quality. This pain may be aggravated by taking a deep breath or by performing any activities. Hip pain may also be present if blood is pooling in the lower abdominal cavity. Clinically, a pulsatile mass may or may not be palpated. It is advised that no hard palpation be performed on the abdomen until an aneurysm is ruled out because of fear of causing sudden rupture if the dissection is advanced. Diagnosis is with immediate TEE, CT with angiography, or MRA. Treatment consists of open surgery or endovascular methods. However, in patients that present with a descending aortic dissection, medical management using β-blockers to control blood pressure is sometimes chosen. Complications include pericardial tamponade, shock, organ failure, or death.

PERIPHERAL ARTERIAL DISEASE (PAD)

Peripheral arterial disease (**PAD**) occurs when there is **obstruction or narrowing of an artery** that interferes with blood flow, typically in the lower extremities. This can be due to atherosclerosis, trauma, or inflammation. Patients will frequently complain of pain, achiness, or tiredness in their legs or calves after walking a short distance, which is relieved with rest (intermittent claudication). Patients may also state that they have burning, numbing, and tingling sensations in their extremities. Some male patients may complain about erectile dysfunction. Clinically, there may be obvious signs of obstructed blood flow, such as pallor, atrophic skin, and hair loss. Dependent rubor may be noted, and pain may become worse when legs are elevated. Peripheral pulses may be decreased or absent if occlusion is present. In severe cases, arterial ulcers may be present with development of gangrene.

An ankle-brachial index (ABI) of <0.9 (either a resting or exercise ABI) is used to diagnose PAD. Doppler ultrasound will identify decreased blood flow through the arteries. Angiography confirms the diagnosis and provides visualization of the narrowed vessels before surgery. Patients should also be assessed for CAD. Treatment includes risk factor modification (e.g., quitting smoking), exercise, cholesterol control medications, antihypertensives, antiplatelet medications, and blood glucose control. Cilostazol and pentoxifylline help treat symptoms of claudication. Endovascular therapy (e.g., stents, balloons) or open bypass surgery may be indicated. Critical limb ischemia is a possible complication, which can lead to infections/amputations.

ARTERIAL AND VENOUS THROMBOSIS AND EMBOLISM

An **arterial thrombosis** is a blood clot located within an **artery**. A **venous thrombosis** is a blood clot located within a **vein**. This is a stationary clot that can grow large enough to cause occlusion of the vessel. An **embolism** is the term used for the thrombus once it breaks free and begins moving through the **vascular system**. This embolism will eventually travel to an artery or vein that is too small to accommodate its size, resulting in an occlusion of the artery or vein with possible life-threatening results.

Treatment is centered on prevention for high-risk patients (e.g., arteriosclerosis, hypercoagulable state, immobility), such as risk modification, exercise, and wearing compression stockings (e.g., for venous insufficiency, varicose veins). Daily aspirin therapy (81 mg), or other anticoagulants, can provide antiplatelet activity that prevents platelets from forming a clot. Suspect a **deep vein thrombosis (DVT)** if the patient presents with pain, swelling, and redness in the calf with a positive Homan sign. Treat with heparin (LMWH, UFH, or fondaparinux) and oral warfarin to prevent a PE. Heparin can be discontinued after therapeutic INR is reached for 24 hours (usually 4 to 5 days). If a thrombus does form and becomes an embolism, emergency treatment is necessary. For example, an arterial embolism can be fatal, but "clot buster" thrombolytic medications or even surgery to remove the clot may improve the patient's prognosis. Vena cava filters can be used in patients with a high risk for emboli. Complications depend on where the clot is located and include angina, MI, stroke, ischemia to limbs, pulmonary embolism, and postphlebitic syndrome.

PHLEBITIS AND THROMBOPHLEBITIS

Phlebitis is inflammation that is present in a vein and is usually superficial. It is gradual in onset and develops into a reddened, often streaky area that follows the path of a vein. It often occurs at an IV site, and the area may be painful, swollen, indurated, and warm. If the **phlebitis** is superficial, warm compresses, elevation of the affected limb, and compression can help to resolve the problem. If recurrent phlebitis is occurring in the deeper vessels, an anticoagulant may be prescribed to prevent formation of a blood clot. **Thrombophlebitis** occurs when a **blood clot** forms within the inflamed vein. Patients complain of pain that may be gradual or sudden in onset, and the affected area may be red, swollen, or indurated. It is seen most often in more sedentary patients and in patients with a component of Virchow's triad (intimal injury, stasis or turbulent blood flow, and a hypercoagulable state). A hypercoagulable state may be seen with some malignancies. A superficial thrombophlebitis may extend and become a deep vein thrombosis (DVT).

For both phlebitis and superficial thrombophlebitis, anticoagulants are typically not required, and they can be treated with NSAIDs, elevation, and hot/wet compresses. Compression stockings are particularly helpful in cases involving the lower extremity. In more severe cases, treatment consists of anticoagulants (e.g., low molecular weight heparin, fondaparinux) to prevent extension and recurrence, and to decrease the risk of embolism. Prevention is crucial in treatment with compression stockings, leg elevation, and decreasing the amount of time spent immobile.

VARICOSE VEINS AND CHRONIC VENOUS INSUFFICIENCY

Varicose veins occur due to faulty valves within the **distal veins**, leading to distension and stretching of the veins. Because the valves are not functioning properly, blood tends to pool in the extremities and cause further distension of the veins. Patients will complain of aching pain or heaviness in the legs that worsens after standing or sitting for extended periods of time. They may also experience pruritus and burning sensations around the veins, cramps, and restless legs. The veins will be visibly distended, bulging, and contorted. This may lead to **chronic venous insufficiency** (impaired venous return), causing the skin to be reddish and darkly pigmented with edema, and ulcers may form due to venous stasis.

Symptoms are similar to varicose veins, with pain that is worse when legs are dependent. The best treatment of varicose veins is prevention. This includes avoiding standing for prolonged periods of time, exercising regularly to keep weight under control, and wearing compression stockings or maintaining leg elevation to promote venous return from the lower extremities. Medical treatments include sclerotherapy, laser vein ablation, vein stripping, or, in severe cases, complete removal of the varicose veins (phlebectomy). Surgery is typically ineffective for chronic venous insufficiency, and treatment is centered around lifestyle modification, compression, elevation, and topical wound care.

GIANT CELL ARTERITIS

Giant cell arteritis, or **temporal arteritis**, is an inflammatory process that affects the **vessels**, most commonly the temporal artery, but may also involve other medium-sized arteries of the head and neck. It typically affects those >50 years old and is more prevalent among females. This condition can lead to occlusion of the temporal artery, resulting in blindness, so diagnosis and treatment should be started quickly. The most common symptom is a severe headache. This can be accompanied by a fever, malaise, fatigue, or weight loss. Approximately 50% of patients who are diagnosed with giant cell arteritis will also have a diagnosis of polymyalgia rheumatica.

Diagnosis consists of erythrocyte sedimentation rate, C-reactive protein, biopsy (this is the standard), MRI, PET, and Doppler. Because of the nature of the illness, treatment is started before the biopsy results are available. Treatment consists of high-dose prednisone, usually 40–60 mg per day. Follow up with the patient 3 days after starting prednisone, as the headache should improve within that time. Continue prednisone for at least 1 month, and then taper. If symptoms return as the dose of prednisone is tapered, the dosage can be increased. Most patients require steroid treatment for about 2 years to monitor and protect the patient from the long-term effects of steroids. Low-dose aspirin is usually given to reduce the chance of blindness, TIA, and stroke. Chest x-rays or other imaging studies are done annually to assess for aortic aneurysm, as a significant number of patients develop this. Complications include blindness, stroke, peripheral vascular disease, and an increased risk of aortic aneurysm.

VALVULAR DISEASE

AORTIC STENOSIS

Aortic stenosis (**AS**) is a very common valve disease. Most patients are asymptomatic until they reach middle age. Aortic calcifications (aortic sclerosis) are frequently seen in those >55 years old. AS can be due to a **congenital disorder of the valve** (e.g., bicuspid valve) or **rheumatic fever**. When AS patients become symptomatic or severe, the classic symptoms of syncopal episodes, chest pain, and heart failure may be present. Patients may complain of chest pain, fatigue, and shortness of breath with activity. Symptoms of CHF (SOB, dyspnea on exertion, orthopnea, and PND) can be present when the disease is advanced, and prognosis is usually poor by the time these symptoms are present, especially if the patient does not respond to medications. On exam, a systolic ejection murmur that is crescendo/decrescendo in nature during the middle to late portion of the cardiac cycle can be heard. This murmur will radiate superiorly to the carotid arteries and is best heard when the patient is sitting upright and leaning forward. There may also be an early systolic ejection click. Pulsus parvus, or a weakened pulse, may be palpated.

Diagnosis consists of echocardiogram for initial diagnosis, and sometimes a transesophageal echo is needed. Medications can't reverse AS, but they can decrease symptoms. Common medications used include antihypertensive medications, diuretics, medications to help with heart rate control, and β-blockers for angina. To correct AS, aortic valve replacement is needed. If the patient is not a good candidate for surgery, percutaneous valve replacement or percutaneous balloon valvuloplasty are options. Balloon or surgical valvotomy is used to repair congenital AS. Complications include arrhythmias, angina, syncope, heart failure, embolization, and cardiac arrest.

AORTIC REGURGITATION

Aortic regurgitation (**AR**), also called **aortic insufficiency**, occurs when blood flows back into the left ventricle during diastole due to the insufficiency of the aortic valve to close tightly. It can be an acute or chronic condition and can have many causes, including endocarditis, hypertension, rheumatic heart disease, syphilis, Marfan syndrome, and congenital causes. If **acute**, patients will complain of sudden, severe SOB, possible chest pain, and signs of heart failure. If **chronic**, there is an asymptomatic time followed by progressive fatigue, SOB with activity, and palpitations. On exam, a high-pitched, decrescendo diastolic murmur will be heard, increasing when patients are seated and leaning forward and in full expiration. A widened pulse pressure will also be detected. Corrigan sign, a water hammer pulse, may be present. Quincke pulse, an alternating erythema and paleness in the nail beds with each heartbeat, may also be seen. De Musset sign, patients visibly nodding the head with each heartbeat, may be evident. An Austin Flint murmur may be present; this is a mid-diastolic, low-pitched rumbling over the cardiac apex due to the mitral valve leaflets vibrating. Patients may have all or only a few of these findings. Diagnosis is made by echo, which can help classify the regurgitation as mild, moderate, or severe. Treatment includes vasodilators, other medications, or valve repair/replacement. Complications include heart failure, cardiogenic shock, and death.

MITRAL STENOSIS

Mitral stenosis is characterized by blood flow being obstructed through the left atrium to ventricle by way of the damaged **mitral valve**. It is fairly common, and most cases are female. The typical etiology is rheumatic fever presenting in the third or fourth decade of life; however, it can be congenital. Patients may complain of a cough, hemoptysis, or hoarseness that will not go away because of recurrent pressure being applied to the laryngeal nerve or bronchi due to an enlarged left atrium. On exam, findings include an opening snap, a loud S1 (unless stenosis is severe), and a low-pitch, diastolic rumble that is best heard at the apex when the patient is in the left lateral position. The murmur increases with exercise and decreases with the Valsalva maneuver (which decreases preload). Symptoms of CHF may be present, with dyspnea on exertion, crackles, and rales heard in the lungs, as well as fatigue. Symptoms are worse during pregnancy because of the increased blood volume and the strain this puts on the mitral valve.

Diagnosis includes echocardiography, TEE, or occasionally cardiac catheterization. Atrial fibrillation may be detected on ECG. Treatment can include diuretics, β-blockers, and calcium channel blockers. Secondary rheumatic fever prophylaxis is needed (follow current guidelines), and endocarditis prophylaxis is required in some patients (e.g., those with a prosthetic valve, previous infective endocarditis). Anticoagulation should be used in patients who have had an embolus or AFib. Mitral valve surgery is indicated in symptomatic patients or patients with severe stenosis (mitral valve area less than 1.5 cm^2). Options include surgical or percutaneous valvotomy, or mitral valve replacement. Complications include AFib, thrombus/embolus, heart failure, pulmonary hypertension, pulmonary edema, and infective endocarditis.

MITRAL REGURGITATION

Mitral regurgitation (**MR**), also called **mitral insufficiency**, occurs when the mitral valve begins to degenerate. It can be due to rheumatic fever, myxomatous degeneration (MVP), congenital disorders, endocarditis, or dilatation of the left ventricle. Dysfunction of the papillary muscles, coronary artery disease, MI, and ischemia can also lead to MR. The symptoms of MR may be acute or chronic. Patients may complain of SOB with activity, orthopnea, fatigue, and weakness. A holosystolic high-pitched, blowing murmur can be heard over the cardiac apex, radiating into the left axilla, and is best heard in the left lateral position. An S3 may also be heard. Patients may exhibit signs of pulmonary edema with rales, crackles, and dyspnea.

Diagnosis is made by echo. Cardiac catheterization may be used to evaluate certain echo findings before surgery. A chest x-ray may show pulmonary edema, left ventricular hypertrophy, and left atrial enlargement. An ECG may show AFib and left atrial/ventricular enlargement. Treatment includes vasodilators, diuretics, and β-blockers for symptomatic patients. Anticoagulation is needed for patients with AFib or mitral annular calcifications. Surgical mitral valve repair or replacement is necessary in acute MR, or if chronic MR symptoms progress or worsen. If MR is due to papillary muscle dysfunction, patients may present in cardiogenic shock if a papillary muscle has ruptured. This is a life-threatening emergency with a very poor prognosis. Complications include infective endocarditis, arrhythmias, thrombus/embolus, and stroke.

MITRAL VALVE PROLAPSE

Mitral valve prolapse (**MVP**) is more common in females, and is a condition in which the **mitral valve leaflets** are bulging into the atrium during systole. It is usually due to myxomatous degeneration of the leaflets or chordae tendineae, which is typically idiopathic, or can be congenital in nature with inherited connective tissue disorders (e.g., Marfan syndrome) or by autosomal dominant inheritance. It is frequently seen in multiple members of a family. Most patients are asymptomatic, but patients may complain of chest pain, SOB with activity, fatigue, or palpitations. On exam, a mid to late systolic ejection click can be heard possibly with a high-pitched, mid to late systolic murmur. This is best heard at the apex and with the patient in the left lateral position. The murmur is accentuated with the Valsalva maneuver or with standing.

Confirm the diagnosis with an echo (2D TTE). Diagnostic echo findings are leaflet displacement ≥2 mm and leaflet thickness of ≥5 mm. Typically, no treatment is needed since most patients are asymptomatic. However, symptoms may be treated with β-blockers. Endocarditis prophylaxis is no longer recommended for MVP. If the patient is asymptomatic, reevaluate every 3–5 years with physical exam and echo. Complications include mitral valve regurgitation, arrhythmias, and endocarditis.

TRICUSPID STENOSIS

Tricuspid stenosis is not very common and involves narrowing of the **tricuspid valve opening**, causing blood flow obstruction between the right atrium and right ventricle. Stenosis is usually due to rheumatic fever, and therefore, it usually involves the aortic and mitral valves also. Other less common etiologies include carcinoid tumors, systemic lupus erythematosus (SLE), or endocarditis. Patients with tricuspid stenosis may be fatigued and frequently feel cold. They may notice a fluttering sensation in the neck or palpitations. If the condition is advanced, they may feel abdominal pain and bloating due to hepatomegaly. On exam, other symptoms of right-sided CHF may be seen (e.g., pitting edema), and a bounding pulse may be palpated in the neck over the carotid arteries. An opening snap may be auscultated with a mid-diastolic rumble. The murmur is louder and longer with leg raising and inspiration (maneuvers that increase venous return), and therefore softer with Valsalva and standing (maneuvers that decrease venous return).

Diagnosis is confirmed with an echo (TTE), which can measure the amount of blood flow and determine the severity of the stenosis. Chest x-ray and ECG may show right atrial enlargement. Treatment includes antiarrhythmics, diuretics, and salt restriction, but requires surgery to repair or replace the valve if right heart failure or low cardiac output is present. Right atrial enlargement and arrhythmias are complications.

TRICUSPID REGURGITATION

Tricuspid regurgitation, also called **tricuspid insufficiency**, is more common than tricuspid stenosis. Each time the right ventricle contracts, there is blood flow backward through the **tricuspid valve** into the right atrium during systole. It can be **primary** (organic valve problems) or **secondary** (normal valve, but problems occur due to right ventricular enlargement). Tricuspid regurgitation is typically due to secondary causes (e.g., pulmonary hypertension, mitral or pulmonary stenosis). Etiologies include endocarditis, rheumatic fever, MI, right ventricular overload/dilatation, and congenital anomalies. Ebstein's anomaly, a congenital condition, can result in an abnormally formed tricuspid valve, resulting in enlargement of the right atrium and CHF. Patients may complain of fatigue, SOB with activity, abdominal bloating, and swelling in their extremities that is not completely relieved with elevation. On exam, the symptoms of right-sided CHF may be observed (e.g., ascites, peripheral edema, jugular venous distension). A harsh, high-pitched, pansystolic murmur can be auscultated at the LLSB, and the murmur increases upon inspiration. While chest x-ray and ECG may show ventricular enlargement, echo is the diagnostic tool of choice. It also helps to evaluate severity. Treatment includes diuretics to remove fluid, digoxin, ACE inhibitors, and, if severe, annuloplasty or valve repair/replacement. Complications include ascites, heart failure, and thrombus/embolus.

PULMONARY STENOSIS

Pulmonary stenosis is narrowing of the **pulmonary outflow tract** that causes blood flow obstruction between the right ventricle and the pulmonary artery during systole. It is most often due to congenital abnormalities and usually remains asymptomatic until the patient is an adult. It may be seen along with other cardiac abnormalities (e.g., Tetralogy of Fallot). Infants may exhibit failure to thrive and poor weight gain. It rarely occurs as a result of rheumatic fever or carcinoid. Patients may complain of fatigue, SOB with activity, chest pain, and syncope. Cyanosis may exist if a right-to-left shunt is also present. A normal S1 followed by a systolic click and a mid-systolic murmur will be present, and the murmur tends to increase with deep inspiration. A wide split S2 can be present with a right ventricular heave. Diagnosis is made per Doppler echo to assess the valve's anatomy, determine the location of the stenosis, and check the right ventricle. Chest x-ray may show a prominent main pulmonary artery. Surgery is sometimes necessary to repair the valve. Balloon valvuloplasty is the treatment of choice and involves stretching the valve with a balloon in order to widen the opening. Complications include endocarditis, arrhythmias, and heart failure.

PULMONARY REGURGITATION

Pulmonary regurgitation (**PR**), also called **pulmonary insufficiency**, is when blood flows backwards from the **pulmonary artery** to the right ventricle. It most commonly occurs in patients with pulmonary hypertension. Occasionally it is due to endocarditis, congenital abnormalities, rheumatic heart disease, or carcinoid syndrome. There are usually no symptoms with this condition unless it becomes advanced. If right-sided heart failure does occur, patients may complain of SOB with activity (most common), fatigue, light-headedness, palpitations, chest pain, and syncope. On exam, a low-pitched murmur, which may increase with breathing, may be heard. When PR is due to pulmonary hypertension, pressure rises in the pulmonary artery, and a Graham Steell murmur can be heard. This murmur is a high-pitched blowing decrescendo murmur and is best heard at the LUSB. There can be a split S2, and a right-sided S3 or S4 may be heard and is accentuated during inspiration. If pulmonary hypertension is not present, there will be a low-pitched crescendo-decrescendo murmur. Diagnosis is made per echo. Right axis deviation may be noted on ECG due to right ventricular hypertrophy/dilatation as well as an RBBB. Usually the symptoms are not severe enough to warrant treatment with replacement of the pulmonary valve, but surgery can be done if patients are extremely symptomatic. Most treatment will focus on correcting the underlying problem, such as pulmonary hypertension. Right-sided heart failure is rare, but is a complication of PR.

OTHER FORMS OF HEART DISEASE
BACTERIAL ENDOCARDITIS

Bacterial endocarditis can be classified as **subacute** (insidious onset) or **acute** (rapid onset). A further distinction is whether it is present in a **native valve** or **prosthetic valve**, or due to IV drug abuse. A patient with heart disease affecting the valves is at risk for developing endocarditis; this includes those with congenital heart disease or valvular disease and those who have prosthetic valves. IV drug abusers, those who have had invasive procedures/surgery, and those who have had prior endocarditis are also at risk. Almost all patients with endocarditis will have a new, regurgitant-type murmur. Splinter hemorrhages may be evident in the nail beds with Osler nodes (tender nodules in finger/toe pads) and Janeway lesions (nontender lesions on palms/soles). Roth spots (retinal hemorrhages) may be evident on funduscopic exam, and patients may show other signs of emboli being present, such as hematuria and renal dysfunction.

After blood cultures are drawn, empiric antibiotic therapy is started for acutely ill patients, and IV vancomycin 15–20 mg/kg every 8–12 hours is typically used. Nafcillin and gentamicin are used empirically in IV drug users. Appropriate antibiotics are started once culture and sensitivity results are in, and continued for 2–8 weeks. These patients require prophylactic antibiotics for future dental or invasive procedures or surgery that involve the gingiva, respiratory tract, or infected skin or musculoskeletal tissue. Prophylaxis is given 1 hour before the procedure, and oral options include: amoxicillin 2 g or, if allergic to penicillin, clindamycin 600 mg or azithromycin 500 mg. Complications include MI, heart failure, emboli, stroke, or organ damage.

ENDOCARDITIS (DIAGNOSTIC CRITERIA)

The **modified Duke criteria** for endocarditis state that a patient must have 2 major criteria, 1 major and 3 minor criteria, or 5 minor criteria in order to have a definite diagnosis of endocarditis. The **major criteria** are: two positive blood cultures (BCs) with typical endocarditis organisms, two positive BCs taken 12 hours apart, three or more positive BCs taken 1 hour apart, a single positive BC for *Coxiella burnetii*, evidence of endocardial involvement on an echocardiogram (e.g., vegetation), myocardial abscess, partial dehiscence of a prosthetic valve, or the presence of new valvular regurgitation. The **minor criteria** are predisposing risk factors (e.g., heart disease, IV drug use), a fever >100.4 °F, vascular features (e.g., emboli, hemorrhage, Janeway lesions), immunologic features (e.g., glomerulonephritis, Osler nodes, Roth spots, rheumatoid factor), or a positive BC that does not meet major criteria. The BCs should be drawn three times, 1 hour apart, with the samples taken at different sites. The most likely organisms to cause endocarditis are *Staphylococcus aureus*, streptococci (e.g., *Streptococcus viridans*), and enterococci. The transthoracic echocardiogram (TTE) is typically used first, but a transesophageal echo may be necessary for accurate visualization of the valves.

ACUTE RHEUMATIC FEVER

Acute rheumatic fever (**ARF**) can occur approximately 2–3 weeks following a group A streptococcal (GAS) infection. It usually affects children 5 to 15 years old, and is no longer as common in the United States. Approximately 60% of cases with carditis affect the mitral valve, followed by a combined aortic and mitral valve involvement. Patients usually first complain of a migratory polyarthralgia of the large joints, and have a fever. For diagnosis of initial ARF, 2 of the major Jones criteria must be present, or 1 major and 2 minor criteria:

- **Major**
  - Carditis
  - Erythema marginatum
  - Subcutaneous nodules
  - Chorea
  - Migratory arthritis of the large joints
- **Minor**
  - Polyarthralgia
  - Erythrocyte sedimentation rate >60 mm/h or C-reactive protein >3.0 mg/dL
  - Fever ≥ 101.3 °F
  - Prolonged PR interval on ECG

Evidence of prior GAS infection includes a rising antibody titer (e.g., antistreptolysin O or anti-DNase B), a positive throat culture, or positive rapid antigen test. Treatment includes bed rest, penicillin or amoxicillin, aspirin or other NSAID, and steroids (instead of aspirin for moderate to severe carditis). Steroids are continued for 2–3 weeks and then tapered. aspirin can be started as prednisone is tapered, and continued for 2–4 weeks after steroids are discontinued. Haldol may be given to control the movements of chorea. Rheumatic fever can be deadly and can lead to permanent heart disease, CHF, and arrhythmias. The risk for recurring ARF is greatest in the first 5 years; therefore, antibiotic prophylaxis is recommended for 5 years or until the patient reaches 18 years of age. Complications include valvular regurgitation, stenosis (usually mitral or aortic), and heart dysfunction.

ACUTE PERICARDITIS

Acute pericarditis occurs when the **pericardial sac** becomes inflamed. This is often idiopathic, but is most commonly due to a viral infection. A bacterial, fungal, or parasitic infection can also cause this condition, as well as tuberculosis. Autoimmune/inflammatory disorders (e.g., lupus, rheumatoid arthritis, rheumatic fever), metabolic disorders (e.g., renal failure/uremia, hypothyroidism), cardiovascular disorders (e.g., MI, aortic dissection), drugs (e.g., penicillin, doxorubicin), and cancer can also cause pericarditis. Patients will complain of pleuritic chest pain that is worse upon inspiration and relieved by sitting up and leaning forward. The pain is precordial or substernal and may radiate to the neck or trapezius ridge, usually to the left side. Patients may have dyspnea and a nonproductive cough. A pericardial friction rub is the hallmark finding on exam.

Diagnosis is based on physical exam and imaging findings. A chest x-ray may detect a large cardiac silhouette, and an echocardiogram is used to detect a pericardial effusion. An ECG can show serial changes, initially with ST elevation and PR depression. Leukocytosis may be present if viral. Treatment is with NSAIDs (typically aspirin), colchicine (which reduces the rate of recurrent pericarditis), and possibly steroids, all used to reduce inflammation. If an effusion is >250 mL, a pericardiocentesis is performed. If severe, a pericardial window may be created surgically to reduce the tension on the pericardial sac; or it may even be necessary to perform a pericardiectomy, in which the pericardial sac is partially or completely removed. Complications include recurrent pericarditis and cardiac tamponade.

PERICARDIAL EFFUSION

A pericardial effusion occurs when an abnormal amount of fluid accumulates within the **pericardial space**. Normal pericardial fluid is about 20–50 mL. Pericardial effusion can occur due to a viral infection, tuberculosis, a malignant tumor, radiation to the chest cavity, or trauma. Patients with pericardial effusions do not always complain of chest pain. They can have a cough, SOB, dyspnea, palpitations, and syncope. If the cause is infectious, they may have a fever. On exam, tachycardia may be present, and distant cardiac sounds with a pericardial rub may be heard. An echo is the method of choice for diagnosing a pericardial effusion. Early effusions first collect posteriorly. Chest x-ray will show cardiomegaly with a globular, water-bottle shape. ECG changes will be nonspecific and may show a low-voltage QRS complex. Treatment can include NSAIDs (e.g., aspirin, ibuprofen), colchicine, antibiotics, and possibly steroids to treat the inflammation; but a pericardiocentesis is frequently needed to drain off the fluid. In severe cases, the pericardial sac can be partially or completely removed from around the heart. A pericardial biopsy may also be needed to determine the cause of the effusion. Complications include cardiac tamponade and death.

CARDIAC TAMPONADE

Cardiac tamponade is an emergency condition in which fluid accumulates in the **pericardial sac**, leading to cardiac constriction that prevents the ventricles from adequately filling, and thus, decreasing cardiac output. It can occur with malignancy (most common), pericarditis, acute MI, a dissecting thoracic aortic aneurysm, recent cardiac surgery, or trauma. Beck's triad is classic for acute cardiac tamponade: muffled heart sounds, hypotension, and increased jugular venous pressure. Patients may have dyspnea, tachycardia, tachypnea, and chest pain. Pulsus paradoxus, which is a >12 mm drop in systolic pressure during inspiration, can be present. Also, the pulse pressure may be narrowed.

Cardiac tamponade is a clinical diagnosis, and prompt diagnosis is key. In patients with suspected cardiac tamponade, perform an immediate echocardiogram. An ECG can show electrical alternans, and a chest x-ray can show a water-bottle-shaped cardiomegaly. A Swan-Ganz catheter to measure pressure within the heart will reveal that all of the pressures are virtually equal. It is an emergency situation, and an immediate pericardiocentesis should be performed to remove the fluid off the heart. Also, a pericardial window or pericardiectomy may be performed. Use inotropes (e.g., dobutamine) and IV fluids as needed to stabilize the patient. Complications include death, shock, and pulmonary edema.

Review Video: Cardiac Tamponade
Visit mometrix.com/academy and enter code: 920182

LIPID DISORDERS

TYPES OF CHOLESTEROL/LIPOPROTEINS AND GUIDELINES FOR LIPID CONTROL

The following are types of cholesterol and guidelines for lipid control:

- **Chylomicrons** are the least dense lipoprotein; they transport dietary triglycerides and cholesterol.
- **Very low-density lipoproteins (VLDL)** are made in the liver and are rich in triglycerides.
- **Intermediate-density lipoproteins (IDL)** result from VLDL and chylomicron metabolism.
- **Low-density lipoproteins (LDL)** are rich in cholesterol and are the most atherogenic.
- **High-density lipoproteins (HDL)** are the smallest and transport cholesterol to the liver.
- **Hyperlipidemias** are classified as primary or secondary. Rule out secondary causes (e.g., DM, sedentary lifestyle, alcohol overuse).
- **Screening**: Fasting serum lipid profile (total cholesterol, triglycerides, HDL-C, calculated LDL-C, VLDL).

Treatment goals for hyperlipidemia are based upon CHD risk. They are as follows:

- **Low risk** (0–1 risk factors): LDL goal is <160 mg/dL. Lifestyle changes should begin with LDL ≥160. Medications should be started with LDL ≥190 (optional if LDL 160–189).
- **Moderate to high risk** (2+ risk factors with 10-year risk ≤20%): LDL goal is <130. Lifestyle changes should begin with LDL ≥130. Medications should be started with LDL ≥130 (if 10-year risk 10–20%) or LDL ≥160 (if 10-year risk <10%).
- **Highest risk** (10-year risk >20%): LDL goal is <100. Lifestyle changes should begin with LDL ≥100. Medications should be started with LDL ≥130 (optional if LDL 100–129).

TREATMENTS TO CONTROL CHOLESTEROL LEVELS

There are a number of medical treatments available to control cholesterol levels:

- **Statins (HMG-CoA reductase inhibitors)** are the first choice for lowering LDL; they have been shown to decrease cardiovascular morbidity and mortality. They can decrease LDL-C (by 25–50%), triglycerides, apolipoprotein B, and total cholesterol. Recommended if: atherosclerotic cardiovascular disease (ASCVD); LDL-C ≥190; age 40–75 if DM and LDL-C 70–189; or if age 40–75 and LDL-C 70–189 and estimated 10-year risk of ASCVD ≥7.5%. Side effects include myalgia, myositis, and increased liver enzymes. Statins are classified as low-, medium-, and high-intensity.
- **Niacin (nicotinic acid)** decreases LDL, increases HDL, and is very effective at decreasing triglycerides. It also reduces risk of cardiovascular disease (CVD). Side effects include flushing, itching, gout, and peptic ulcers. Taking with food and 325 mg aspirin (30 minutes before) decreases flushing.
- **Bile acid sequestrants** can decrease LDL, can increase HDL, and may or may not be helpful with decreasing triglycerides. Side effects include constipation, gas, and decreased fat-soluble vitamin and drug absorption.
- **Fibrates** can decrease LDL, triglycerides (by 50%), apolipoprotein B, and total cholesterol; and can increase HDL-C (up to 20%). Side effects include myalgia, myositis, hepatitis, gallstones, and potentiate warfarin.
- **Cholesterol-absorption inhibitor (ezetimibe)** can decrease LDL, can lower apolipoprotein B, and may or may not be helpful with decreasing triglycerides. Side effects include increased liver enzymes when used in conjunction with a statin.
- **PCSK9 monoclonal antibodies** are for those with familial hypercholesterolemia.
- **Omega-3 fatty acids** help decrease triglycerides.

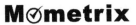

Dermatologic System

ERYTHEMA MULTIFORME

Erythema multiforme (**EM**), once thought to be a milder form of Stevens-Johnson syndrome, is actually an **inflammatory reaction**, usually due to a viral infection or sometimes a medication, that causes an acute, self-limited rash with characteristic target lesions that usually present first on the extremities and then begin to resolve within 1 week. There are two forms: **EM minor** (localized eruption with little to no mucosal involvement) and **EM major** (mucosal involvement but <10% epidermal detachment).

STEVENS-JOHNSON SYNDROME AND TOXIC EPIDERMAL NECROLYSIS

Both Stevens-Johnson syndrome (SJS) and toxic epidermal necrolysis (TEN) are severe **hypersensitivity reactions** that usually occur due to a medication reaction (usually antibiotics, NSAIDs, or anticonvulsant medications) or sometimes due to an infection. Immunocompromised patients are more likely to develop this. Patients will have vague, flu-like symptoms for a few days, followed by development of a progressing rash beginning on the face and trunk, usually with extensive mucosal involvement, and epidermal detachment (<10% for SJS and >30% for TEN). The following features are often present: acute onset of fever, a history of drug exposure often 1–4 weeks before symptoms, diffuse erythema that progresses to vesicles and bullae, necrosis of the epidermis, positive Nikolsky sign (epidermal detachment when pressure is applied). Hospitalization is necessary to treat SJS or TEN with fluid replacement, wound care, and supportive therapy. If the syndrome is severe, treatment in a burn unit, IV immunoglobulin (IVIG), and skin grafting may be necessary. Complications include skin infections, skin issues (scarring, discoloring, and permanent hair loss), sepsis, ocular disease, organ damage, and death.

FOLLICULITIS

Folliculitis is inflammation around the **hair follicle** due to an infection or non-infectious cause. The most common causes are frequent shaving, occlusion, hot/humid weather, and chronic inflammatory skin conditions. The most common causative organism is *Staphylococcus*. *Pseudomonas* is the most likely cause of hot tub folliculitis. Folliculitis can be superficial or deep, mild and self-limiting, or reoccurring. Patients will have pruritic or painful, small, erythematous pustules surrounding the hair. These pustules may break open and crust over. Deep lesions form nodules. Folliculitis can occasionally involve a large area and cause swelling and extreme pain.

Diagnosis is made upon clinical evaluation. If folliculitis is chronic or resistant to treatment, further evaluation is needed, including cultures, Gram stain, KOH preparations, or biopsy. Warm compresses can help relieve the symptoms, and folliculitis, if superficial, will usually resolve spontaneously without medical treatment after a few days with use of antibacterial soap and good hand-washing practices. Topical antibiotics (e.g., mupirocin, clindamycin 1%) can be used as first-line treatment. If folliculitis is severe, or caused by *Staphylococcus* or MRSA, then oral antibiotics (e.g., cephalexin, dicloxacillin, clindamycin) are necessary to treat the condition. If available, always follow culture and sensitivity reports. Complications include cellulitis, skin damage (spots and scarring), and permanent hair loss.

ONYCHOMYCOSIS

Onychomycosis or **tinea unguium** is a fungal infection of any part of the **fingernails or toenails**. This can cause pain and discomfort, and can possibly lead to issues walking, especially in the elderly or those with diabetes. The nail appears thick (due to hyperkeratosis), deformed, and white or yellow, and onycholysis (separation from the nail bed) may occur. Diagnose by direct microscopy with a KOH preparation. A fungal culture may be used if microscopy is unsuccessful. Treatment with topical agents is usually not very effective, while newer oral agents (e.g., terbinafine, itraconazole) have better outcomes. Complications include cellulitis and ulcers, especially in diabetics.

PARONYCHIA

Paronychia is a soft tissue infection of the **nail fold** and is the most common infection of the hand. Infection often occurs after trauma to the area by moisture, physical, or chemical damage. It can be acute (usually due to staphylococci) or chronic (usually fungal). The nail bed becomes red, swollen, and painful, and yellow-green pus begins to collect and form an abscess. Diagnose clinically. Treatment includes warm soaks (if early infection), antibiotics, and incision and drainage if an abscess forms. If the infection reoccurs after treatment, suspect a fungal cause. Complications include this infection occasionally spreading beyond the nail fold.

IMPETIGO

Impetigo is a common **bacterial skin infection** caused by streptococci, staphylococci, or both, that enter through a break in the skin. It is highly contagious and is the most common bacterial infection in children. Impetigo can be nonbullous or bullous and appears as multiple vesicles or pustules filled with clear, yellow fluid that easily burst. These leave behind a red, raw area of irritation and a honey-colored crust. The rash is most common on the face and lips but may spread to other areas. Mupirocin ointment is recommended for treatment, but oral antibiotics (e.g., cephalexin, clindamycin) may be needed for severe cases or cases involving MRSA.

ERYSIPELAS

Erysipelas is a **superficial skin infection** caused by streptococci, usually group A streptococci. Patients may note a recent trauma or pharyngitis and may experience a prodrome of malaise, fever, and chills. Erysipelas appears as a well-circumscribed, painful area of marked erythema and inflammation. This is different from cellulitis, as it is more raised and has definite borders. Diagnose clinically and treat with oral or IM penicillin or, if allergic to penicillin, cephalexin or erythromycin. Complications include abscess, scarring, sepsis, and gangrene.

CELLULITIS

Cellulitis is an **acute bacterial infection** causing inflammation of the skin and subcutaneous tissues. It is commonly caused by staphylococci or streptococci that enter the skin through a portal of entry (e.g., cut, insect bite, wound). Patients complain of a spreading, painful area of erythema, inflammation, and warmth. Diagnosis can be made clinically; however, further investigation is warranted if systemic symptoms are present (e.g., fever, chills, tachycardia) or if signs of more serious infection are present (e.g., violaceous bullae, hemorrhage, gas in the tissue). Treat empirically with antibiotics and, as always, follow the antibiotic guidelines for your area. Abscesses, if present, should be incised and drained. Hospitalization and proper consultations (e.g., surgery) are needed for patients with signs of serious infection. Complications include abscesses, gangrenous cellulitis, necrotizing fasciitis, septic shock, or death.

LICE

Lice are parasites that live on humans, on the head, body (on clothes), or pubic area. They can only crawl and have a lifespan of about 30 days. A female lays about 300 nits (eggs) in her lifetime. Nits hatch in 6–9 days and mature about 7 days after hatching. Itching is the main complaint. Diagnose through direct or microscopic observation. Treatment involves environmental controls (most important) and medicine (e.g., pyrethrin shampoos or creams, malathion) that must be repeated in 7–10 days. There is increasing resistance to lindane.

SCABIES

Scabies are mites (*Sarcoptes scabiei hominis*) that burrow under the skin, usually seen in the webbed spaces, flexor surface of the wrist, belt-line, and pubic areas. Diagnose microscopically through a burrow scraping. Treat with topical permethrin cream, lindane lotion (if ≥2 years old), or oral ivermectin (second-line). It is important to treat close contacts simultaneously.

SPIDER BITES

Clinically significant spider bites in the US include bites from the black widow and brown recluse. **Black widow spiders** have a red, hourglass shape on the ventral abdomen. Their bites are neurotoxic and can cause immediate pain, diaphoresis, cramping, and in the worse cases, headache, hypertension, nausea, and vomiting. **Brown recluse spiders** have a violin-shaped pattern on their cephalothorax. Their venom is cytotoxic and hemolytic, causing pain hours after the bite, as well as inflammation and ischemia. Ulceration usually occurs 7–14 days after the bite. Treatment of spider bites is supportive, with wound care and pain medication. Antivenom is occasionally used for black widow bites, but reserved for severe cases. In brown recluse spider bites, cool compresses are helpful to impede the venom, which is temperature dependent. Antibiotics and skin grafts may be necessary.

CONDYLOMA ACUMINATUM

Condyloma acuminatum is a sexually transmitted **genital wart** that is usually benign and involves human papillomavirus (HPV) type 6 or 11. There are about 40 types of HPV, which spreads through sexual contact. HPV type 16 and 18 are responsible for the majority of cervical, anal, oropharyngeal, vaginal, and penile cancers. There is an HPV vaccine available against HPV 6, 11, 16,18, 31, 33, 45, 52, and 58; it is a series of 2 injections at 0 and 6–12 months (recommended at 11–12 years old, but can be from 9 to <15 years old) or 3 injections at 0, 2, and 6 months if 15–26 years old. The lesions are pink or gray and can become pedunculated. Genital warts are diagnosed through histopathology and treated topically or through excision. Complications include disfigurement and cancerous transformation.

VERRUCAE

Verrucae (**warts**) are common, benign epidermal lesions caused by HPV (usually type 1–4, 27, 29) that can spontaneously regress in 1–2 years. They are usually asymptomatic, but can be painful, especially plantar warts. Diagnose clinically and treat topically (e.g., salicylic acid), or through excision, cryosurgery (liquid nitrogen), or medication (e.g., cimetidine).

MOLLUSCUM CONTAGIOSUM

Molluscum contagiosum is due to a **poxvirus** and causes grouped, pink, dome-shaped **lesions** with central umbilication and a central plug. These are highly contagious by direct and indirect contact, but they are benign and can spontaneously resolve in 1–2 years. This is common in children and young adults. Diagnose clinically and treat with cryosurgery, curettage, or topical agents.

ACTINIC KERATOSIS AND SEBORRHEIC KERATOSIS

Actinic keratosis is a slow-growing, **precancerous skin lesion** that is due to UV light exposure. It typically appears after the fourth decade of life, but may appear sooner if the patient is fair-skinned or lives in an area of intense UV exposure. It can progress to invasive squamous cell carcinoma about 10% of the time. Lesions are rough, keratotic, and pink, red, or brown. Confirm diagnosis with a skin biopsy. Treatment varies depending on the number of lesions and includes surgery, cryosurgery (e.g., liquid nitrogen), resurfacing procedures, and medical treatment (e.g., topical 5-fluorouracil, imiquimod, photodynamic therapy). Prevention is key, and the primary complication is progression to invasive squamous cell carcinoma.

Seborrheic keratosis is another common **skin lesion** in older patients, but it is completely **benign**. It is a slow-growing, wart-like epithelial lesion that appears stuck on the skin. The lesions vary in color from white to black, but are usually tan to brown. They can be found on any skin area except the palms and soles. Diagnosis is confirmed with a shave biopsy, which can also be used to remove the lesion. No treatment is necessary, but these can be removed (e.g., cryotherapy, electrodesiccation, curettage) for cosmetic reasons. There are no complications.

MELANOMA

Malignant melanoma is the most serious form of **skin cancer** and can be fatal. It develops in the **melanin cells** of the skin and can metastasize. It is more likely to occur in those who are fair skinned, those who have a high exposure to UV light, and those who have a positive family history of melanoma. Regular checks with a dermatologist and vigilant use of proper covering and sunscreen are necessary to help prevent melanoma. Melanoma can develop in a mole or may be a new lesion on the skin. Warning signs include changes to the shape, size, or color of a nevus or lesion. The lesion may have asymmetry, irregular borders, uneven color, and a diameter >6 mm, and may be elevated. Diagnosis is made per histopathology from an excisional biopsy. The lesion is staged (stage I-II: primary and localized; stage III: regional metastasis; stage IV: distant metastasis) and further categorized using the Clark levels and Breslow thickness classification. A sentinel lymph node biopsy may be needed to see if the cancer has spread to adjacent lymph nodes. Diagnostic studies should be done to ensure there have not been any metastases of the melanoma. Treatment consists of surgical excision, to include a small amount of surrounding normal tissue (the margin size depends on the thickness of the lesion). Radiation and chemotherapy are used palliatively with advanced melanoma. Complications include metastases and death.

BASAL CELL CARCINOMA

Basal cell carcinoma (**BCC**) is the most common and slowest-growing form of skin cancer. It is an epithelial tumor of keratinocytes in the stratum basale (the deepest level of the epidermis) that is caused by excessive exposure to UV light. These usually appear on the head, face, and neck, and patients who develop BCC are likely to have more in the future. The lesions are usually pearly white to pink in color, may have a waxy appearance, and can be flat or scaly in appearance. These tend to recurrently bleed and crust over. There may be a depressed area in the center with surface telangiectases. Diagnosis is by a shave or punch biopsy and histology. Treatment of basal cell carcinoma involves removal of the lesion by a specialist. It can be surgically excised or removed with curettage and electrodessication, cryotherapy, or antineoplastic creams (such as 5-fluorouracil or imiquimod), or by using photodynamic therapy. Patients should be educated on the importance of protecting the skin from sun exposure. Sunscreen with a high SPF level should be used whenever patients are outside. Complications include increased risk for other types of skin cancer, disfigurement, and spreading of cancer (rare).

SQUAMOUS CELL CARCINOMA

Squamous cell carcinoma (**SCC**) is the second most common type of **skin cancer**, after BCC. It involves keratinocytes and invades the **dermis**. It is usually found on the head and neck (sun-exposed areas), can spread/metastasize, and can be fatal if left untreated. Though not as deadly as melanoma, SCC is more likely to cause serious complications when compared to BCC. SCC risk increases in patients with increased UV light exposure (especially fair-skinned patients), in men, in those with actinic keratosis, in the immunocompromised, and in those with a history of human papillomavirus (HPV). Patients often present describing a sore or ulcer that doesn't heal. SCC lesions can appear anywhere on the body and can be crusty or scaly, occasionally nodular, and may appear red or white when forming on mucous membranes. Diagnosis is made per histopathology. Treatment is similar to BCC and includes removal of the lesion with excision, curettage and electrodessication, Mohs microscopic surgery, or cryotherapy. For high-risk lesions, a more aggressive approach may be used, including radiation for metastases. The skin should always be protected from sun by shielding or applying sunscreen with a high SPF rating. Complications include metastases to lymph nodes and organs, disfigurement, and death (uncommon).

CONTACT DERMATITIS

Contact dermatitis is an **inflammatory response** to an allergen or irritant. This can be caused by numerous agents, such as lotions, soaps, nickel, poison ivy, or poison sumac. The skin rash associated with contact dermatitis often occurs quickly following exposure to an irritant, and the rash is more painful than pruritic. (In contrast, the rash associated with an allergen is a delayed hypersensitivity reaction, which, once sensitized, typically occurs within 1–2 days of exposure, and this rash is usually extremely pruritic.) With contact dermatitis, the skin becomes red and edematous with papules and vesicular lesions. In chronic exposure, the skin can become hyperpigmented with lichenification, plaques, fissures, and hyperkeratosis. Diagnosis is made mostly per history/physical. Finding and eliminating the possible trigger(s) can also be diagnostic. For cases that don't easily resolve, patch testing may be effective. Treatment consists of discontinuing exposure to the causative substance, cool compresses, topical corticosteroids, and antihistamines (e.g., hydroxyzine or diphenhydramine can be taken if the dermatitis is due to exposure to an allergen). If contact dermatitis is severe, oral steroids can be given to reduce the inflammation. Complications include neurodermatitis (lichen simplex chronicus—thick, leathery skin from chronic scratching) and infection.

DIAPER RASH

Diaper rash is a form of **contact dermatitis** and commonly occurs in babies wearing diapers or in incontinent adults. It is caused by exposure of the skin to the moisture of urine and waste material. If severe, the rash can have an accompanying bacterial or fungal infection. The skin with prolonged moisture against it will become very inflamed, red, tender, and possibly broken or cracked. Often there is irritation in the convex surfaces of the infant's body. This irritation can be simple erythema, lesions, papules, or erosions. If a fungal infection develops because of the moisture, there may be small red papules, or satellite lesions, surrounding the inflamed area. Diagnosis is made clinically. The goal of treating diaper rash is to keep the skin clean and dry. Leaving the skin open to air and avoiding a wet diaper against the skin will help to relieve the rash. Barrier creams and ointment containing zinc oxide can help to prevent further irritation of the skin. An antifungal or antibacterial cream may be necessary if a secondary infection occurs. Persistent fungal diaper rashes can be a sign of an underlying immune condition or type 1 diabetes. Complications include candidal or bacterial infections.

ATOPIC DERMATITIS (ECZEMA)

Atopic dermatitis, or eczema, is a **skin rash** that is more prevalent in children than adults, though it can occur at any time in life. However, it usually presents before 5 years of age. The exact cause is unknown, but it is thought to be immune-mediated. It is frequently seen in families, and along with asthma or hay fever. Patients have extremely pruritic, dry skin with reddish to dark-colored areas with scales, weeping, and lichenification. They may have excoriations and papules that crust over after opening. The pruritus can be aggravated by temperature changes, hot showers or baths, or allergens (e.g., cigarette smoke). Atopic dermatitis most often occurs over the antecubital fossa and behind the knees, though it can occur anywhere on the body. Diagnosis consists of these essential features:

- Pruritus
- Visible dermatitis (acute, subacute, or chronic)
- Typical distribution patterns (infants and children with facial, neck, or extensor involvement; history of flexural lesions at any age; sparing of the groin and axilla)
- Chronic and relapsing nature

Treat with lubricating creams and oils immediately after bathing, topical corticosteroid creams or ointments, or immunomodulators (e.g., tacrolimus), and avoid irritants and triggers to the outbreaks. Complications include neurodermatitis, skin infections, blepharitis, and sleep issues.

NUMMULAR ECZEMA

Nummular eczema is a form of eczema that causes coin-shaped patches on the skin. Unlike atopic dermatitis, it is uncommon in children. It usually appears in males in the sixth or seventh decade of life. There is no definitive cause, but it does tend to be aggravated by strong soaps and detergents, anything that dries the skin, and extremes in temperature. It begins as vesicles and papules that coalesce to form the characteristic erythematous, discoid plaque. They usually start on the legs, are very pruritic, are often symmetric, and tend to be dry and scaly. The rash can resemble a fungal infection or ringworm, but tends to recur. Diagnosis is made per history and physical. Treat with mid-to-strong corticosteroid creams or ointments and baths, followed by immediate moisturizer use. With a severe outbreak, short-term oral steroids may be necessary, as well as UVB phototherapy. Coal tar preparations can help with an outbreak, but they tend to stain clothes. Treat with

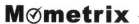

appropriate antibiotics if a secondary skin infection develops. Avoid the triggers that cause flare-ups to help decrease the severity and frequency of outbreaks. Complications include skin infections and scars.

DYSHIDROSIS

Dyshidrosis, or dyshidrotic eczema, is a form of eczema that causes vesicular lesions to form on the **palms and soles**. This condition typically occurs between ages 10 and 40, and the exact cause is not known. It seems to occur more frequently during stressful times, and may be linked to exposure to metal salts. There is an increased incidence in those patients with atopy (a familial hypersensitivity to allergens). Dyshidrosis is a chronic condition with no known cure. Signs and symptoms include extremely pruritic vesicular lesions (that may form bullae) on the palms of the hands and soles of the feet. These can break open and crust over. As the lesions are resolving, the skin becomes very dry and cracked, which can be painful, and desquamation occurs. Secondary skin infections can also occur. Diagnosis is made upon clinical assessment: pruritus, recurrence, acute onset, and deep-seated bullae or vesicles on the soles and palms or the lateral finger. High-potency topical corticosteroid creams or ointments, cold compresses, antihistamines, antibiotics for secondary infections, UV light phototherapy, and immunosuppressants may treat symptoms and decrease the severity of the flare-ups. Complications include limited use of hands and feet, skin infections, and cellulitis.

PSORIASIS

Psoriasis is a very common, chronic, inflammatory disease affecting 1–2% of the US population. The cause is unknown, but current theories support an autoimmune origin and/or genetics. Psoriasis results from an **accelerated skin reproduction cycle** and **lymphocyte infiltration**. Lesions show parakeratotic cells, scales, and a thinned or absent stratum granulosum. It occurs most frequently on elbows, knees, scalp, intergluteal cleft, glans penis, and lumbosacral areas. Other triggers can include stress, skin irritation, sunlight, alcohol consumption, AIDS, chemotherapy, or other autoimmune conditions.

There are a variety of forms of psoriasis, including plaque-type, arthritic, nail, inverse, guttate, pustular, and erythrodermic psoriasis. Guttate psoriasis can be confused with pityriasis rosea, but pityriasis rosea, which is self-limited, begins with a herald patch and has a Christmas-tree distribution. The most common form of psoriasis, which is called **chronic plaque psoriasis**, accounts for about 75% of cases. With chronic plaque psoriasis, there are erythemic, raised, sharply defined plaques with thick, silvery scales. The lesions are usually symmetrically distributed and often on extensor surfaces. The plaques can be asymptomatic or pruritic. Diagnosis is made by history and clinical assessment. Treatment includes topical treatments (e.g., steroid creams and ointments, retinoids, salicylic acid, emollients, vitamin D3 analogs), phototherapy, and systemic treatments (e.g., methotrexate, cyclosporine, adalimumab, etanercept, infliximab, ustekinumab). Complications include secondary infections, psoriatic arthritis, cardiovascular disease, metabolic syndrome, MI, lymphoma, depression, and kidney disease.

LICHEN PLANUS

Lichen planus is a recurrent skin condition that appears to be immune-mediated. The exact cause is unknown, but it has been associated with hepatitis C and certain medications (e.g., penicillamine, NSAIDS, β-blockers). The appearance of the lesions may be remembered with the **5 P's**: pruritic, purple, planar (flat-topped), polygonal papules and plaques that usually form in a row. It most commonly occurs around the flexural surfaces of the ankles or wrists. Oral lesions occur in about 50% of cases, and these can burn; and Wickham striae are usually noted (a fine network of lines on the surface of lichen planus lesions). Once the lesions fade, they may leave a darker pigmented area or scar. Diagnosis is made per clinical evaluation; however, a skin biopsy may be needed. On history and physical, note medications that may induce this disorder. Lichen planus usually resolves spontaneously within 1 year, but symptoms can be controlled with topical steroid creams or ointments, topical or oral retinoids, antihistamines, UV light therapy, or immunomodulating medications. If severe, oral or intralesional steroids may be necessary. Complications include infection, permanent alopecia, and increased risk of skin cancer.

BURNS

Burns are damage to the skin or tissue due to thermal, chemical, radiation, or electrical causes. They are classified as first-, second-, or third-degree burns. They are also described according to the **total body surface area (TBSA)** that is affected. **First-degree burns** only affect the epidermis; they appear red and are painful. **Second-degree (partial-thickness) burns** affect part of the dermis; they can be superficial or deep, with redness and blisters, and are very painful. **Third-degree (full-thickness) burns** extend down into the subcutaneous tissue/fat; they are whitish, blackened, and without sensation. Sometimes a designation of a **fourth-degree burn** is used when the burn involves deep fascia, muscles, and bones. When assessing a patient with burns, it is important to first stop the burning process and begin with the **ABCs** (airway, breathing, circulation). Assess for an inhalation injury and carbon monoxide poisoning if there is soot or burns around the mouth or nose.

RULE OF NINES

By using the rule of nines, one can quickly determine the TBSA affected (see figure below). Also, for small burns, remember the patient's palm is 1% of the TBSA. Patients with TBSA >10% need IV fluids, and if ≥20%, will require IV fluid resuscitation. Patients should be referred to a burn center for a burn of any thickness that is >20% TBSA; second-degree >10% TBSA; third-degree >5% TBSA; or second- or third-degree burns of critical areas (e.g., joints, face, hands, feet, genitalia); electrical/lightning burns; chemical burns; or inhalation injury. Small burns may be treated with silver sulfadiazine.

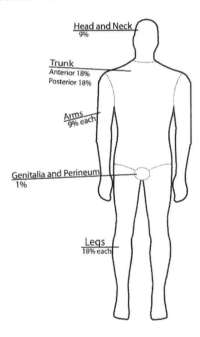

Head and Neck
9%

Trunk
Anterior 18%
Posterior 18%

Arms
9% each

Genitalia and Perineum
1%

Legs
18% each

BULLOUS PEMPHIGOID

Bullous pemphigoid is a chronic, autoimmune **blistering disease** that usually affects the elderly. The cause is unknown, but possible triggers include medications, trauma, radiation, and other diseases (e.g., psoriasis, lichen planus, DM, rheumatoid arthritis [RA]). Patients complain of a pruritic, blistering rash. Tense bullae appear on the trunk and flexural surfaces, and in intertriginous areas, but usually spare the mucous membranes. Nikolsky sign is negative. Diagnosis is made by skin biopsy and immunofluorescence studies. It is important to differentiate bullous pemphigoid from pemphigus vulgaris (flaccid bullae that usually involve the oral mucosa), which has a worse prognosis. Treatment includes topical or oral steroids. Complications include scarring and possible death in the elderly.

URTICARIA

Urticaria, or **hives**, are pruritic, well-circumscribed, red, raised areas of the skin. The wheals are transient and are due to a variety of causes, including allergic reactions to foods or allergens, medications, exercise, cold or heat, stress, medical conditions (e.g., autoimmune disease, hypothyroidism, hyperthyroidism), or infections. Urticaria can be **acute** (<6 weeks), **recurrent**, or **chronic** (>6 weeks). Urticaria may result from IgE-mediated (type I hypersensitivity reaction) or non-immune-mediated mast cell and basophil activation. Chronic urticaria can be due to any of the above causes; however, it is often idiopathic or associated with chronic medical conditions (e.g., SLE, lymphoma), cholinergic causes (e.g., stress, heat), or autoimmune disorders. A thorough history is necessary; however, it may be difficult to determine the exact trigger. Determine if any bronchospasm or angioedema is present, as these require urgent treatment (albuterol or epinephrine respectively).

Diagnosis is clinical, but further tests are necessary for chronic urticaria (e.g., allergy skin testing, routine labs). Avoid triggers and treat with second-generation antihistamines (e.g., loratadine, cetirizine, fexofenadine), as these cause less sedation than first-generation antihistamines (e.g., diphenhydramine, hydroxyzine). This is especially important in the elderly, as the first-generation antihistamines can cause confusion and urinary retention. Complications include bronchospasm, angioedema, and anaphylaxis.

LIPOMAS AND EPITHELIAL INCLUSION CYSTS

Lipomas are benign, slow-growing fatty tumors and are the most common **soft tissue tumor**. They are usually found subcutaneously, are not fixed to fascia, and are soft and painless. Diagnosis is clinical; however, further investigation is necessary if the tumor grows rapidly or is fixed to fascia (rule out a liposarcoma). Treat with excision by fully removing the tumor, including the capsule, if symptomatic or large. **Epithelial** or **epidermal inclusion cysts** form when epithelial tissue implants in the dermis; they are typically found on the face, neck, and trunk. They are usually solitary, skin-colored to yellow, dome-shaped lesions with a central punctum, and they contain a foul-smelling, cheesy material. Diagnose clinically; however, a biopsy or fine-needle aspiration may be helpful in diagnosis. If not infected, treat with either watchful waiting or with complete excision, including the capsule. If infected, treat with appropriate antibiotics (e.g., dicloxacillin, clindamycin).

Endocrine System

DISEASES OF THE THYROID GLAND

PARATHYROID HORMONE

Parathyroid hormone (**PTH**) is secreted by the four parathyroid glands, which sit posterior to the thyroid gland. Release of PTH is controlled by the pituitary gland's secretion of **parathyroid stimulating hormone**. The function of PTH is to control the body's **calcium and phosphorus balance**. When the calcium levels are low, PTH secretion is increased; when calcium levels rise, PTH secretion is suppressed. PTH causes release of calcium from bones into the circulating bloodstream, renal reabsorption of calcium, renal excretion of phosphorus, and conversion of vitamin D to its active form (1,25-dihydroxyvitamin D).

Hyperparathyroidism can be from primary or secondary causes. **Primary hyperparathyroidism** is most commonly caused by a parathyroid adenoma that causes increased amounts of PTH to be released. With some types of cancer, there can be ectopic sources of parathyroid tissue that will secrete excess PTH. Multiple endocrine neoplasia (MEN) syndromes can affect multiple endocrine glands, including the parathyroids, and lead to hyperparathyroidism. **Secondary causes** include chronic kidney disease and vitamin D deficiency. Accidental removal of the parathyroid glands during thyroid surgery can cause **hypoparathyroidism**. Hypomagnesemia can cause there to be a decreased amount of PTH secreted by the glands. Rarely, there can be genetic causes of deficiencies in PTH secretion (e.g., DiGeorge syndrome).

HYPERPARATHYROIDISM AND HYPOPARATHYROIDISM

Hyperparathyroidism occurs when there is **overproduction of parathyroid hormone (PTH)**. Normal range is 10–55 pg/mL. This occurs more often in women and those over 50 years old. Hypercalcemia (total calcium >10.4 mg/dL) is the most common finding in hyperparathyroidism. Patients may complain of signs of hypercalcemia, which can be remembered as "bones, stones, groans, and moans." This refers to **bone pain** due to demineralization, **kidney stones**, **abdominal groans** (nausea, vomiting, constipation, loss of appetite), and **psychiatric moans** (nervous system issues: muscle weakness, fatigue, lethargy, depression, confusion). Polyuria can occur with renal failure. Cardiac arrhythmias, hypertension, and even coma can occur. Calcium levels >12 mg/dL may be due to cancer, and therefore cancer must be ruled out, especially if calcium levels rise rapidly. Treat with parathyroidectomy of affected glands.

Hypoparathyroidism is the **deficiency of PTH**. This is more common in women and is usually due to accidental damage during thyroid/neck surgery, radioactive iodine treatment for hyperthyroidism, radiation, or autoimmune causes. As calcium levels drop, patients may complain of paresthesias of the fingers, toes, and perioral area. Patients will show other signs of neuromuscular irritability, with muscle aches, hyperreflexia, carpopedal spasm (tetany), laryngospasm, and facial grimacing. A positive Chvostek sign (unilateral spasm of the facial muscles when the facial nerve is tapped) and a positive Trousseau sign (carpal spasm when upper arm is compressed with a blood pressure cuff) may be present. Irritability, confusion, fatigue, seizures, brittle hair and nails, and personality changes may occur. Diagnose with an ionized calcium level (<4.7 mg/dL), reduced PTH, and elevated phosphate. Treat with calcium and vitamin D supplements. Patients with renal failure must also reduce the amount of phosphate in their diet. Patients with tetany are treated with IV calcium gluconate.

HYPERTHYROIDISM AND GRAVES' DISEASE

Hyperthyroidism (**thyrotoxicosis**) is a disease of **excess thyroid hormone production and secretion**. It can have many causes, including Graves' disease, thyroiditis, toxic multinodular goiter (Plummer disease), and toxic adenoma. **Graves' disease** is an **autoimmune disease** and is the most common cause of hyperthyroidism in the US. Exophthalmos and pretibial myxedema are usually present with Graves' disease, whereas these two symptoms are not seen with regular hyperthyroidism. Common signs and symptoms of thyrotoxicosis include irritability, nervousness, tremors, muscle weakness, palpitations, hypertension, atrial fibrillation (especially in the elderly), frequent bowel movements, heat intolerance, increased sweating, and weight loss with an increase in appetite. Hyperreflexia, fine or brittle hair, warm, moist skin, menstrual irregularity, and a goiter may be present.

Diagnose clinically and with thyroid function tests. Low TSH, with high total T3 and high free T4, confirms hyperthyroidism. With Graves' disease, thyroid-stimulating immunoglobulins (TSIs) are positive, as well as other antibodies. Radioactive iodine scanning can help differentiate between the causes of hyperthyroidism. Thyrotoxicosis can be treated with antithyroid drugs (e.g., methimazole, propylthiouracil [PTU]), β-blockers (e.g., atenolol) for hyperadrenergic symptoms, iodine, and thyroidectomy. Graves' disease is usually treated with radioactive iodine. Toxic multinodular goiter and toxic adenoma are treated with either radioactive iodine or surgery. Complications include dysrhythmias, hypertension, CHF, osteoporosis, thyroid storm, and pregnancy issues including miscarriage.

THYROID STORM

Thyroid storm (**thyrotoxic crisis**) is a very rare, but life-threatening condition in which the thyroid secretes massive amounts of **thyroid hormones** at one time, causing an acute state of **thyrotoxicosis**. This can be due to a tumor, excessive manipulation during surgery, infection, trauma, or a complication of Graves' disease. Those who take excessive doses of thyroid hormones, or suddenly discontinue antithyroid medications, may also experience a thyroid storm. Signs and symptoms include high fever, extreme irritability, nausea, vomiting, diarrhea, dehydration, CHF, arrhythmias, disorientation, and delirium. This can progress to the point of seizures, coma, or death.

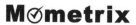

Diagnosis is clinical. Since this is a medical emergency, treatment should not be delayed while waiting for the thyroid panel results. A patient presenting with symptoms of thyroid storm should have immediate treatment: supportive measures, β-blockers to treat increased adrenergic tone, thioamides (e.g., methimazole, PTU) to stop new thyroid hormone synthesis, iodine to stop the release of thyroid hormones, bile acid sequestrants to slow liver recycling of hormones, and glucocorticoids to decrease T4 to T3 conversion (this also assists with adrenal insufficiency). Note that thioamides (anti-thyroids) can cause agranulocytosis in 0.2–0.5% of patients. PTU helps inhibit peripheral T4 to T3 conversion but has been linked to severe liver injury/acute liver failure (black box warnings); therefore, use with caution. Once the crisis has passed, radioactive iodine or thyroidectomy may be used in patients with contraindications to antithyroid drugs. Complications include hypotension, shock, coma, and death.

SUBACUTE THYROIDITIS

Subacute thyroiditis is a self-limited disease that causes **inflammation of the thyroid gland**. Most commonly, subacute thyroiditis is caused by a viral infection (e.g., coxsackie, mumps, influenza, adenovirus). Also, it can occasionally occur with certain medications (e.g., lithium, amiodarone) or is possibly due to an autoimmune cause (e.g., subacute lymphocytic thyroiditis, subacute postpartum thyroiditis). Patients will usually have a fever with a painful, tender, asymmetrically or symmetrically enlarged thyroid gland. They may remember having symptoms of an upper respiratory infection before the thyroid symptoms began. In addition to the localized tenderness, patients may describe symptoms of either hyper- or hypothyroidism. Usually, patients are initially in a hyperthyroid state, followed by a period of hypothyroidism, and then return to a euthyroid state.

Diagnosis is clinical, using thyroid function tests (TSH, free T4, serum thyroglobulin) and other labs. Lab tests will show an elevated WBC and ESR. Thyroid antibodies may be positive, but will not be as high as with Graves' disease. A fine-needle biopsy may be done, especially if a solitary nodule is found. Patients are treated with high-dose NSAIDs (usually ibuprofen or naproxen; avoid aspirin) and sometimes steroids to decrease the inflammation within the thyroid gland. Antibiotics do not have a role here because of the condition's viral etiology. The TSH and T4 levels should be monitored every 4 weeks for resolution, as this can take several months. Around 95% of cases will resolve on their own in 18 months without complications. In the other cases, hypothyroidism will be permanent.

HYPOTHYROIDISM

Hypothyroidism, a **deficiency of thyroid hormones**, is more common in women and is most commonly due to autoimmune factors (e.g., Hashimoto thyroiditis) in the US. However, worldwide, **iodine deficiency** is the most common cause of hypothyroidism. Hypothyroidism may be **primary** (due to diseased thyroid) or **secondary** (diseased hypothalamus or pituitary). For example, pituitary tumors can also cause a decrease in TSH secretion, which will lead to secondary hypothyroidism.

Symptoms are often nonspecific. Patients may complain of fatigue, weakness, loss of concentration/memory, cold intolerance, constipation, weight gain, and a decreased appetite. Patients may have myxedema (a nonpitting edema of the face, periorbital area, hands, and feet), a hoarse voice, dry and coarse skin, and dry, brittle hair with hair loss. Hypertension and bradycardia may be present, as well as paresthesias in the hands along the median nerve. Lab results with hypothyroidism will show an elevated TSH as the pituitary gland tries to stimulate more production of the thyroid hormones. Triiodothyronine (T3) and thyroxine (T4) are the primary thyroid hormones. Test for free T4, which will be decreased (T3 is not sensitive to hypothyroidism). With Hashimoto thyroiditis, thyroid peroxidase antibodies will be present. Treatment includes thyroid replacement hormone (levothyroxine) and careful monitoring of the thyroid hormone levels to reach therapeutic dosage. Complications include goiter, depression, weight gain, peripheral neuropathy, myxedema coma, infertility, miscarriage, high cholesterol, and heart failure.

HASHIMOTO THYROIDITIS

Hashimoto thyroiditis is a **chronic autoimmune-mediated form of hypothyroidism** and the most common cause of hypothyroidism in the US. The body's immune system attacks the **thyroid tissue**, preventing the normal secretion of thyroid hormones. Patients may complain of the usual symptoms of hypothyroidism, including fatigue, cold intolerance, weight gain with a decreased appetite, forgetfulness, dry skin, and a puffy face, as well as a goiter. Female patients may also have menorrhagia. Thyroid hormone levels may be normal early in the disease. The TSH level will be elevated, though, and the thyroid hormone levels will begin to decrease as the disease progresses. Anti-thyroid peroxidase (anti-TPO) antibodies can also be tested to determine an autoimmune etiology, but the autoantibodies may be negative 10–15% of the time. In this case, a biopsy will confirm the diagnosis.

Treatment involves typically lifelong thyroid hormone replacement therapy and possibly surgery. TSH and free T4 levels are regularly tested, measured every 6–8 weeks after initiation and medicine adjustments, until normal levels are achieved. After that, follow up with patients every 6–12 months. To avoid maternal and fetal sequelae, treatment and careful monitoring must be continued through pregnancy. Complications of this disease include goiter, heart failure, depression, decreased libido, pregnancy and fetal issues, and myxedema coma.

DISEASES OF THE ADRENAL GLAND

ADRENAL INSUFFICIENCY

Adrenal insufficiency can be primary or secondary, and chronic or acute. **Primary adrenal insufficiency (Addison's disease)** is chronic, has an insidious onset, and is due to autoimmune factors, infections (e.g., TB), or disease within the adrenal gland causing a decrease in cortisol secretion from the gland. **Secondary adrenal insufficiency**, which is more common, involves a decrease in adrenocorticotropin hormone (ACTH) production from the pituitary; therefore, aldosterone levels are not affected. Causes include a pituitary adenoma, steroid use, or discontinuation of steroids. **Adrenal crisis** is a life-threatening emergency of **acute adrenal insufficiency** usually due to rapid corticosteroid withdrawal or a stressful event (e.g., illness, accident). With adrenal insufficiency, patients may complain of fatigue, weakness, and dizziness, and may have orthostatic hypotension, weight loss, nausea, and vomiting. The skin may become hyperpigmented in primary disease. With acute adrenal crisis, patients can present with signs of shock, nausea/vomiting, hypotension, and abdominal pain.

Diagnose with a high-dose ACTH stimulation test. Autoantibodies against 21-hydroxylase can help diagnose the cause. Addison's disease is treated with cortisol replacement therapy (e.g., hydrocortisone). If the patient is aldosterone deficient, replace with the mineralocorticoid fludrocortisone. With secondary adrenal insufficiency, the cause is the focus of treatment (e.g., resection of a pituitary adenoma). When adrenal crisis is suspected, treat with immediate IV hydrocortisone. It is important that patients are slowly weaned off steroids to prevent adrenal insufficiency/adrenal crisis. Complications include adrenal crisis, shock, coma, and death.

CUSHING SYNDROME AND CUSHING DISEASE

Cushing syndrome results when **cortisol levels** are increased. Most commonly, this is due to steroid treatment with **prednisone**. Endogenous causes include a pituitary adenoma producing excess amounts of adrenocorticotropic hormone (ACTH), which leads to elevated cortisol (termed **Cushing disease**) or a primary tumor of the adrenal gland causing increased cortisol secretion. Forms of cancer (e.g., lung, carcinoid) can present with ectopic sources of ACTH secretion. Patients will develop proximal muscle weakness, muscular atrophy, truncal obesity with thin arms and legs, round facies, buffalo hump, and purple striae usually across the abdomen. Patients may bruise easily and have non-healing sores; women may be affected with hirsutism and oligomenorrhea or amenorrhea. Osteoporosis can occur, as can glucose intolerance.

For diagnosis, a patient should be screened with one of the following: 24-hour urine free cortisol ×3, low-dose (1 mg) dexamethasone suppression test, midnight serum, or salivary cortisol. Once Cushing syndrome is established, determine the cause using an ACTH and simultaneous cortisol measurement (elevated indicates adrenal adenoma or carcinoma) or a high-dose (8 mg overnight, or 2-day) dexamethasone suppression test (differentiates between pituitary cause and ectopic ACTH cause). Patients should be weaned off prednisone if possible. Removal of a pituitary adenoma can decrease ACTH production. Removal of an adrenal adenoma or other ectopic source of hormone secretion can decrease cortisol levels. Complications include hypertension, CVD, DM, osteoporosis, risk of adrenal crisis, and psychosis.

DISEASES OF THE PITUITARY GLAND

GIGANTISM AND ACROMEGALY

Gigantism and acromegaly both occur from **excessive production of growth hormone (GH)**, usually due to a pituitary adenoma. **Gigantism**, which is very rare, occurs in children, before the epiphyseal plates close, while **acromegaly** occurs in adults after epiphyseal fusion. In children, GH helps with bone growth and development. Therefore, gigantism results in **excessive long bone growth**. In adulthood, the epiphyseal plates are fused, and the bones are no longer able to grow. With excess GH, more calcium is laid down on the bone, causing **bony enlargement**. Signs and symptoms include prominent forehead and jawbones (prognathism); large hands, feet, nose, and lower lip; a deep voice; arthritis; and possible headaches. Patients may develop left ventricular hypertrophy, CHF, hypertension, and cardiac arrhythmias. IGF-1 (insulin-like growth factor 1), which is more consistent throughout the day than GH, and an oral glucose tolerance test checking for GH non-suppression, are helpful in making the diagnosis. MRI is used to check for pituitary tumors. Treatment is aimed at treating the cause. Removal of a pituitary adenoma will decrease or stop the production of GH. However, if this does not occur, pituitary radiation and medication may help (e.g., somatostatin analogs, dopamine analogs, or GH receptor antagonists). Complications include diabetes, hypertension, cardiomyopathy, osteoarthritis, sleep apnea, carpal tunnel syndrome, spinal cord compression, uterine fibroids, and colon polyps.

HYPOPITUITARY DWARFISM

Hypopituitary dwarfism occurs in children who suffer from **decreased production of growth hormone (GH)**; this may be due to congenital or acquired causes (e.g., pituitary adenoma, brain injury), or it may be idiopathic. GH secretion can be decreased in adults, resulting in increased fat and decreased muscle mass, but this will not affect bone growth since the epiphyseal plates have fused. Children who have decreased secretion of GH will be very short in stature because of inadequate bone development. **Dwarfism** is categorized by the Little People of America (LPA) as a person being less than 4'10" tall due to a medical or genetic condition. Patients with hypopituitary dwarfism fall below the 3rd percentile in height, but will have normal body proportions, and will usually have delayed tooth development. There are no intellectual deficits associated with this.

Diagnosis is multifactorial, including history, physical, labs (e.g., low levels of insulin-like growth factor 1 [IGF-1] and IGF-binding protein 3), and imaging studies (e.g., bone age, MRI). Rule out other causes (e.g., Turner syndrome, familial short stature, malnutrition). If due to decreased GH, and not a primary skeletal disorder, the child can be treated with human growth hormone to try to stimulate growth. Surgery may be necessary to remove a pituitary adenoma if that is the cause. Complications include panhypopituitarism, delayed puberty, and complications associated with GH replacement (e.g., fluid retention, pseudotumor cerebri, slipped capital femoral epiphysis, myalgia, and arthralgia).

DIABETES INSIPIDUS

Diabetes insipidus (**DI**) is a disease caused by an impairment in the secretion of or response to **antidiuretic hormone (ADH)**, also called **vasopressin**, resulting in excessive thirst and urination. There are two main types: **central** (decreased production/secretion of ADH from the hypothalamus/pituitary) or **nephrogenic** (resistance to the effects of ADH by the kidney, which may be caused by lithium use). DI can occur because of decreased levels of ADH, damage to the hypothalamus gland where ADH is produced, damage to the pituitary gland where ADH is stored, or primary kidney damage that prevents the kidneys from functioning properly.

Signs and symptoms include polyuria, polydipsia, and nocturia. The patient may present with dehydration, hypernatremia, and low levels of ADH. Labs show an increased urinary output (>3 L/24 hours), poorly concentrated urine (<200 mOsm/kg), and a urinary specific gravity of ≤1.005. Water deprivation testing can be used to differentiate central DI (osmolality rises after ADH is given) from nephrogenic DI (osmolality stays the same after ADH is given). An MRI is used to rule out a pituitary tumor/adenoma. A low-sodium diet and desmopressin (intranasally or orally) are treatments of choice for central DI. Hypothalamic/pituitary tumors can be surgically removed or debulked, if possible. With nephrogenic DI, correct the cause, and treat with sodium and protein restriction along with adequate water intake. Sometimes thiazide diuretics (e.g., HCTZ), amiloride, and NSAIDs are used in both central and nephrogenic DI. Electrolyte imbalances and dehydration may cause many symptoms, including hypotension, tachycardia, and dysrhythmias.

DIABETES MELLITUS
TYPE 1 DIABETES MELLITUS

Type 1 diabetes mellitus (**type I DM**), previously termed juvenile or insulin-dependent DM, is autoimmune in nature and destroys **pancreatic islet cells**, causing greatly **decreased insulin production**. Type I is often diagnosed early in life, before age 30, but may develop after age 30, and symptoms may appear fairly suddenly. There is ≤6% risk in those with a positive family history with one parent with type I DM, an almost 30% risk in those with two parents, and a ≤50% concordance rate in twins. Patients with type 1 DM classically have symptoms of polyuria, polydipsia, and polyphagia. There can be weight loss even though patients are eating more, and patients may complain of weakness and fatigue. Diagnosis is made when fasting plasma glucose (FPG) levels are ≥126 mg/dL, when a 2-hour PG is ≥200 mg/dL during an oral glucose tolerance test (OGTT) (75 g), or when HbA1c is ≥6.5%. These three tests require a second positive result to confirm the diagnosis. However, diagnosis is automatically established if the patient has classic hyperglycemic or hyperglycemic crisis (e.g., ketoacidosis) symptoms along with a random PG ≥200 mg/dL. Lifelong insulin treatment is required for type I DM. Complications include diabetic retinopathy, diabetic neuropathy, micro- and macrovascular conditions (e.g., atherosclerosis, MI), and infection.

> **Review Video: Diabetes Mellitus: Complications**
> Visit mometrix.com/academy and enter code: 996788

TYPES OF INSULIN TO CONTROL GLUCOSE LEVELS WITH TYPE 1 DIABETES MELLITUS

The different types of insulin available for controlling glucose levels with type 1 diabetes mellitus are:

- **Rapid-acting** (lispro/aspart)
  - Onset of action: 12–30 minutes
  - Peak action: 30 minutes–3 hours
  - Duration of action: 3–5 hours
- **Short-acting** (regular insulin)
  - Onset of action: 30 minutes
  - Peak action: 2.5–5 hours
  - Duration of action: 4–24 hours
- **Intermediate-acting** (NPH insulin)
  - Onset of action: 1–1.5 hours
  - Peak action: 6–10 hours
  - Duration of action: 14–24 hours
- **Long-acting** (glargine)
  - Onset of action: 3–4 hours
  - Peak action: No peak
  - Duration of action: Approximately 24 hours (range 11–32 hours)

Rapid-acting: Typically taken right before meals and combined with longer-acting insulin.
Short-acting: Typically taken 30 minutes before meals and used with longer-acting insulin.

Intermediate-acting: Combined with rapid- or short-acting insulin to continue coverage; given bid.
Long-acting: Can be combined with rapid- or short-acting insulin, as necessary; given qd or bid.

> **Review Video: Diabetes Mellitus**
> Visit mometrix.com/academy and enter code: 501396

TYPE 2 DIABETES MELLITUS

Type 2 diabetes mellitus (**type 2 DM**) is an endocrine/metabolic disorder that results in **impaired secretion and peripheral response to insulin**. There is a strong genetic predisposition towards developing type 2 DM and a 90% twin concordance. Risk factors include age ≥40; positive family history; being overweight/obese; history of gestational diabetes; hypertension; and African American, American Indian, Hispanic/Latino, or Asian American descent. Many patients are asymptomatic. Patients may present with classic symptoms of polyuria, polydipsia, polyphagia, weight loss, and signs of hyperglycemia (e.g., blurred vision, paresthesias, yeast infections).

Diagnosis can be made in a patient presenting with classic symptoms of hyperglycemia and a random blood glucose ≥200 mg/dL. In an asymptomatic patient, diagnosis is made with a fasting blood glucose ≥126 mg/dL, a 2-hour PG ≥200 mg/dL during an OGTT (75 g), or when HbA1c is ≥6.5%. Treatment includes a comprehensive medical evaluation and preventive monitoring: annual fundoscopic and foot exams, as well as annual screening for atherosclerotic CVD, peripheral neuropathy, and albuminuria. Dietary modification, weight reduction, and exercise are steps to slow the progression and improve glycemic control. At diagnosis, metformin therapy should be initiated with the previously mentioned lifestyle changes. HbA1c should be rechecked every 6 months, and every 3 months if not meeting treatment goals (e.g., HbA1c <7.0%, preprandial PG 80–130 mg/dL, postprandial <180 mg/dL). If treatment regimen is unsuccessful, add another oral or injectable medication or change to insulin. Consult endocrinologist. Complications include cardiovascular disease, neuropathy, diabetic retinopathy, nephropathy, and infections (especially of the foot).

ORAL MEDICATIONS TO CONTROL GLUCOSE LEVELS WITH TYPE 2 DIABETES MELLITUS

There are a number of medications to control glucose levels for type 2 diabetes mellitus:

- **Biguanides (insulin sensitizers; e.g., Metformin)**: These are the initial medications of choice for type 2 DM. They decrease hepatic gluconeogenesis, decrease intestinal absorption of glucose, and increase peripheral glucose uptake/use. They can decrease HbA1c and decrease LDL cholesterol. They should be avoided in liver or renal disease, in those with CHF, and before receiving IV contrast. Side effects include nausea, vomiting, diarrhea, and lactic acidosis.
- **Sulfonylureas (insulin secretagogues; e.g., first generation: acetohexamide, chlorpropamide, tolazamide, tolbutamide; second generation: glipizide, glimepiride, glyburide)**: This class stimulates insulin release from pancreatic β cells and has a great glycemic-lowering effect. Dosed once a day. They should be avoided in severe renal or hepatic impairment and are contraindicated in those with a sulfa allergy. They have been associated with an increased risk of cardiovascular death. Side effects include weight gain and hypoglycemia, but there are fewer side effects with second-generation medications.
- **Meglitinides (short-acting insulin secretagogues; e.g., repaglinide, nateglinide)**: These work similarly to sulfonylureas and can be used if allergic to sulfonylureas. Preprandial dosing.
- **α-glucosidase inhibitors (intestinal enzyme inhibitors; e.g., acarbose, miglitol)**: This class of drugs is best given with the first bite at meals. It works by delaying intestinal glucose absorption and so helps decrease postprandial glucose surges. It should be avoided in intestinal, liver, or renal disease. Side effect is flatulence.

- **Thiazolidinediones (insulin sensitizers; e.g., pioglitazone, rosiglitazone):** This class has been shown to slow the progression of DM, decrease triglycerides, and increase HDL cholesterol. Maximum effect in 12–16 weeks. Side effects include edema, macular edema, weight gain, anemia, CHF, and hepatotoxicity (rare). It should be avoided in liver disease and CHF. Access to rosiglitazone is limited due to an elevated risk of MI.
- **Dipeptidyl peptidase 4 inhibitors (e.g., alogliptin, linagliptin, saxagliptin, sitagliptin):** DPP-4 inhibitors work by prolonging the effects of incretin hormones (hormones that stimulate insulin secretion due to meals). Side effects include arthralgias and hypersensitivity reactions.
- **Sodium-glucose cotransporter 2 inhibitors (e.g., canagliflozin, dapagliflozin):** SGLT-2 inhibitors work by increasing urinary glucose excretion. Side effects include genital mycotic infections, UTIs, and hypotension. Contraindicated in severe renal impairment; they have been associated with lower limb amputation.

Eyes, Ears, Nose, and Throat

EYE DISORDERS

BLOWOUT FRACTURE

A blowout fracture is a fracture of the **orbital floor** and involves the maxillary bone and the posterior medial floor of the orbit. It occurs due to **excessive facial trauma**. These patients will report trauma and complain of significant pain. Diplopia may be present because of restriction of the extraocular muscles. The eyelid may be edematous with crepitus present on palpation. A potential complication of a blowout fracture is entrapment of the orbital contents within the maxillary sinus. If this occurs, the eye may have a sunken appearance, or enophthalmos. Diagnosis is made per history and confirmed with imaging studies, usually CT scan. A blowout fracture will typically heal on its own with regular follow-up to ensure proper healing is occurring. Patients should be advised to avoid blowing their noses. Oral antibiotics may be given to decrease the risk of orbital infection. In some cases, such as with restrictive diplopia or enophthalmos, surgery may be necessary to repair the orbital wall. Complications include inferior rectus muscle entrapment leading to ischemia, nerve damage to the infraorbital nerve, and enophthalmos.

CORNEAL ABRASION

A corneal abrasion is caused by minor trauma to the surface of the eye, resulting in a scratching of the **cornea**. Patients will complain of pain and tearing of the eye, and may even complain of blurred vision. First rule out penetrating trauma and infection, and exclude the diagnosis of open globe before proceeding. To diagnose a corneal abrasion, topical anesthetics should be instilled in the eye. Fluorescein is then administered in the eye, and a UV light is used to examine the eye. The area of the cornea that is affected will light up brightly, indicating the area of abrasion. The eye should be gently irrigated to ensure there are no lingering foreign objects that can continue to cause damage. Topical antibiotics (most often ophthalmic fluoroquinolones [e.g., ofloxacin] or trimethoprim/polymyxin B ophthalmic) are used until asymptomatic, as well as topical anesthetics. Anticholinergics (e.g., cyclopentolate HCl 1%) are used in large abrasions. This condition should heal within 2–3 days of treatment. Recently, patching has been called into question. Patching may not benefit patients and may delay healing time, but it is often used in patients with large abrasions. Do not patch if patient has a high risk of infection. Patients with contact lenses should be examined for corneal infiltrates or ulcers, and if these are found, should be referred to an ophthalmologist immediately. Contact wearers without infiltrate or ulcer should be treated with ofloxacin or ciprofloxacin drops 4 times a day for *Pseudomonas* coverage. Complications include bacterial keratitis, corneal ulcer, and loss of vision.

HYPHEMA

Hyphema is blood in the **anterior chamber** of the eye. It is most frequently caused by blunt trauma to the eye, but can also occur following eye surgery or certain medical disorders, such as sickle cell anemia. A hyphema is very obvious because blood will be visible underneath the cornea and cause the iris to be blocked. There may also be conjunctival hemorrhages present. Treatment involves strict activity restrictions with avoidance of all

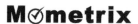

strenuous activities. Aspirin and other anticoagulant medications should be avoided to decrease the risk of additional bleeding. If the hyphema is managed on an outpatient basis, patients should be re-evaluated every couple of days to assess for rebleeding. Bleeding can reoccur 3–6 days following the initial eye trauma and may be worse than the initial bleeding that caused the hyphema. Most hyphemas spontaneously resolve within 4 days. Complications include increased intraocular pressure, vision disturbances, and glaucoma, especially later in life.

ORBITAL CELLULITIS

Orbital cellulitis is a soft-tissue infection posterior to the **orbital septum**, whereas **preseptal cellulitis** (periorbital cellulitis) only involves the **preseptal structures**. Orbital cellulitis is a serious condition and must be managed urgently to prevent further complications. It is usually due to sinusitis caused by *Streptococcus, Staphylococcus,* or *Haemophilus influenzae* type B. Dental or other infections may also be the cause. Patients will have a painfully swollen red eye/eyelid, sometimes severe enough to cause the eye to be swollen shut with drooping (ptosis). Patients may have blurred vision along with a fever and headache. Proptosis (bulging eye) and ophthalmoplegia (eye muscle paralysis) are hallmark signs of orbital cellulitis. On exam, the extraocular movements may also be restricted, depending on the amount of edema. A CT scan should be done to determine severity, to rule out the presence of a foreign body, and to assess any damage to the optic nerve. Also order a CBC (complete blood count), blood cultures, and culture of a nasal swab. Patients should be hospitalized and treated with appropriate IV antibiotics. Immunocompromised patients may develop a fungal orbital cellulitis. Once the infection is controlled with IV antibiotics, patients can be discharged home on oral antibiotics for 2 to 3 more weeks with close follow-up. Complications include intracranial expansion, vision loss, and cavernous sinus thrombosis.

BLEPHARITIS

Blepharitis is an inflammation or infection of the **eyelid and eyelashes**. There are two types: **staphylococcal blepharitis** and **seborrheic blepharitis**, with seborrheic being the more common. In addition to the eyelids and eyelashes, blepharitis can affect the eyebrows and scalp. Patients may complain of burning of the eyes and matting of the eyelashes. The eyes may be irritated with a gritty feeling. They can also appear red. Include questioning in the history regarding possible allergens or use of retinoids. Note any history of eczema or acne.

Diagnosis is made per clinical assessment, usually pink or reddened eyelid with crusting. Under otoscope, if a hard, crusty material is visible in eyelashes, this most often indicates staphylococcal blepharitis, whereas if the material in the eyelashes looks like oily, flaky material, this is more compatible with seborrheic blepharitis. Treating blepharitis involves debriding the lid margin of the matted material, usually using a cotton applicator. Warm compresses may be helpful. Topical antibiotics may be given and should be applied in the morning and at bedtime to prevent blurred vision from interfering with activities. Antihistamine eye drops do not help to relieve the symptoms of blepharitis by either cause. However, if the irritation is allergic in origin, then the drops will have an immediate effect. Lubricating eye drops will not help. Patients, especially in unilateral cases, need to be evaluated for sebaceous cell malignancy.

CHALAZION

A chalazion is caused by the inflammation of a **sebaceous gland** (meibomian gland) on the eyelid. It is not the same thing as a sty—a sty will also involve hair follicles and is more superficial appearing. Chalazia are commonly found in patients with rosacea or blepharitis. A chalazion usually occurs on the **upper eyelid**. There may be gradual swelling that increases over the course of a few days to a few weeks. The lesion may appear red and inflamed, and patients may complain of pain. Eventually, it becomes a painless nodular lesion. Diagnosis is made by clinical assessment. Warm compresses may help to relieve the pain and promote absorption of the oil that is trapped in the sebaceous gland. If a bacterial infection is superimposed on the chalazion, an ophthalmic antibiotic may be prescribed. If the chalazion is large and there is no sign of infection, an injection of triamcinolone (Kenalog) directly into the mass may help to relieve the inflammation and promote healing. In rare cases, surgical incision of the mass may be necessary if it persists and is not resolving

92

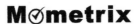

with more conservative treatments. Patients who experience recurring chalazia should be assessed for carcinoma.

ECTROPION AND ENTROPION

An ectropion is a condition in which the **lower eyelid turns outward**. This usually occurs during the aging process due to laxity of the muscles within the eyelid. The ectropion causes dryness and irritation of the eye. A paralysis of the facial nerve can cause this to occur because of the loss of neuromuscular control of the facial muscles on the affected side. Scarring due to trauma or burns can also cause an ectropion. Repair of the ectropion is accomplished through surgery to tighten the muscles of the lower eyelid. An **entropion** is a condition in which the **lower eyelid turns inward**. This is most commonly caused by the aging process due to muscle laxity causing the lower eyelid to involute. Facial nerve palsy and scarring can also cause this condition. Patients will complain of irritation of the eye, with tearing and the sensation of a foreign body being in the eye due to the eyelashes rubbing on the sclera. Treatment is by surgical correction.

HORDEOLUM

A hordeolum, or **sty**, is a condition in which an eyelash follicle becomes infected. Patients may complain of tenderness around the area. The small abscess will appear red and swollen. It will eventually come to a head, and purulent discharge may be expressed from the small infection. Treatment of a hordeolum generally consists of frequent application of warm compresses to draw the abscess to a head so that the infectious material can be expressed. The hordeolum may not drain and can resolve on its own. If the condition becomes severe, if complicated by preseptal cellulitis, or if patients develop recurrent hordeola, oral antibiotics (e.g., cephalexin) may be given to eradicate the infection. Oral doxycycline may be used in adults if recurrent and/or multiple lesions, or if significant/chronic meibomitis (inflammation of the meibomian glands, which can lead to a chalazion). It is important to remember that children should not be given tetracycline antibiotics due to alterations that can occur in tooth or bone development, unless >8 years old and if it is a severe or life-threatening infection. Tetracyclines should also not be given to females who are or may become pregnant (Category D) because of the risk of birth anomalies. Complications include lid deformity and progression to a chalazion.

CATARACT

Cataracts are a disease involving opacification of the **lens** and are the leading cause of **treatable blindness** in the world. They typically present as either congenital or senile cataracts. **Congenital cataracts** are usually due to intrauterine infections, metabolic disorders, or genetic factors. An irregular red reflex is the typical initial clinical finding. TORCH titers (toxoplasmosis, other infections, rubella, cytomegalovirus, herpes simplex virus) and a VDRL (Venereal Disease Research Lab) test for syphilis should be drawn. Surgical intervention before 17 weeks of age is recommended to prevent and minimize visual impairment, including irreversible amblyopia ("lazy eye") and sensory nystagmus (involuntary, rapid eye movements), which is especially seen in bilateral congenital cataracts. **Senile cataracts** involve a gradual thickening of the lens and present with gradual, progressive visual impairment (typically night vision and near vision issues). Patients often complain of a glare. Treatment involves unilateral or bilateral surgical lens extraction. The main complication is blindness.

PTERYGIUM

A pterygium is a triangular raised lesion that grows on the **surface of the eye**. It most commonly occurs on the nasal side of the cornea and may appear red. Patients usually seek treatment for this because of cosmetic appearances, but it can grow to obstruct the visual fields. This occurs if it extends over the cornea. Occasionally, it can be irritating to the eye. Diagnosis is made by clinical assessment. Care should be made to differentiate it from any neoplastic conditions. Treatment involves surgical removal of the pterygium, though this is usually reserved for cases in which the lesion affects the visual fields or is irritating. Surgery may be necessary to replace a portion of the conjunctiva. An antimetabolite may also be applied during surgery to prevent recurrence of the lesion. Almost one-half of patients who develop a pterygium will go on to develop the lesion again. There are usually no long-term effects of decreased visual acuity following surgery if the lesion is not encroaching upon the cornea.

MACULAR DEGENERATION

Macular degeneration is the most common cause of **irreversible central blindness** in the Caucasian population. It is rare in other races. There are two types of macular degeneration: dry and wet. **Dry macular degeneration** is more common and occurs when drusen (yellow deposits) accumulate deep in the eye under the retina. It begins in middle age and progresses slowly, causing a loss of central vision, eventually leading to blindness. It can, however, develop into wet macular degeneration. **Wet macular degeneration** occurs when capillaries break through the retina and grow behind the macula of the eye. This form of the disease progresses more rapidly to blindness (days to weeks). Any vision loss that occurs over a period of weeks or days requires urgent ophthalmic evaluation. Drusen may be seen under the retina on fundoscopic exam, even before there is any visual loss. Center vision deficits may be seen on visual field exam.

There is no definitive cure for macular degeneration. However, vitamin C, vitamin E, zinc, copper, and β-carotene may slow the process of dry macular degeneration. Medications (ranibizumab, aflibercept, or bevacizumab) and surgery may improve vision in wet macular degeneration. There is a genetic link with this disease, and prevention is important. Eating leafy green vegetables high in carotenoids, quitting smoking, and protecting the eyes from UV light can reduce risk. Complication: Dry macular degeneration can suddenly turn to wet macular degeneration, resulting in rapid vision loss.

RHEGMATOGENOUS RETINAL DETACHMENT

Rhegmatogenous is the most common form of **retinal detachment** and is a medical emergency. Refer to an ophthalmologist immediately. Rhegmatogenous retinal detachment occurs when there is a **tear in the retina**, allowing the vitreous humor to enter the space behind the retina and causing a detachment of the retina from the posterior eye. The most common cause of this type of retinal detachment is the aging process, which leads to shrinkage of the vitreous humor. This causes pulling on the retina, leading to a tear or hole in the retina. Patients will describe floaters and flashes of light with an associated decrease in vision. The loss of vision will occur in a curtain-type fashion, where the vision appears as a dark curtain descending over the visual field, usually starting at the upper periphery and marching downwards. This occurs as the torn retina flaps down. Patients complaining of floaters who present with monocular decreased visual fields should be referred to an ophthalmologist immediately. This condition is a surgical emergency and needs to be treated immediately. Delay of even one day can result in some degree of permanent visual loss after surgical repair.

TRACTIONAL RETINAL DETACHMENT

A tractional retinal detachment occurs in conditions that cause scarring within the **vitreous humor**, such as diabetic retinopathy. This is the second most common type of **retinal detachment**. The fibrous strands that make up a scar cause traction to be applied to the retina. This traction results in separation of the retina from the posterior eye. Onset is usually gradual. Some patients may have floaters or flashes of light in their vision, along with the curtain-type vision loss, as seen with rhegmatogenous retinal detachment. More commonly, there will be visual loss with a description of blind spots in the vision. Treatment usually involves removing the vitreous humor, thereby removing the fibrous scar material. Gas or an oily substance may be injected into the eye to prevent recurrence of this condition. The best treatment is prevention by maintaining adequate control of blood sugar levels in diabetics to prevent the development of diabetic retinopathy. There is a chance of permanent visual loss with this condition, despite aggressive treatment.

EXUDATIVE RETINAL DETACHMENT

An exudative retinal detachment occurs when fluid builds up **behind the retina**. This can occur with multiple medical conditions, including various collagen-vascular diseases, posterior scleritis, neoplasms of the eye, infections, preeclampsia, and congenital abnormalities. This condition results in visual loss, with patients complaining of experiencing blind spots in their vision. They may also experience floaters or flashes of light in their vision. Surgery is not always necessary to treat this condition. Treatment of the underlying condition is usually sufficient to prevent permanent visual loss. With chronic medical conditions that cause an exudative retinal detachment, achieving adequate medical control of the condition can result in reversal of the detachment as the fluid behind the retina dissipates. Urgent treatment of the cause of the retinal detachment is

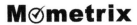

necessary to prevent permanent visual loss. Some patients may develop a chronic problem with this condition, and then surgery to prevent fluid accumulation behind the retina is necessary.

DIABETIC RETINOPATHY

Diabetic retinopathy is the leading cause of **blindness** in the US in diabetics <65 years old. It begins as tiny **microaneurysms in the retina**. Exudates form in the retina as these aneurysms rupture. Patients frequently have no visual loss at this stage. As retinopathy progresses, the exudates become larger, and the rupturing aneurysms can lead to swelling of the **macula**. Patients may or may not have a decrease in visual acuity. Focal laser photocoagulation is done at this stage to decrease the **macular edema** by cauterizing the leaking microaneurysms. The final stages of diabetic retinopathy occur when new vessels are developed around the optic nerve. These vessels are very fragile and are easily ruptured, which leads to bleeding within the retina and vitreous humor. As scar tissue forms, the fibrous strands of the scar may cause a **tractional retinal detachment**. Focal laser photocoagulation can be performed to decrease the rupture of these new vessels, but visual loss is common with this condition, and blindness frequently occurs. Annual eye exams are critical to managing this disease.

HYPERTENSIVE RETINOPATHY

Uncontrolled blood pressure is the cause of **hypertensive retinopathy**. As pressure rises within the body's arteries, the small arteries in the eye are also affected. This results in narrowing of the **retinal arteries** and a decrease in blood flow to the structures of the eye. Patients may or may not notice a decrease in their visual acuity. On exam, possible changes include narrowed retinal arteries, copper wiring from sclerosis of the vessels, arteriovenous nicking, cotton-wool spots (retinal ischemia), retinal hemorrhages, and possible optic disc swelling. A swollen optic disc (papilledema) can result with malignant hypertension, a hypertensive emergency in which the diastolic blood pressure is >120 mmHg. Treatment of hypertensive retinopathy involves controlling the blood pressure with diet, exercise, and medications. **Malignant hypertension** is an emergency condition and should be treated immediately, but slowly over 24–48 hours. Visual loss that results from hypertensive retinopathy may be permanent, but control of the blood pressure can prevent additional damage. Hypertensive encephalopathy, stroke, and hemorrhage are additional possible complications.

CONJUNCTIVITIS

Conjunctivitis ("**pink eye**") is an inflammation or infection of the conjunctiva of one or both eyes. It can be caused by bacteria, virus, allergy, or an irritant. Patients will complain of a gritty, irritating, itching sensation in the eye, which is red from hemorrhage of small vessels. Vision is usually not affected. With **bacterial conjunctivitis**, there is a copious mucus discharge, and patients may have problems with the eye being matted closed in the morning. **Viral and allergic conjunctivitis** typically cause a watery discharge. This is a diagnosis of exclusion, based on clinical assessment. The following should be ruled out: sty, ulceration, and blepharitis. If bacterial conjunctivitis is suspected, treatment consists of erythromycin 5 mg/g ointment ophthalmically, applying a 1 cm ribbon 4–6 times per day for 5 to 7 days; or trimethoprim-polymyxin B ophthalmically, 1 drop every 3 hours (max 6 drops/day) for 7 to 10 days; or other ophthalmic antibiotics. If there is no response to antibiotic drops, the patient should be referred to an ophthalmologist. Viral conjunctivitis only requires symptomatic relief. Patients should avoid rubbing the eye. Frequent hand washing can decrease transmission of the condition. Allergic conjunctivitis can be treated with ophthalmic antihistamines, but this condition may be chronic in patients who suffer from recurrent environmental allergies. Corneal injury may occur, resulting in vision impairment.

DACRYOCYSTITIS/DACRYOADENITIS

Dacryocystitis is a condition in which the **lacrimal sac** becomes inflamed. This inflammation can be due to a blockage at some point in the tear drainage system or a stone that has formed within the lacrimal sac. Patients will complain of pain along the inside corner of the eye. The area will appear red and swollen and may extend from the inner canthus of the eye to the upper nose or nasal bridge. If the dacryocystitis is chronic in nature, tearing is the most prevalent complaint. Diagnosis is made by clinical assessment. CBC may show elevated WBCs, and occasionally CT scans are ordered to show anatomy and surrounding areas of lacrimal sac. To treat this inflammation and infection, antibiotics can be given. Depending upon the severity, patients may require hospitalization for IV antibiotic therapy. If severe, incision and drainage may be necessary to treat an abscess. Once the inflammation and infection have resolved, surgery may be necessary to correct the blockage. If a stone is present within the lacrimal sac, this will need to be surgically removed to prevent future blockages leading to abscess formation. Complications include cellulitis, sepsis, meningitis, fistula, and abscess. **Dacryoadenitis** is the inflammatory enlargement of the lacrimal gland and presents as redness and swelling of the upper eyelid with an S-shaped ptosis (drooping of the upper eyelid).

PRIMARY OPEN-ANGLE GLAUCOMA

Primary open-angle glaucoma is the most common form of **glaucoma**. It is asymptomatic, progressive, and irreversible, and causes optic nerve damage. It is more common in patients over 40, in African Americans, and in patients with a positive family history. Screening is vital since patients are asymptomatic; however, patients may notice peripheral visual field loss later in the disease. Diagnose by measuring intraocular pressure and corneal thickness, visual field testing, and ophthalmoscopy. Increased cupping of the optic disc and thinning of the neural rim may be seen on fundoscopic exam. Treatment begins with ophthalmic eye drops: ophthalmic β-blockers (e.g., timolol), prostaglandin analogs (e.g., latanoprost), α-2 agonists (e.g., brimonidine), and carbonic anhydrase inhibitors (e.g., brinzolamide). Miotic agents (e.g., pilocarpine) that work on the muscarinic receptors of the eye to increase fluid flow may also be prescribed. Laser and traditional surgical treatments are usually reserved for when medical management fails to produce adequate results in decreasing the ocular pressure. Refer to an ophthalmologist for monitoring and chronic treatment. Permanent vision loss is the primary complication.

ANGLE-CLOSURE GLAUCOMA

This affects approximately 10% of patients who have glaucoma. There are several types of **primary angle-closure glaucoma**: subacute, acute (medical emergency), and chronic. The angle through which fluid drains from the eye is narrowed, resulting in an increase in ocular pressure. This is treated with surgery by creating an opening behind the iris through which the fluid can flow from the eye, resulting in a decrease in ocular pressure. In **subacute** and **chronic angle-closure glaucoma**, the closure is usually gradual and can be asymptomatic unless there is an attack. **Acute angle-closure glaucoma** results in the sudden onset of blurred vision with visual halos, pain/headache, red eye, and nausea and vomiting. This is a medical emergency and requires immediate treatment/referral to an ophthalmologist. The cornea may be edematous when examined, and ocular pressure readings are extremely elevated with this condition. Ophthalmic medications (e.g., pilocarpine, timolol, travoprost) can be given to reduce the corneal edema and intraocular pressure. Laser surgery (iridotomy) is necessary to open the angle so that fluid can flow from the eye to cause a decrease in the ocular pressure. Complications include optic nerve damage and vision loss.

STRABISMUS

Strabismus is a condition in which the **extraocular muscles** are weakened, leading to a gaze deviation in one eye. It differs from a "lazy eye," or amblyopia, because there is no loss of visual acuity associated with a strabismus. The condition is labeled by the direction in which the gaze is affected:

- **Hypertropia** occurs when the gaze is diverted upward.
- **Exotropia** when the gaze is deviated outward.
- **Esotropia** when the gaze is deviated inward ("cross-eye").
- **Hypotropia** when the gaze is deviated downward.

A wide, flattened nose with a skin fold at the inner canthus can cause the appearance of esotropia and is called **pseudoesotropia**. This usually resolves with age. Eye muscle strengthening can be performed to help straighten the gaze in mild cases of strabismus. If this fails or if the strabismus is severe, surgery may be necessary to draw the affected muscles tighter in order to straighten the gaze.

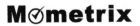

PAPILLEDEMA

Papilledema is **optic disc swelling**, typically bilateral, secondary to increased intracranial pressure. Symptoms may include headache, nausea/vomiting, pulsatile tinnitus, blurred vision, and double vision. However, visual symptoms are often absent. Fundoscopic exam can show disc margin blurring, venous congestion with hemorrhages, exudates, and cotton-wool spots (indicates nerve fiber damage) around the disc. Initial findings typically present nasally. Test the visual field for enlargement of the blind spot. Order an urgent head CT or MRI with contrast to rule out a mass lesion. Once normal imaging is established, perform a lumbar puncture to assess opening pressure and to rule out neoplastic or infectious causes. Causes include brain tumor, head trauma/hemorrhage, meningitis, encephalitis, and idiopathic intracranial hypertension (pseudotumor cerebri). Treat the underlying cause. Blindness is the main complication.

EAR DISORDERS

LABYRINTHITIS

Labyrinthitis is an inflammatory condition affecting the **labyrinth of the inner ear**. It usually occurs following a viral infection, such as a cold or the flu. Bacterial infections of the upper respiratory system, trauma to the head or ear, or benign tumors of the ear may also cause this condition. Vertigo is the main symptom that patients will experience. This can be quite severe, with nausea and vomiting, along with a complete loss of balance. Patients may have hearing loss, a headache, or tinnitus with this condition. The symptoms can be positional or may occur at rest. Diagnosis is made by clinical assessment, using imaging to rule out other disorders if needed. It is important to obtain an audiogram. Labyrinthitis is usually treated with bed rest, hydration, and anti-vertigo medications, such as meclizine. Viral labyrinthitis is also often treated with a tapering dose of corticosteroids, like prednisone. Antibiotics will be given if the condition is caused by a bacterial infection. For symptom relief, antihistamines, antiemetics, and benzodiazepines are commonly used, but should be used short-term. Complications are not usually common, but include tinnitus and hearing loss (especially in cases of meningitis).

VERTIGO

Vertigo is the sense that the room is spinning. It can originate from a **central** (central nervous system [CNS]) or **peripheral cause**. CNS causes include anemic or hemorrhagic episodes, tumors, trauma, or multiple sclerosis. Peripheral causes include labyrinthitis, Ménière disease, vestibular neuronitis, and benign paroxysmal positional vertigo (BPPV). In the US, vertigo is commonly caused by BPPV. It causes short-term positional vertigo accompanied by nystagmus (rhythmic movement of the eyes) and usually nausea. This is a clinical diagnosis, which can be confirmed with an abnormal Dix-Hallpike maneuver (a test that elicits vertigo and nystagmus). Small stones (otoliths) within the labyrinth cause this condition, and the Epley maneuver can be used to change the position of the stones. Medications are not effective since they do not address the causative factor. Complications are rare after repositioning maneuvers, but include worsening vertigo and otoliths causing a canal jam.

OTITIS MEDIA

Otitis media (**OM**) is an infection of the **middle ear** and is the second most common childhood illness after upper respiratory infections (URI). It is most commonly bacterial or viral, and it affects children more often than adults because of the straight anatomic structure of the auditory canal and eustachian tube, which promotes the accumulation of fluid behind the tympanic membrane. The most common cause of otitis media in children is infection with *Streptococcus pneumoniae, Haemophilus influenzae,* or *Moraxella* (*Branhamella*) *catarrhalis*. The incidence of infection with the first two organisms is on the decline, however, because of immunizations now available.

Signs and symptoms include ear pain and fever, and symptoms of an upper respiratory infection may also be present. On otoscopic exam, a bulging tympanic membrane with purulent effusion may be evident. There should be decreased movement of the membrane with insufflation. Treat with antibiotics if patient age is >6 months with severe otalgia, otalgia >48 hours, or temperature >39 °C, or if bilateral non-severe acute OM (AOM). Antibiotics may be started, but since many cases resolve on their own, a conservative approach can be taken if patient is 6–23 months or older with a unilateral non-severe AOM. In this case, observe and start antibiotics if symptoms worsen or if there is no improvement within 48–72 hours of symptom onset. Amoxicillin is the drug of choice (unless used in the last 30 days) for uncomplicated OM without penicillin allergy. The most common dose is 500 mg every 12 hours (if >40 kg). High-dose amoxicillin is an option in pediatrics (if age is >3 months and <40 kg) of 40–45 mg/kg every 12 hours. High-dose amoxicillin-clavulanate is the antibiotic of choice for children in a daycare setting. Drug resistance varies across the US, so current guidelines for any specific area should be followed. Complications include mastoiditis, labyrinthitis, and hearing loss.

> **Review Video: Otitis Media**
> Visit mometrix.com/academy and enter code: 328778

CHOLESTEATOMA

A cholesteatoma is an abnormal growth of squamous epithelium in the **middle ear** that can cause permanent hearing loss. It can be congenital but is typically caused by **chronic tympanic membrane retractions** or from a **tympanic membrane perforation** (either traumatic or due to tympanostomy tubes). The patient with a history of ear infections, who presents with painless ear drainage (hallmark sign), hearing loss, and occasionally dizziness, should be evaluated for a cholesteatoma. Diagnosis is made on physical exam and by CT scan. Evaluation might include a hearing and balance test. Refer to an otolaryngologist since surgical removal is necessary, unless medically contraindicated. If left untreated, a cholesteatoma can lead to permanent hearing loss through bone deterioration, abscess formation, meningitis, and even death.

OTITIS EXTERNA

Otitis externa (**OE**) is an infection of the **external ear canal**. It is usually caused by *Pseudomonas* bacteria or *Staphylococcus aureus* infections. Occasionally, OE can be due to a fungal infection. OE is often referred to as "swimmer's ear" because of the prevalence in those who spend a lot of time in the water. Significant ear pain that is exacerbated with movement of the external ear is the main symptom. Patients may have enlargement of the preauricular lymph nodes. Exam of the ear canal will reveal edema and erythema of the ear canal, possibly with purulent discharge.

Diagnosis is made by clinical assessment and history. The mainstays of treatment with OE involve cleaning the ear, treating the inflammation, controlling pain, and avoiding contributing factors. After cleaning of the ear, the ear is treated with topical antibiotics with or without corticosteroids, antiseptics, or acidifying agents. For drops, tilt head towards opposite shoulder, pull superior part of auricle up, and instill drops. The patient should side lie for 5 minutes or use a cotton ball in the ear. If swelling is severe, a wick is placed in the ear canal to facilitate instillation of the solution. The wick may remain for 2–3 days. Aminoglycoside eardrops can also be used, but care should be taken to ensure the tympanic membrane is intact because of the risk of ototoxicity with these medications. Complications include necrotizing (malignant) external otitis, mastoiditis, and periauricular cellulitis.

MASTOIDITIS

Mastoiditis is an infection of the **mastoid bone** of the skull and usually occurs following **otitis media**, especially in patients younger than 5 years old. It is typically due to *Streptococcus pneumoniae*. In the past, mastoiditis was relatively common and was the leading cause of death in children. Since the advent of antibiotics and prompt treatment of otitis media infections, the incidence of mastoiditis has greatly declined. Patients, if old enough, may complain of severe pain in the ear and behind the ear. There may be swelling and erythema in the area that causes the affected ear to stick out from the head. Patients may have a high fever and headache. A CT of the temporal bone will show an opacification of the mastoid air cells due to the infection. Treatment includes tympanocentesis with culture and sensitivity, with aggressive IV antibiotics in order to penetrate the bone tissue and treat the infection. Once IV antibiotics are effective (afebrile for 48 hours), the patient will continue on oral antibiotics for 14 days to completely eradicate the infection. Myringotomy may be needed to remove fluid and ventilate the ear. If medical treatment is not effective, a mastoidectomy may be

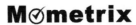

performed. Complications include hearing loss, facial nerve palsy (cranial nerve VII), brain abscess, and meningitis.

MÉNIÈRE'S DISEASE

Ménière's disease (**idiopathic endolymphatic hydrops**) is a condition affecting the **labyrinth of the ear**. The labyrinth is made up of bony and membranous portions. The membranous portion contains a fluid called **endolymph**. It is thought that Ménière's disease results when the membranous portion of the labyrinth ruptures, causing the endolymph to mix with **perilymph**, a fluid separating the membranous portion from the bony portion. Signs and symptoms include tinnitus, vertigo, and loss of hearing. Some patients experience a feeling of pressure within the affected ear(s). These symptoms are often not constant, but rather occur intermittently. Diagnosis is made by clinical assessment. Sensorineural hearing loss, tinnitus, and occasional episodes of vertigo, as well as the occasional aural fullness, are the usual qualifiers for a diagnosis. Other diagnoses should be ruled out. There is no cure for Ménière's disease. The symptoms can be decreased, though, with dietary restrictions on sodium, caffeine, and alcohol. Quitting smoking may help decrease the severity of symptoms. Gentamicin eardrops may help decrease the vertigo. With severe cases, the labyrinth can be surgically removed, but this will result in hearing loss in the ear. Benzodiazepines, antihistamines, and antiemetics are often used for acute episodes of symptoms. Complications include intractable vertigo and hearing loss.

NASAL/SINUS DISORDERS
ALLERGIC RHINITIS

Allergic rhinitis affects the **nose and eyes**. It occurs in individuals with allergies to **environmental irritants** such as pollen, animal dander, trees, and dust. Symptoms vary from minor allergic reactions to urticaria (hives) and throat constriction. The onset of symptoms can often be associated with exposure to an environmental irritant. Signs and symptoms include rhinorrhea (runny nose), itchy and watery eyes, mild cough, sneezing, facial itching, and sore throat. Patients may complain of a headache, possibly over the sinuses, with a feeling of pressure due to increased mucus production. Fatigue, irritability, reduced performance, and possibly depression can be side effects.

Diagnosis is made by clinical assessment, history, and findings. Allergic shiners, a nasal crease, boggy nasal turbinates, and cobblestoning of the posterior pharynx may be noted on physical exam. Allergy skin testing and allergen-specific serum IgE tests are useful. Treatment includes environmental controls to specific triggers, medication, and immunotherapy (subcutaneous or sublingual). Intranasal steroid sprays or antihistamines with decongestants are the most effective maintenance therapies. Antihistamines decrease the release of histamine and suppress the allergic symptoms; however, they have sedative side effects. Therefore, second-generation antihistamines are usually preferred (loratadine, cetirizine, fexofenadine). Complications include sinusitis, otitis media, palatal changes, apnea, and asthma.

SINUSITIS (ACUTE AND CHRONIC)

Sinusitis (**rhinosinusitis**) is inflammation of the nasal passages and paranasal sinuses that is symptomatic. Mucus cannot drain because of the edematous sinuses, producing an excellent environment in which bacteria can thrive, leading to a sinus infection. It is classified as **acute sinusitis** if symptoms last <30 days and **chronic** if >90 days. Signs and symptoms include a current or resolving upper respiratory infection (URI) and a headache (generally over the frontal, ethmoid, or maxillary sinuses). Complaints of positional increases in the headache, a fullness or pressure within the head, stuffy nose, fever, and aching in the teeth may also be present.

Diagnosis is made per clinical assessment. It is important to attempt to distinguish bacterial from viral sinusitis. Sinusitis is likely **bacterial** if the patient presents with sinusitis symptoms for ≥10 days, especially if symptoms are severe, with high fever, facial pain, and purulent nasal discharge. Since URIs typically last only 5–7 days, also consider bacterial sinusitis when, 7 days following a URI which was improving, there is a sudden return with worsening symptoms. Treatment will be decided based on whether the sinusitis is of bacterial or

99

viral origin. For both viral and bacterial sinusitis, symptoms can be improved with analgesia, mucolytics, decongestants, steroids, nasal irrigation, and antihistamines. First-line treatment for acute bacterial sinusitis includes 14 days of high-dose amoxicillin (80–90 mg/kg/day), clarithromycin, or azithromycin. Chronic sinusitis is typically treated with daily nasal irrigation, nasal steroids, and 3–6 weeks (or more) of antibiotics. Drug resistance varies across the US, so clinicians should be aware of local resistance trends. Complications include meningitis, cavernous sinus thrombosis, orbital cellulitis, and abscess.

MOUTH/THROAT DISORDERS

PHARYNGITIS

Pharyngitis is an inflammation of the **pharynx**, causing a sore throat. It is most commonly caused by a **viral infection**. The most common bacterial cause of pharyngitis is **group A streptococci (GAS)**. Patients will complain of a very sore throat that may or may not be accompanied by other cold symptoms. Cold symptoms are usually present with viral forms of pharyngitis. A fever, headache, and soft palate petechiae may also be present. Children with GAS pharyngitis may also have nausea and vomiting. On exam, cervical and tonsillar lymph nodes will be enlarged, and the oropharynx will appear edematous/erythematous, possibly with white exudates present. Centor criteria are symptoms that may be present and are used to guide the clinician: tonsillar exudates, absence of cough, fever (may be by history), 3 to 14 years of age, and anterior cervical adenopathy. Patients with ≥4 Centor criteria have a 51–53% risk and are likely to have GAS. For patients that have ≥2 Centor criteria, use a rapid antigen detection test (RADT) to diagnose GAS. Those with <2 Centor criteria, unless they have a high risk for infection, are usually treated as having viral pharyngitis.

Culture confirms diagnosis (90–99% sensitive), but as RADT is very sensitive (70–90%), culture is not often ordered. Treatment of viral pharyngitis is supportive, with warm salt water, antipyretics, and analgesics. Penicillin is the drug of choice for GAS pharyngitis—for example, penicillin VK, penicillin G benzathine (an IM form), and amoxicillin (preferred in children due to better taste tolerability). Complications include glomerulonephritis, rheumatic fever, scarlet fever, toxic shock syndrome, otitis media, sinusitis, cellulitis, and peritonsillar abscess.

EPIGLOTTITIS

Epiglottitis is an acute inflammation of the **epiglottis** and can be a fatal medical emergency. The causative agent in adults is usually *H. influenzae, H. parainfluenzae, Streptococcus pneumoniae,* or group A streptococci. In children, the causative agent is typically *Haemophilus influenzae* type b (Hib). Whereas the incidence of epiglottitis has decreased in children due to the Hib vaccine, the incidence in adults has remained the same. Patients can decline rapidly, so airway management is of utmost importance. Throughout patient care, it is key to avoid agitating the patient.

Signs and symptoms include sore throat, odynophagia/dysphagia (painful swallowing/difficulty swallowing), drooling, and a classic tripod sitting position (sitting up on hands, tongue out, and head forward). If epiglottitis is suspected, one should NOT attempt to visualize the epiglottis directly with a tongue depressor during PE, because this may cause more inflammation and could close the airway. Stridor, muffled voice, and a history of diabetes mellitus are indicators for the likelihood of airway intervention. Diagnosis by radiograph (which shows the classic thumbprint sign) is being replaced by nasopharyngoscopy/laryngoscopy in the operating room, which allows for direct visualization. Treatment with third-generation cephalosporins, like ceftriaxone (Rocephin), are used due to the increasing resistance to ampicillin; amoxicillin/clavulanic acid is another option. If penicillin/cephalosporin allergic, chloramphenicol can be used. Close contacts should be treated prophylactically with rifampin. Complications include meningitis, pneumonia, pulmonary edema, and death.

APHTHOUS ULCERS

Aphthous ulcers, also known as **recurrent aphthous stomatitis (RAS)**, or **canker sores**, occur only within the soft tissues of the **oral cavity**. They can appear on the lips, oral mucosa, gums, or tongue. Canker sores are not contagious, typically start in childhood, and often resolve in the third decade of life. There is commonly a positive family history. They have no definite known cause, but irritants in the oral cavity, such as strongly acidic foods, may contribute to aphthous ulcers. Also, smoking cessation, stress, food allergies, and sodium lauryl sulfate (which is contained in many dental products) may contribute to RAS. Patients will complain of a painful area in the oral cavity with some local swelling. Exam will reveal a shallow, oval or round, yellowish or grayish ulcer that is well-demarcated with an erythematous halo. The ulcer is usually about 2–4 mm in width, and there is typically no bleeding present. Diagnosis is made per clinical assessment and history. Treatment involves topical corticosteroids, and oral vitamin B12 may help reduce RAS recurrences. Avoid predisposing factors and items that irritate the ulcer, such as acidic foods and drinks and rough, hard foods. Over-the-counter topical numbing medications may be helpful in decreasing the pain. Aphthous ulcers generally resolve spontaneously within 7–10 days. Scarring is the main complication but is uncommon.

DENTAL ABSCESS

A dental abscess is an infection that forms around the roots of a tooth, or teeth, or in the gum tissue. Infection within the **dental pulp** (periapical) is more common in children, while an abscess in the **surrounding tissue** (periodontal) is more common in adults. Dental abscesses are polymicrobial. Patients will develop severe pain in an isolated area of the mouth. The cheek will be swollen, and the gingiva will be warm and appear red and swollen. Also, the lymph nodes in the neck on the affected side may be enlarged. A fever and headache may be present. The abscess may rupture, but treatment is still necessary. Diagnosis is made per clinical assessment. Treatment includes antibiotics, usually amoxicillin-clavulanate, and drainage of the abscess. Antibiotic treatment is very important to prevent systemic spread of the infection. Refer to a dentist or an oral surgeon. Complications include deep tissue infections, osteomyelitis, sinusitis, Ludwig angina (a rapidly spreading cellulitis), and cavernous sinus thrombosis.

ORAL LEUKOPLAKIA

Oral leukoplakia is a white patchy lesion found in the **oral cavity**. It can be caused by tobacco use (either smoking or chewing), alcohol use, chronic irritation, vitamin deficiency, candidiasis, or endocrine disturbances, and is considered a premalignant form of oral cancer. Another form of the condition is **hairy leukoplakia** (typically along the borders of the tongue), which is seen in HIV-positive patients or others with suppressed immune systems and is associated with the Epstein-Barr virus. Patients with oral leukoplakia will complain of a painless white patch in their mouth. This patch can be on the oral mucosa, the tongue, or the gums. It is a slightly raised, rough patch that is white or grayish in color and cannot be rubbed off. There may occasionally be leukoplakia lesions or nodules that appear pink or red in color, and these lesions have a strong potential for malignancy.

Diagnosis is made by clinical assessment and confirmation by biopsy. Treatment involves surgical excision of the lesion. There is a chance that patients can develop these lesions again, especially if they continue to smoke or use smokeless tobacco. Quitting smoking and tobacco use is the best way to prevent future lesions. Oral cancer is a possible complication.

ORAL CANDIDIASIS

Oral candidiasis, or **oral thrush**, is a fungal infection (typically *Candida albicans*) affecting the **oral mucosa**. It is usually not contagious and commonly occurs in those who wear dentures. It can also occur in newborns, diabetics, patients who take steroids (especially inhalation steroids), immunocompromised patients, and those undergoing head or neck radiation. It may also occur in those taking antibiotics due to alterations in the natural flora of the mouth. Patients will have white plaques over the oral mucosa, which can be scraped off with a tongue depressor to reveal red, raw areas. The lesions may or may not be painful to patients. Diagnosis is most often made by clinical assessment, but if confirmation is needed, cultures can be taken. Topical or oral antifungals (e.g., nystatin, clotrimazole, fluconazole) are used to treat oral candidiasis. Resistance to the azole drugs is an increasing concern. Patients should be reminded to daily clean their dentures thoroughly. For patients using inhaled steroids, care should be taken to completely rinse their mouth after each treatment. There are usually no complications in the immunocompetent, but in the immunocompromised, candidiasis can spread to the bloodstream, esophagus, heart valves, etc. Also, it can lead to malnutrition if eating becomes difficult.

MUMPS/PAROTITIS

Mumps is a systemic viral infection involving the **salivary glands**. It generally affects the **parotid salivary glands**, which are the largest. **Parotitis** is a general term for inflammation of the parotid glands, which may be caused by bacteria, HIV, autoimmune disorders, etc. **Mumps** is caused by a paramyxovirus and is transmitted through airborne respiratory particles and saliva. It generally affects children more than adults, but the live, two-dose MMR vaccine has decreased the incidence of the disease. The incubation period is 12–24 days. Patients may complain of facial pain with a fever, headache, and rash. The affected side of the face will appear swollen, like "chipmunk cheeks." Mumps/parotitis can affect the testes in boys, which may lead to infertility. Diagnosis is clinical, and serology testing can confirm. Patients should be isolated for 5 days from onset of symptoms, and the local health department should be contacted. Treatment is supportive. Ice or heat applied to the cheeks may help with pain relief, as can acetaminophen or ibuprofen for pain and fever relief. Chewing may be painful, so soft, non-acidic foods should be given with plenty of fluids. Aseptic meningitis/encephalitis, orchitis, and pancreatitis are possible complications.

SIALADENITIS

Sialadenitis is an infection of the **salivary glands**. It differs from parotitis, or mumps, in that it involves a blockage of the flow of saliva, causing bacteria to grow within the **ducts**. This leads to a **bacterial infection**, usually caused by *Staphylococcus aureus*. The salivary glands most commonly affected are the parotid glands in the cheek and the submandibular glands under the chin. Patients will complain of pain in the affected area. Purulent drainage may flow into the mouth, causing a foul-smelling and foul-tasting sensation. Patients may have a fever and headache. Diagnosis is usually made by clinical assessment, but CT may be useful if stones are suspected but not palpable. Treatment is usually accomplished with appropriate antibiotic therapy and hydration. If infection is severe, the gland may need to be drained, with culture and sensitivity testing performed on the extracted pus. If a stone is causing a blockage of the ductwork leading from the salivary gland, this will need to be surgically removed. Complications include abscess formation, and patients may develop a chronic form of sialadenitis that causes recurrent flare-ups of the condition.

PERITONSILLAR ABSCESS

A peritonsillar abscess can occur as a complication of **bacterial tonsillitis**. The causative organism is usually group A β-hemolytic streptococci. An abscess can develop in the soft tissue surrounding the **tonsil** and lead to a severe infection. Patients will have severe throat pain with enlarged lymph nodes on the affected side. Signs and symptoms include fever, headache, difficulty swallowing, muffled voice ("hot potato" voice), difficulty closing the mouth, drooling, neck swelling, ipsilateral ear pain, and trismus. Trismus can help distinguish an abscess from tonsillitis/cellulitis. Diagnosis is made by clinical assessment—deviation of the uvula and tonsil displacement. Immediately refer the patient to an otolaryngologist. Needle aspiration with culture of the fluid drained confirms the diagnosis.

Treatment may be handled on an outpatient or inpatient basis. Treatment involves hydration, incision and drainage (with culture, if not previously performed), then appropriate antibiotics. High-dose IV penicillin, cephalosporins, and amoxicillin-clavulanate (if mononucleosis is ruled out) are good initial choices. As always, local patterns of susceptibility should be taken into consideration. If MRSA is common, or if severe or not responding, use clindamycin or vancomycin. Patients may require future surgery to remove the tonsils and prevent recurrence of this infection. Complications include airway obstruction, sepsis, aspiration pneumonia, carotid artery pseudoaneurysm and rupture, thrombophlebitis (of the jugular vein), mediastinitis, and necrotizing fasciitis.

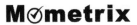

Gastrointestinal System/Nutrition

ESOPHAGEAL DISORDERS

ESOPHAGITIS

Esophagitis is inflammation of the **mucosal tissues of the esophagus**. There are several forms, including reflux, infectious, eosinophilic, pill, and radiation/chemoradiation-induced esophagitis. **Reflux esophagitis** (the most common type) occurs when the lower esophageal sphincter (LES) becomes lax and does not remain closed properly, letting stomach acids reflux into the esophagus. This causes inflammation, which can eventually lead to ulceration. Patients may complain of GERD-type symptoms, with a burning or bad taste in the mouth/throat, pain over the chest/into the throat (which may mimic cardiac pain), and possibly a mild cough. They may experience nausea/vomiting. If esophageal ulceration occurs, patients will have severe pain. If the ulcer is bleeding, vomiting of blood may occur (which may have a coffee-ground appearance), or the patient may have a positive stool guaiac. Patients may become anemic.

Treat reflux with proton pump inhibitors (PPIs are first line; typically treat 4–8 weeks) or histamine-2 receptor antagonists (H2RAs), sucralfate, or occasionally cisapride (associated with serious cardiac arrhythmias/death). Treat the underlying cause of infectious esophagitis (e.g., nystatin, acyclovir). Treatment of eosinophilic esophagitis involves elimination diets, steroids, and PPIs. Avoid offending medications and instruct patients on proper pill-taking methods (8 oz. of water). Radiation-induced inflammation may take several months to heal after treatment is stopped, and may be treated with viscous lidocaine and sucralfate. Lifestyle modifications may also help (avoid spicy foods, fried foods, caffeine, and alcohol; discontinue smoking). Since the cause of esophagitis varies, diagnosis is often made clinically or with endoscopy and possible cytology or biopsy. Complications include erosive esophagitis leading to bleeding, strictures, Barrett's esophagus, and aspiration pneumonia.

ESOPHAGEAL STRICTURE

Esophageal stricture is a **narrowing of the esophagus** due to intrinsic narrowing, extrinsic restriction, or lower esophageal sphincter (LES)/dysmotility issues. There are a variety of causes, including reflux, infectious, caustic ingestion, congenital, medication- or radiation-induced, and cancer. The majority of cases are reflux-induced strictures due to LES issues or dysmotility issues that result in scarring. This scarring can cause the LES to be narrowed, which prevents food from passing into the stomach properly. Suspect achalasia if liquids are also an issue. Patients may complain of difficulty swallowing (dysphagia), odynophagia, a sensation that food is stuck in their throat, heartburn, and chest pain. Diagnosis is made with a barium esophagram or upper GI endoscopy. Treatment involves use of proton pump inhibitors (PPIs) and dilating the sphincter to widen it. This can be accomplished during an esophagogastroduodenoscopy (EGD) by passing dilators, which gradually increase in diameter, through the sphincter. A balloon procedure can also be performed during EGD to widen the sphincter. A risk with both of these procedures is tearing of the esophagus, requiring surgical repair. If these treatments fail to relieve the symptoms, surgery may be needed to correct the sphincter. Complications include perforation, bleeding, bacteremia due to endoscopy, Barrett's esophagus, and recurrent strictures.

ESOPHAGEAL ACHALASIA

Esophageal achalasia is a disorder of the **esophagus** that affects **motility**. It may be primary or secondary to other conditions. Achalasia is most common in middle-aged and older adults and can also be a genetic trait. Achalasia can be present in esophageal tumors, Zenker's diverticulum, Chagas disease, nutcracker esophagus, and diffuse esophageal spasms. Patients present with dysphagia with both solids and liquids. Other symptoms might include pain, chest pain, heartburn, cough, or a slight regurgitation of food. Diagnosis includes barium swallow to rule out a mass or tumor. Diagnosis is confirmed when there is incomplete lower esophagus sphincter relaxation and aperistalsis in the lower portion of the esophagus per manometry. Laboratory results may show anemia or malnutrition. The most effective treatments are pneumatic dilation and surgical myotomy. Other options are Botox injections, and medications aimed at esophageal sphincter relaxation.

MALLORY-WEISS TEAR OR SYNDROME

Mallory-Weiss tear or syndrome is a non-penetrating, longitudinal laceration of the **esophageal mucosa** that occurs in the distal portion of the esophagus or proximal portion of the stomach. The tear can be caused by forceful vomiting or coughing, or by chronic alcohol use. Patients may be light-headed and describe an episode of vomiting or coughing followed by hematemesis (vomiting bright red blood). They may report dyspepsia and pain in the chest or abdomen, or if this has been going on for a period of time, they may experience melena (dark, tarry stools from upper GI bleeding). An esophagogastroduodenoscopy (EGD) will be done to confirm diagnosis, and cauterization may be performed if the bleeding has gone on for more than a few hours. Esophageal clips or endoscopic band ligation may also be performed. Most tears do not need to be surgically corrected and heal spontaneously as early as 96 hours. Antacids can be given to prevent further irritation of the tear. If there has been significant blood loss, a transfusion may be necessary to correct a volume-depletion anemia. Complications include shock, anemia, need for a blood transfusion, and dehydration.

ESOPHAGEAL VARICES

Esophageal varices most often occur along with **cirrhosis of the liver**, but any form of **liver disease** can lead to their development. With liver disease, blood flow through the liver is obstructed and slowed. This causes portal hypertension (pressure that builds up in the portal vein), which causes collateral vessels to form to bypass the portal system. This causes veins around the esophagus and upper stomach to swell and engorge (varices). Bleeding varices may occur when the portal-systemic pressure gradient reaches 10–12 mmHg and are fatal in approximately 20% of patients. If varices bleed, patient will present with sudden, painless, and often massive vomiting of blood. If bleeding is less severe, melena can be present. Also, patients may be asymptomatic from the esophageal varices themselves but will show signs of liver disease (e.g., jaundice, ascites, edema, easy bruising, malaise). They may have a history of alcoholism, though not all forms of cirrhosis are caused by alcohol. Diagnose with endoscopy. If varices bleed, immediate endoscopic banding along with administering IV octreotide (a somatostatin analog) is the treatment of choice. Sclerotherapy is second-line. If bleeding cannot be controlled or recurs, a TIPS (transjugular intrahepatic portosystemic shunt) procedure can be used. Nonselective β-blockers (e.g., propranolol) may be given to prevent rupture of varices. Complications include shock, uncontrolled bleeding, and death.

GASTRIC DISORDERS

GASTROESOPHAGEAL REFLUX DISEASE (GERD)

Gastroesophageal reflux disease (GERD) is a chronic condition in which gastric contents reflux into the **esophagus**, more than is physiologically normal, causing burning pain and possibly tissue damage. The esophagus, stomach, or lower esophageal sphincter (LES) dysfunctions, causing gastric and sometimes duodenal contents to reflux into the esophagus. Patients usually complain of experiencing heartburn ≥2 days a week along with regurgitation and dysphagia. Occasionally, atypical symptoms—a hoarse voice, coughing, wheezing, or noncardiac chest pain—are present, which warrants further investigation.

Diagnose clinically if symptoms are typical and respond to therapy. Endoscopy (EGD) and, if normal, 24-hour pH monitoring are also used to establish a diagnosis. Esophageal manometry is helpful when evaluating for surgery. Treatment includes lifestyle modifications, acid-suppressing therapy, and surgery. Lifestyle modifications include elevating the head of the bed, avoiding eating 2–3 hours before bedtime, avoiding causative foods (e.g., coffee, chocolate, alcohol, tomato-based foods) or medications (e.g., anticholinergics, β-agonists, calcium channel blockers), and weight loss. Antacids, H2-receptor antagonists (e.g., famotidine, cimetidine), and proton pump inhibitors (PPIs; e.g., omeprazole, lansoprazole) can be used for acid suppression. Antacids work better for mild symptoms, H2-receptor agonists work better for moderate symptoms, and PPIs work best for severe symptoms and erosive esophagitis. Treatment is typically 4–8 weeks. Surgery (usually fundoplication) may be indicated for those with serious esophagitis not fully responding to PPIs, and those with extraesophageal issues (e.g., hiatal hernia, respiratory/ENT side effects of GERD). Complications include esophagitis (50% of patients), ulcers, strictures, and Barrett esophagus with an increased risk of adenocarcinoma.

PEPTIC ULCER DISEASE

Peptic ulcer disease (**PUD**) occurs in the **stomach or duodenum** and has several causes. The most common causes are use of **nonsteroidal anti-inflammatory medications** (NSAIDs: ibuprofen, naproxen, aspirin) and infection with ***H. pylori* bacteria**. Excessive acid production in the stomach due to a tumor can also break down the gastric mucosa and cause ulcers. Patients may complain of a burning or gnawing epigastric pain, usually right after eating if a gastric ulcer, or 2–3 hours after eating if it is a duodenal ulcer. The pain may be relieved with eating, as food coats the stomach, although spicy foods can aggravate the pain. Patients may also feel bloated and have nausea/vomiting, heartburn, and chest pain. With bleeding of the ulcer, stools may be tarry (melena), and there may be blood in vomitus (hematemesis). Further investigation is needed if patients have anemia, bleeding, early satiety, or weight loss.

Confirm diagnosis through endoscopy and test for *H. pylori*. Treatment is focused on treating the underlying cause. Discontinue NSAIDs and treat *H. pylori* infections with a combination of antibiotics and a proton pump inhibitor (PPI). Dietary changes to reduce acid secretion are recommended (avoid alcohol, caffeine, tobacco). Acid production is suppressed through PPIs (e.g., omeprazole, lansoprazole) or H2RAs (e.g., cimetidine, famotidine). Surgery is necessary and recommended within 12 hours if the ulcer has perforated. Complications include perforation, hemorrhage, gastric outlet obstruction, and a future risk for gastric cancer if *H. pylori* was responsible for the ulcer(s).

GASTRIC CANCER

Gastric cancer is the fourth leading cause of **cancer death** in the world as of 2015, according to the World Health Organization (WHO). It is highest in Eastern Asia and Central/Eastern Europe. The incidence increases with age and accounts for almost 30,000 new cases in the US per year. It can be caused by infection with ***Helicobacter pylori* bacteria**, which causes chronic inflammation in the gastric mucosa, leading to development of cancerous cells (typically adenocarcinoma) in the **stomach lining**. Eating a diet high in salt (e.g., processed meats, smoked and pickled foods) as well as smoking have been linked to stomach cancer. Alcohol use may also play a role in the development of gastric cancer. Most symptoms are similar to GERD-type symptoms (e.g., dyspepsia, nausea/vomiting) and treated at home with antacids. Therefore, most patients are not aware they have stomach cancer until the disease has progressed to an advanced stage and other physical symptoms appear. Other symptoms include abdominal pain not relieved by antacids, unintentional weight loss, chronic feeling of fullness, and tarry stools if bleeding is occurring. Diagnose with endoscopy and biopsy. Tumor markers CEA and CA 19–9 may be elevated (in 45–50% and ~20% of patients respectively). Treatment is with surgical removal of the malignant tissue (partial or total gastrectomy) and possibly radiation and/or chemotherapy. Complications include a high rate of recurrence and death. 5-year survival rate is 30%.

PYLORIC STENOSIS

The **pylorus** is a muscular valve that serves as the opening between the stomach and the first part of the small intestine, known as the **duodenum**. **Pyloric stenosis** occurs in infants when the pylorus muscles thicken and enlarge, narrowing the opening and subsequently blocking food from reaching the duodenum. This inhibits the transport of food from the stomach to the small intestine and may cause almost complete obstruction. Though there is no definite known cause, it is thought that it may be genetic in nature. This is more common in firstborn males and usually presents at 3–6 weeks of age. The infant will have gradually worsening vomiting after meals; vomiting becomes projectile. The child will act fussy and still hungry after eating, and may have a slower degree of weight gain. Dehydration will eventually develop, as well as constipation. On exam, an olive-shaped mass can be palpated in the abdomen due to the enlarged pylorus. Diagnose with an ultrasound and check for metabolic alkalosis. Treatment is by surgical correction (pyloromyotomy) of the pyloric sphincter and correction of metabolic alkalosis with chloride and potassium. This is usually a very successful surgery that results in full recovery from the condition.

GALLBLADDER DISORDERS

CHOLELITHIASIS, BILIARY COLIC, AND CHOLANGITIS

Cholelithiasis is the development of **gallstones** in the gallbladder from cholesterol (80%) and other bile byproducts (20% are pigment stones: black or brown). These can block the ducts leading from the gallbladder, causing **cholecystitis** (inflammation of the gallbladder) or **cholangitis** (infection of the bile ducts). Most patients with cholelithiasis are asymptomatic (~60–80%). Symptoms can vary depending on which duct is blocked by the stone. Ducts leading to the pancreas can cause acute pancreatitis, with severe abdominal pain radiating to the back and vomiting. Blockage of ducts leading to the liver can result in jaundice (as in cholangitis). Generally, if a stone blocks the cystic duct, patients may experience **biliary colic**: nausea/vomiting, right upper quadrant (RUQ) abdominal pain that may refer to the right scapular tip (Collins sign), and bloating until the stone falls back into the gallbladder and the pain subsides. Patients may have several flare-ups of pain/biliary colic and may be advised to have elective surgery. **Cholangitis** presents with the classic triad (Charcot triad) of fever, RUQ pain, and jaundice.

Diagnose cholelithiasis with ultrasound. Medical treatment options include oral bile salt therapy (i.e., ursodeoxycholic acid) and extracorporeal lithotripsy, especially if stones are small (<1 cm) and cholesterol-based. Cholecystectomy to remove the gallbladder/gallstones, or removal of a stone from a duct, may be necessary. Patients who do not undergo surgery for correction of this condition should be advised to avoid fatty foods that can aggravate the problem and contribute to enlargement of the gallstones or development of new stones. Treat uncomplicated cholangitis with antibiotics, and—if acute or severe—emergent ERCP (endoscopic retrograde cholangiopancreatography), PTC (for biliary drainage), or emergent surgery. Complications of cholelithiasis include ascending cholangitis, cholecystitis, and pancreatitis.

CHOLECYSTITIS (ACUTE AND CHRONIC)

Cholecystitis is an inflammatory condition of the **gallbladder** that can be **acute** or **chronic**. Bile normally passes from the gallbladder to the small intestine to aid in digestion, but there is a **disruption** in this flow with cholecystitis. This usually occurs due to a **gallstone** (≥95% of cases; 80% are cholesterol stones and 20% are pigment stones) in the **cystic duct** causing bile to build up, leading to inflammation, swelling, and possibly a bacterial infection (cholangitis). **Chronic cholecystitis** refers to long-standing inflammation and recurrent episodes of biliary colic that causes progressive fibrosis of the gallbladder.

Cholecystitis risks include being older, female, pregnant, or obese, taking HRT/birth control, or having rapid weight loss. Patients often have prior attacks of biliary colic (i.e., without abdominal physical exam findings) before presenting with cholecystitis. Cholecystitis usually begins with severe, constant epigastric pain that lasts longer than colic (usually >6 hours) and localizes to the RUQ, often occurring after a fatty meal. Patients may guard, have pain aggravated by taking a deep breath during RUQ abdominal palpation (positive Murphy sign), or complain of referred right shoulder pain. Also, there may be nausea, vomiting, and fever (usually no fever in chronic cholecystitis). Diagnose through transabdominal ultrasound, which is 90–95% sensitive and about 80% specific. Scintigraphy is an alternative, and a CT may be necessary to view other structures. Treat with a cholecystectomy, usually done laparoscopically. Complications include cholangitis, empyema of the gallbladder, gangrene, perforation/peritonitis, sepsis, and pancreatitis.

LIVER DISORDERS

HEPATITIS A, B, AND C (ACUTE AND CHRONIC)

Viral hepatitis is an infectious disease that causes hepatic inflammation. It includes hepatitis viruses A, B, C, D, and E. There are various routes of transmission: fecal-oral (Hep A), blood (Hep B & C), needle (Hep D), and water (Hep E). Hep A and E both cause **acute** infections lasting <6 months. Hepatitis B, C, and D can become **chronic** (may take decades) and may also develop into cancer. Hep D only occurs with Hep B. Most of the hepatitis cases in the US are from Hep A, B, and C. The incubation period varies from 15 to 180 days depending on the type (lowest incubation time for Hep A and E; longest for Hep B, C, and D). The prodromal phase begins with anorexia, nausea/vomiting, malaise, fever, and occasionally urticaria and arthralgias. Next, the icteric phase begins with dark urine, pale-colored stools, jaundice, and possibly RUQ pain with hepatomegaly. Finally comes the convalescent phase, when jaundice/symptoms resolve and liver function tests (LFTs) return to normal.

Hep A is transmitted through the fecal-oral route by infected individuals and can be contracted through contaminated food (especially raw/undercooked) and water. Symptoms generally resolve spontaneously within 2 months. **Hep B** is blood-borne and is contracted through contact with blood and body fluids of infected individuals (often sexually transmitted). **Hep C** is also contracted through blood and body fluids. It is the most serious form of viral hepatitis (75–85% develop chronic infection), and it is the leading cause of liver transplants. Diagnose acute disease through positive serology tests: IgM anti-HAV (indicates Hep A); HBsAG and IgM anti-HBc (indicates Hep B); anti-HCV (indicates Hep C); anti-HDV (indicates Hep D); anti-HEV (indicates Hep E). Chronic Hep B: IgG anti-HBc becomes positive. Chronic Hep C: both the anti-HCV and HCV-RNA will remain positive ≥6 months after the initial infection. Treatment involves supportive care. Treat chronic Hep B with pegylated interferon (PEG-IFN), entecavir, or tenofovir. Treat chronic Hep C with PEG-IFN and ribavirin. There are currently vaccines for Hep A, B, and E. Complications of Hep B, C, and D include fibrosis, cirrhosis, hepatic failure, and liver cancer.

CIRRHOSIS

Cirrhosis is a chronic, usually irreversible disease of the **liver** where, due to injury, normal tissue is replaced with **nodules and fibrotic tissue** (scarring). It is usually caused by **chronic viral hepatitis** (usually Hep C, but also Hep B with or without Hep D) or **alcoholic liver disease**. Often signs and symptoms are not present for years, until cirrhosis is in the late stage. These include fatigue, weight loss, jaundice, easy bruising and bleeding, pruritus, ascites, spider angiomas, gynecomastia, and confusion.

Diagnose through liver function tests (LFTs), coagulation studies, serologic tests for hepatitis, imaging studies (e.g., ultrasound), and liver biopsy. Treat the underlying cause, treat complications as they arise, and offer supportive care. Lifestyle changes include discontinuing alcohol and drugs that harm the liver (e.g., NSAIDs, erythromycin, ketoconazole) and nutritional support (e.g., vitamin D, zinc, folate). Treat esophageal varices and portal hypertension with β-blockers, and a TIPS procedure (transjugular intrahepatic portosystemic shunt) may be necessary to control complications of portal hypertension. Screen patients with an ultrasound for hepatocellular carcinoma every 6 months. Assess the severity of the disease with the Child-Turcotte-Pugh and MELD (Model for End-Stage Liver Disease) scoring systems. A liver transplant may be necessary if disease is severe (in general, refer for a liver transplant evaluation if MELD score ≥15). Complications include portal hypertension, pulmonary hypertension, esophageal varices, ascites, spontaneous bacterial peritonitis, hepatorenal syndrome, hepatic encephalopathy, and liver cancer.

HEPATIC NEOPLASMS

Hepatic neoplasms may be benign or malignant, or may be metastases from other primary tumors. Examples of **benign neoplasms** include hemangiomas (most common benign tumor), focal nodular hyperplasia, and hepatocellular adenoma (usually found in women of child-bearing age using estrogen-based OCPs). Many of these are found incidentally on ultrasound and usually require no treatment. However, when hepatocellular adenomas are ≥5 cm, they are usually resected due to the increased risk of hemorrhage and malignant transformation. **Primary malignant hepatic neoplasms** include hepatocellular carcinoma (HCC), cholangiocarcinoma, and hepatoblastoma (a rare tumor in infants or children). While uncommon, HCC is the most common primary liver cancer and is usually linked to hepatitis C infection. **Liver metastases** are by far the overall most common cause of hepatic neoplasms. They usually arise from the GI tract, breast, lung, pancreas, kidney, or skin. Signs and symptoms of hepatic neoplasms vary and may be absent or vague and nonspecific. They include weight loss, anorexia, fever, nausea/vomiting, fatigue, ascites, edema, and possibly jaundice or abdominal pain. Diagnosis is through imaging studies (ultrasound, CT, MRI) and biopsy. Treatment is tailored toward the specific neoplasm; treatments range from no treatment to resection, radiation, and chemotherapy. Complications include hemorrhage, liver failure, and death.

PANCREATIC DISORDERS
PANCREATITIS (ACUTE AND CHRONIC)

Pancreatitis is inflammation of the **pancreas** and can be acute or chronic. The most common cause is **cholelithiasis** (gallstones causing duct blockage), and next is **excessive alcohol consumption** (in both binge drinkers and chronic alcoholics). Pancreatitis may occur after endoscopic retrograde cholangiopancreatography (ERCP). Certain drugs (e.g., ACE inhibitors, sulfa drugs, tetracycline), infections, cystic fibrosis, trauma, and high calcium or triglyceride blood levels can also lead to pancreatitis. Patients usually recover from the **acute** form within days or weeks. Smoking and alcohol use increase the risk of developing **chronic pancreatitis**, which forms after repeated damage to the pancreas, causing fibrosis, calcification, and ductal damage. The primary symptom of pancreatitis is constant, boring abdominal pain that radiates to the back, which may be relieved by sitting upright and leaning forward. Other symptoms include nausea/vomiting, anorexia, tachycardia, and fever. In the chronic form, diarrhea, weight loss, steatorrhea, and DM may develop later in the disease as pancreatic enzyme production declines.

Diagnose pancreatitis clinically and with serum amylase and lipase levels (3 times the normal range for acute pancreatitis; generally lower in chronic pancreatitis and therefore not as helpful). Lipase is more sensitive and specific than amylase. Imaging studies (e.g., ultrasound, CT, MRCP) are helpful if diagnosis is unclear, and to rule out cancer. Treatment of pancreatitis is mostly symptomatic. Early IV fluids (in the first 12–24 hours) and pain management are necessary. Enteral nutrition (nasogastric tube) usually begins within 48 hrs. Avoid TPN (total parenteral nutrition), which has been linked to infectious complications. Sometimes the damage to the pancreas is severe enough to warrant surgical resection of a portion of the organ. Patients with chronic pancreatitis may require pancreatic enzyme replacement. Complications include pseudocyst formation, infection, hemorrhage, necrosis, perforation, systemic inflammatory response syndrome (SIRS), and organ failure.

PANCREATIC NEOPLASMS

Pancreatic cancer is the 4th leading cause of **cancer deaths** in the US for both men and women. There are two main categories: **exocrine** (most common, >95%; most aggressive) and **endocrine neoplasms**. **Adenocarcinoma** accounts for >90 % of exocrine tumors and usually arises from the duct cells rather than the acinar cells (which produce digestive enzymes). Endocrine neoplasms, also termed **pancreatic neuroendocrine tumors (NETs)** or **islet cell tumors**, are rare, and can be functioning (produce hormones) or nonfunctioning. Both types of pancreatic cancer are usually diagnosed late in the disease process, which partially accounts for the poor prognosis (5-year survival: <5% for locally advanced disease and <2% for metastatic pancreatic cancer). Risk factors for developing pancreatic cancer include chronic pancreatitis, smoking, and obesity. Signs and symptoms include weight loss, pain radiating to the back, jaundice, dark urine, pruritus, and new-onset DM. Physical exam may show a positive Courvoisier sign: the presence of a palpable pancreatic head tumor that can feel like an enlarged gallbladder.

Diagnose with imaging studies (e.g., endoscopic ultrasound, CT, MRI, MRCP, ERCP) as well as with a biopsy. CA 19–9 can be used to track progress of the disease. Treatment depends on the stage and accessibility to the tumor(s). Options include resection (e.g., Whipple procedure, also known as pancreaticoduodenectomy), although most are unresectable at the time of the diagnosis; radiation; and chemotherapy. Complications include metastases, malabsorption, biliary obstruction, liver failure, gastric outlet obstruction, bowel obstruction, and death.

SMALL INTESTINE AND COLON DISORDERS
APPENDICITIS

Appendicitis is inflammation of the **vermiform appendix** and is a medical emergency. Appendicitis can occur due to an obstruction from lymphoid hyperplasia, impacted feces (fecalith), infection, or a foreign body (e.g., undigested seeds). Certain forms of cancer and parasites can also cause inflammation. Blockage of the appendix will lead to swelling, inflammation, infection, and possibly abscess formation. Patients may complain of periumbilical pain that gradually worsens and eventually migrates to the right lower quadrant (RLQ) at

McBurney's point. Nausea, vomiting, anorexia, fever, diarrhea, or constipation may also be present. On exam, patients have rebound tenderness and guarding, and may have a positive Rovsing's, psoas, or obturator sign. Diagnose clinically and confirm with an ultrasound or CT scan. However, do not delay surgery for an imaging study if the patient presents with classic signs and symptoms. CT is preferred for atypical presentations. The WBC count will be elevated, often 11,000–15,000/µL. Appendicitis should be immediately treated with IV antibiotics (usually third-generation cephalosporins) and surgery to prevent eventual rupture and subsequent peritonitis. Appendectomy can usually be performed laparoscopically. Complications include abscess formation, rupture, and peritonitis.

CELIAC DISEASE

Celiac disease is an immune-mediated inflammatory response due to the inability to process dietary gluten, the storage protein of wheat, rye, and barley. This causes a delayed hypersensitivity reaction (48–72 hours) that results in damage to the **small intestine villi** with villous atrophy, which causes malabsorption. There is a genetic predisposition to developing this chronic condition, which mainly affects those of Northern European descent. Signs and symptoms include abdominal pain and bloating, nausea/vomiting, diarrhea, light-colored and very foul-smelling stool, steatorrhea, constipation, fatigue, weight loss, anemia, osteoporosis, muscle weakness and paresthesias, hormonal issues, and dermatitis herpetiformis. It may present as failure to thrive in infants or children.

Diagnosis is made with immunoglobulin A anti-tissue transglutaminase antibody (IgA TTG). If patient is younger than 2 years, combine with the IgG-deamidated gliadin peptide test. Confirmation must be made through multiple biopsy sites of the duodenum. Supporting data are obtained through complete blood count (CBC), comprehensive chemistry panel, vitamin D, vitamin B12, and bone density tests. Treatment involves complete dietary restriction of gluten. Patients often improve within 1–2 weeks of being on a gluten-free diet. Correct vitamin deficiencies. Refer patients to a dietician, and regular follow-ups are recommended for monitoring symptoms. Complications include refractory disease, collagenous sprue, and intestinal lymphomas.

DIVERTICULAR DISEASE

Diverticula are outpouchings in the **intestine** that commonly develop during the aging process. True diverticula (e.g., Meckel diverticula) involve all layers of the GI tract: the mucosa, submucosa, muscularis propria, and serosa/adventitia. However, **colonic diverticula**, which will be discussed here, are pseudo-diverticula and only involve the **mucosal and submucosal layers**. They can occur anywhere along the intestinal tract, but are most common in the sigmoid colon. **Diverticulosis** is asymptomatic diverticula. **Diverticulitis** involves inflammation of the diverticula and possibly occurs when digestive matter becomes trapped within these outpouchings, leading to swelling and possible infection. Diverticula can rupture and bleed if the condition becomes severe. Patients will generally complain of left lower quadrant abdominal pain with changes in bowel habits. Bloating, gas, constipation, diarrhea, nausea/vomiting, and fever may also be present.

Diagnose clinically and confirm with a CT scan. Diverticulitis, if uncomplicated and mild, is generally treated with a clear-liquid diet and possibly broad-spectrum oral antibiotics for 7–10 days (e.g., ciprofloxacin with metronidazole; trimethoprim/sulfamethoxazole with metronidazole; Augmentin; or moxifloxacin). After symptoms improve in 48–72 hours, advance diet as tolerated. If severe or complicated diverticulitis, admit, keep NPO, and treat with IV fluids and IV antibiotics. Diverticulitis usually resolves without surgery, but resection of the affected portion of the intestine may be necessary in severe cases. Avoidance of small particulate matter in the diet, such as foods with seeds (sesame seeds, berry seeds, etc.) and popcorn, is no longer recommended. Complications of diverticular disease include GI bleeding, perforation, abscess or fistula formation, and peritonitis.

IRRITABLE BOWEL SYNDROME

Irritable bowel syndrome (**IBS**) is a functional **GI disorder** causing abdominal pain, altered stool consistency, and/or altered bowel habits. It is very common and may affect up to 20% of Americans. The cause is unknown, but it usually occurs in response to stressors, either psychological or physical, and can be severe enough to be debilitating. Chronic fatigue, dyspepsia, depression, and fibromyalgia are common comorbidities. Patients may complain of intermittent periods of bloating, painful gas, postprandial urgency, mucorrhea, diarrhea, and constipation. Some patients may have predominantly diarrhea (IBS-D) or constipation (IBS-C), while others alternate between the two (IBS-M, "mixed"). A pattern of symptoms may be discernible after people eat certain foods or during periods of stress.

IBS used to be considered a diagnosis of exclusion. Diagnosis is made clinically following the Rome IV criteria: abdominal pain 1 day/week in the last 3 months with 2 or more of the following: related to defecation, associated with change in stool frequency, or associated with change in stool form. Treatment is directed at the symptom. Fiber supplements may help with constipation and diarrhea. Typically, a normal diet may be followed. However, patients may benefit from avoiding foods that lead to bloating (e.g., legumes, cabbage) and avoiding possible triggers like lactose or gluten. Some medications used in IBS include anticholinergics, antispasmodics, antidiarrheals, prokinetics, TCAs, and IBS agents (e.g., lubiprostone, linaclotide). Complications include interference with daily activities and work, hemorrhoids, and malnutrition.

CROHN'S DISEASE

Crohn's disease is a **chronic inflammatory bowel disease** that can affect **any** portion of the digestive tract, from the mouth to the anus. It causes **transmural inflammation** in the mucosal lining of the GI tract, and patients usually experience periods of remission. Crohn's disease is usually diagnosed during the teens or 20s, and there is no cure. The cause is not known, but it is proposed to be due to a bacterial infection, an autoimmune response, environmental factors like smoking, and predisposing genetic factors. Patients with Crohn's disease will complain of abdominal pain and chronic diarrhea with or without blood, fever, a poor appetite, and weight loss. Because Crohn's disease can occur at any point in the digestive tract, symptoms may be more focused on a particular area.

Diagnose through clinical assessment, endoscopy/colonoscopy with biopsy, imaging studies (e.g., CT), and inflammatory markers like CRP and ESR. During endoscopy, "skip" lesions may be noted, as well as granulomas (pathognomonic) on biopsy. Treatment is symptomatic, with the goal being to reduce inflammation within the digestive tract. This can be accomplished with anti-inflammatory drugs (e.g., mesalamine, which is a 5-ASA or aminosalicylate), steroids, antibiotics (e.g., metronidazole, ciprofloxacin), immunomodulators (e.g., methotrexate), and biologics (e.g., infliximab). Antidiarrheals like loperamide are useful, but should be avoided in active colitis due to an increased risk of developing toxic megacolon. Surgery is usually necessary at some point in the course of the disease to treat complications. Complications include anemia, abscesses, fistulas, increased risk of cancer, bowel obstruction, and toxic megacolon.

ULCERATIVE COLITIS

Ulcerative colitis (**UC**) is a **chronic inflammatory bowel disease** that **only** affects the **mucous membranes** lining the rectum and large intestine, causing bloody diarrhea. It begins distally, typically in the rectum, and moves proximally in a continuous pattern with a clearly defined margin. There are periods of flare-ups and remission. The etiology of UC is not understood, but it is thought to be due to multiple factors, including environmental, genetic, and immune-mediated ones. Stress, NSAID use, and drinking milk may exacerbate or trigger UC. Unlike with Crohn's disease, cigarette smoking is actually protective in UC. Patients complain of abdominal pain and cramps with bloody diarrhea, sometimes with mucus/pus, and tenesmus. In severe cases, fever, malaise, anorexia, and weight loss may be present. UC may have extraintestinal signs and symptoms that include uveitis, arthralgias, and aphthous ulcers.

Diagnosis is made with sigmoidoscopy or colonoscopy with biopsy. However, caution should be taken in severe disease due to the risk of perforation from the endoscopy. Test stool for infectious cause. Treat with 5-ASA anti-inflammatory drugs (e.g., sulfasalazine, mesalamine) and steroids. 5-ASAs should be continued after steroids are tapered. There are immunosuppressants (e.g., cyclosporine, tacrolimus) and biologics (e.g., infliximab, adalimumab) available that may help if patients are steroid-resistant or have severe disease. Antidiarrheals and pain relievers may also be helpful. If mucosal damage is severe, hospitalization and surgery

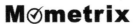

may be necessary to resect the damaged portion of the large intestine. Complications include anemia, perforation, colon cancer, ankylosing spondylitis, and toxic megacolon.

LACTOSE INTOLERANCE

Lactose intolerance develops in those individuals who are lacking in the enzyme **lactase**, which breaks down the disaccharide **sugar** in milk. **Primary lactose intolerance** is an acquired lactase deficiency that occurs after the infant is weaned, and occurs in 75% of the world's population. It is especially high in the Asian, Hispanic, Native American, African American, and African populations, reaching up to 98% in Southeast Asians. **Secondary deficiencies** occur due to damage to the mucosa of the small intestine and are common after viral gastroenteritis. Patients will regain lactase activity as the mucosa heals. Patients may complain of bloating, gas, abdominal pain, nausea, and cramping diarrhea, usually within 30 minutes of consuming dairy.

Diagnosis of true lactose intolerance can be accomplished several different ways, but the hydrogen breath test is typically used. Hydrogen levels are measured in the breath at various intervals before and after patients are given a lactose-rich drink. These should remain low, but will become elevated if lactose intolerant. Another test is the lactose tolerance test, which is rarely used. After fasting overnight, a baseline glucose level is measured, then the patient is given a dairy-rich drink, and blood glucose levels are measured over two hours. If glucose levels remain low, there is a deficiency in lactase. Treatment is with dietary changes to avoid lactose-rich foods and beverages. Typically, yogurt and cheeses are tolerated better, and most patients may ingest up to 375 mL of lactose milk without symptoms. Lactose-free milk, as well as OTC lactase preparations, are available. Calcium supplementation is usually necessary. The primary possible complication is osteopenia.

> **Review Video: Lactose Intolerance**
> Visit mometrix.com/academy and enter code: 672651

INTUSSUSCEPTION

Intussusception is a **telescoping of the intestine** inside an adjacent portion of intestine, causing **bowel obstruction** and possible **ischemia**. It usually occurs in children between 6 months and 3 years, affects boys more often, and is fatal in 2–5 days if untreated. This is rare in adults, usually involves the colon, and is typically due to cancer. There may be a "lead point" or trigger found (e.g., Meckel diverticulum, polyp, lymphoid hyperplasia), usually in adults and older children, that provides an explanation for the intussusception point. In 1998, the rotavirus vaccine RotaShield was introduced and was linked to an increased risk of intussusception. It was promptly removed from the market in 1999, and newer vaccines (RotaTeq and Rotarix) since released have not been linked with intussusception. Symptoms include vomiting, fever, intense colicky pain that may later become constant, and lethargy. Patients may have diarrhea with "currant jelly" stools because of the frank blood that is present, but this is a late finding. On exam, there may be a palpable abdominal mass.

Diagnosis is made with ultrasound; either a target (donut) sign or pseudokidney sign may be noted. Treatment is usually successful with a barium or air enema. This forces the bowel to straighten and slides the telescoped portion of the bowel back to normal. Avoid enemas if a perforation is suspected. If there is damaged or dead tissue, surgery is necessary to resect the ischemic or dead portion of bowel. A laparotomy is usually necessary in adults due to the presence of a lead point. Complications include dehydration, bleeding, infection, gangrene, perforation, shock, and death.

TOXIC MEGACOLON

Toxic megacolon is an acute, transmural **inflammation of the colonic mucosa** that causes dysfunction and severe, nonobstructive dilatation that can be life-threatening. This medical emergency usually occurs in patients who suffer from **inflammatory bowel disease (IBD)**, but may also be seen in Hirschsprung disease, infections, and pseudomembranous colitis due to antibiotic use. Patients may complain of abdominal distension, abdominal pain, and diarrhea, usually have a fever, and may appear dehydrated. Toxic megacolon can progress to the development of symptoms of shock (e.g., hypotension, tachycardia, tachypnea, altered mental status).

Diagnosis is made clinically and with abdominal x-rays that show the dilated colon (>6 cm). This condition can lead to shock and death, so prompt treatment is necessary. WBCs may be elevated with a left shift, the patient may be anemic, and potassium may be decreased if patients are dehydrated. The colon is rested for 24 hours along with decompression (e.g., nasogastric tube, rolling techniques) to try to reduce the distension. If this is not effective, surgery is usually performed to resect the affected section of the colon. Patients should be rehydrated with IV fluids, and electrolyte imbalances should be corrected. IV steroids are given to reduce inflammation within the colon, along with IV antibiotics. Complications include perforation, sepsis, and death.

BOWEL OBSTRUCTION

A bowel obstruction can be caused by **improper function of the intestines** or by a **mechanical obstruction** (something is blocking the way). Improper functioning of the bowel is not caused by a mechanical obstruction, but is due to halted peristalsis, and is referred to as an *ileus* or *paralytic ileus*. It can be due to medications, infection, ischemia, injury, or manipulation during surgery. Mechanical obstructions are divided into **small (SBO)** (which is more common) or **large bowel obstructions (LBO)** and may be partial or complete. Mechanical obstruction of the bowel can occur from tumors, adhesions, volvulus, hernias, foreign objects, or impacted stool. With SBO, patients may complain of abdominal pain and cramping in the absence of regular bowel movements or gas (especially if a complete obstruction). Patients may have vomiting and a full, bloated feeling. With a complete obstruction, a severe form of constipation (obstipation) ensues. On exam, bowel sounds may be high-pitched or tingling in nature early on, but eventually there may be absent bowel sounds. LBOs typically have milder symptoms that progress slower, but with marked abdominal distension. An ileus has diminished bowel sounds and usually less abdominal cramping.

Diagnose with plain x-rays; further studies with CT may be necessary. CTs are the imaging choice for LBOs. Treatment involves bowel rest, nasogastric tube suction to decompress the gut, IV fluids, antiemetics, and antibiotics (that cover gram-negative and anaerobic organisms). If the condition is severe (e.g., signs of ischemia/strangulation/volvulus) or does not improve with conservative management, surgery is necessary. Surgery should not be delayed if there is a complete obstruction. Complications include perforation, peritonitis, sepsis, bowel infarction, gangrene, and death.

POLYPS AND COLORECTAL CANCER

Colonic polyps are slow-growing growths on the **colonic mucosa** that are common and increase with age. They have the potential for **malignant transformation** (<1%), and therefore, patients should be screened for colon cancer starting at the age of 50 and repeated every 10 years. The process of malignant transformation takes approximately 10 years, so this is a very preventable condition. **Colorectal cancer** is the second leading cause of **cancer death** in the US. It usually arises from an **adenomatous polyp**. Risk factors for colorectal cancer include eating processed or red meats, family history, sedentary lifestyle, obesity, and smoking/alcohol use. Patients with **familial adenomatous polyposis (FAP)** have hundreds of polyps, resulting in cancer by the age of 40, so a colectomy is performed when diagnosed. **Lynch syndrome** or **hereditary nonpolyposis colorectal cancer (HNPCC)** results in colorectal cancer by the mid-40s; it is also linked with other cancers, like uterine and ovarian. Patients with a family history of colon cancer must be screened earlier (10 years before the age of the patient's first-degree relative's diagnosis).

There are typically no signs or symptoms of polyps or cancer until the neoplasm becomes large. However, there may be rectal bleeding, pain, cramps, changes in bowel habits, or signs of obstruction if the polyp or mass is large. Diagnosis is made with colonoscopy and biopsy, and further investigation with a CT as necessary. Also test for blood using a fecal occult blood test or fecal immunochemical test. Treat polyps by removal, and treat cancer with resection, radiation, and/or chemotherapy. Colorectal cancer stages are as follows. Stage 0: carcinoma in situ; stage I: local involvement to the submucosal layer; stage II: local involvement to the muscularis propria; stage III: lymph node or regional involvement; stage IV: distant metastases. Monitor progress with CEA levels. Complications of colorectal cancer include bleeding, metastases, and death.

RECTAL/ANAL DISEASES

ANORECTAL ABSCESS AND FISTULA

An anorectal abscess, or localized infection in the **anal or rectal areas**, can have several causes. An **anal fissure** can become infected or an **anal gland** can become blocked, leading to abscess formation. Diverticulitis, Crohn's disease, pelvic inflammatory disease, and anal intercourse can place a patient at risk for developing an anorectal abscess. These can be perianal (most common), ischiorectal, intersphincteric, or supralevator (least common) abscesses. An anorectal abscess will cause patients significant pain with the development of an indurated, inflamed area, and may feel like a hard, hot lump. Patients may have very painful bowel movements and may develop constipation because of the fear of having a bowel movement. If the abscess ruptures, pus may be discharged through the rectum. Diagnosis is made per clinical assessment/digital exam. A CT may be necessary if the lesion is located deep or high, toward the intestines. Treat with incision and drainage (I&D) and pack with iodoform gauze (remove after 24 hours). Sitz baths can help with some of the inflammation, and prescribe antibiotics if the patient is febrile or immunocompromised, or if the infection is severe. If the abscess is deep or extensive, surgery may be necessary.

Anorectal fistulas are tracts that usually run between the **anus and the superficial skin**. This is a common complication of anorectal abscesses and can also occur due to Crohn's disease, diverticulitis, and trauma. There is usually a history of recurrent abscesses followed by complaints of purulent discharge and sometimes pain. Diagnose clinically and with sigmoidoscopy. Treat with surgery. The main complication is fecal incontinence.

ANAL FISSURE

An anal fissure is a small, longitudinal tear in the **epithelial tissue** surrounding the **anal sphincter**. It is caused by excessive stretching of the anal sphincter, as with a large bowel movement. Patients will complain of pain at the anus, especially with bowel movements, usually with a history of constipation, and they may have noticed bright red blood in their stool or on toilet paper following a bowel movement. This can be extremely painful for patients, so a gentle perianal exam should be used to visualize and diagnose. The fissures are usually located in the midline, and most are posterior. Anal fissures usually resolve with supportive treatment. If the fissures are very painful, warm sitz baths may be soothing, as well as a topical anesthetic, which is helpful if the pain is preventing patients from having a bowel movement. To prevent recurrence, stool softeners and a diet high in fiber and fluids should be recommended to keep bowel movements regular and prevent constipation. Chronic anal fissures may be treated with nitroglycerine ointment, topical calcium channel blockers, or botulinum toxin injections. Occasionally surgery (lateral internal sphincterotomy) is necessary to correct the fissure. Complications include bleeding, infection, chronic anal fissures, fistulas, and fecal incontinence.

PILONIDAL DISEASE

A pilonidal disease refers to either a hair-containing cyst, an acute abscess, or a chronic sinus that forms at the base of the **coccyx** that can become infected. It occurs at the superior end of the cleft between the buttocks, at the **sacrococcygeal area**. Pilonidal disease occurs more often in men than women. It is believed to occur due to **ingrown hair** in the region. The pilonidal cyst may form into a typical abscess with a red, indurated area at the base of the spine. Patients may or may not have a fever, but the abscess will be painful. If it opens, pus will drain from the abscess. Diagnosis is made per clinical assessment. No treatment is necessary if it is asymptomatic or there are no signs of infection. If an acute abscess does develop, treat with an incision and drainage (I&D) and pack with gauze, which should be removed in 24–48 hours. Once removed, start warm sitz baths bid to tid. Antibiotics are typically ineffective. Surgical resection may be necessary if there is chronic disease or chronic sinus tracts. Complications include abscess recurrence and chronic sinus tracts; rarely, squamous cell carcinoma has been reported in sinus tracts.

HEMORRHOIDS

Hemorrhoids occur when the **vessels surrounding the anus and rectum** become engorged and swollen. Hemorrhoids commonly occur with excessive straining with a bowel movement (e.g., when constipated), during pregnancy, and with prolonged sitting on the toilet, due to the increased pressure applied to the pelvic floor. They can also occur as a result of anal intercourse, chronic diarrhea, obesity, and as part of the aging process. Hemorrhoids can be internal or external. **Internal hemorrhoids**, which originate above the dentate/pectinate line, are not painful, can bleed, can produce mucus, and will cause patients to have bright red blood on the toilet paper after a bowel movement. Internal hemorrhoids may prolapse, causing itching and pain due to muscle spasms in the sphincter. Internal hemorrhoids are classified as follows. **Grade I**: in anal canal; **Grade II**: protrudes past anal verge with straining but reduces spontaneously; **Grade III**: protrudes past anal verge with straining but requires manual reduction; **Grade IV**: chronically prolapsed. **External hemorrhoids** are painful, may thrombose, and cause hygiene issues.

Diagnosis is made per clinical exam and with anoscopy or sigmoidoscopy to evaluate bleeding. Most hemorrhoids will resolve on their own or with conservative, symptomatic treatment. Stool softeners are recommended. OTC topical ointments, creams, and suppositories are available to help relieve the swelling and pain (e.g., hydrocortisone). Sitz baths and witch hazel pads can also help. In-office procedures include rubber band ligation (most common), infrared coagulation, and sclerotherapy. If severe or recurrent, surgery may be necessary to remove the hemorrhoids. Complications include infection, anemia, thrombosis, and strangulated hemorrhoids.

HERNIAS

A hernia is a protrusion of an organ through the **muscle or fascia** that usually contains it. There are several types. **Hiatal hernias** occur when the upper segment of the **stomach** protrudes through the diaphragm. **Ventral hernias** can occur anywhere there is a weakened area in the **abdominal wall** (e.g., epigastric, primary abdominal, incisional); they cause a section of bowel to protrude through the opening. These are most commonly due to **incisional hernias**, which occur at the site of an **abdominal surgical incision** (more common if incision is vertical). **Spigelian hernias** are rare and occur on the outer edges of the **rectus abdominis muscle**. **Umbilical hernias** occur at the **umbilicus** due to a weakened area of the abdominal fascia, causing the bowel to protrude through the umbilical opening. **Inguinal hernias** are the most common hernia overall; they are more common in males, and they occur through a weakened portion of the **lower abdominal wall**. They can be direct (weakness in the posterior wall of the inguinal canal/Hesselbach triangle) or indirect (more common; pass through the internal inguinal ring and into the inguinal canal). **Femoral hernias** are more common in women; they occur below the **inguinal ligament** and bulge into the thigh. Hernias are diagnosed clinically and are treated surgically. Hiatal hernias may require a Nissen fundoplication procedure, in which the lower esophagus is reinforced. Other hernias are repaired by surgical closure, sometimes using a mesh material at the site of the weakened area to strengthen the wall. Complications include bowel obstruction, incarceration, and strangulation.

VITAMIN/NUTRITIONAL DEFICIENCIES
THIAMINE (VITAMIN B1) AND THIAMINE DEFICIENCY

Thiamin or thiamine (vitamin B1) is a water-soluble vitamin that, like all B vitamins, is used in the **metabolism** of food into usable energy. Thiamine is especially important in carbohydrate metabolism and proper nerve function, and is essential to pyruvate metabolism. **Beriberi** is a condition caused by thiamine deficiency that causes wasting, peripheral neuropathy, and (rarely) heart issues like CHF. Beriberi can be divided into **dry beriberi**, which refers to the nervous system effects, or **wet beriberi**, which refers to the cardiovascular effects of thiamine deficiency. **Wernicke-Korsakoff syndrome** is another disease caused by thiamine deficiency, and is characterized by a classic presentation of confusion, ataxia, and horizontal nystagmus. It is usually seen in chronic alcoholics, but may also appear in extreme malnutrition and after bariatric surgery. With proper treatment, most conditions due to thiamine deficiency are reversible until the late findings of Korsakoff syndrome (e.g., memory loss). Treat with parenteral thiamine until symptoms are gone. Maintaining proper levels of thiamine involves eating thiamine-rich foods, including sunflower seeds, beans, oats, meat (e.g., pork), green peas, and potatoes. Thiamine is metabolized in the liver and excreted in the urine. There are no known cases of thiamine toxicity.

RIBOFLAVIN (VITAMIN B2) AND RIBOFLAVIN DEFICIENCY

Riboflavin, or vitamin B2, is a water-soluble vitamin that acts as a **coenzyme** that is necessary for normal **cell growth, development, and energy production**. Riboflavin also helps in red blood cell production and maintaining healthy mucous membranes. A primary deficiency in riboflavin may be due to malnutrition, though this is rare in industrialized countries. It can also be due to a secondary deficiency caused by chronic diarrhea or a malabsorption syndrome that prevents riboflavin from being absorbed. Riboflavin and thiamine deficiencies are usually seen together. Symptoms of riboflavin deficiency include swelling of the mucous membranes, sore throat, and cracks on the lips or corners of the mouth (angular stomatitis or cheilitis). Seborrheic dermatitis may develop without adequate levels of riboflavin, as can certain types of anemia. Treat with riboflavin replacement through supplements and eating beef (especially high in beef liver), fortified cereals and breads, yogurt, cheese, eggs, and spinach, and drinking milk. If there is an underlying malabsorption disorder causing the deficiency, this should be treated. Riboflavin is metabolized in the liver and excreted in the urine. There are no known cases of riboflavin toxicity.

NIACIN (VITAMIN B3) AND NIACIN DEFICIENCY

Niacin, or vitamin B3, is a water-soluble vitamin that is essential for **cell function and cell metabolism**. Dietary tryptophan can be metabolized to niacin. A niacin deficiency can lead to a condition called **pellagra**. This can occur with malnutrition, due to a lack of niacin in the diet (e.g., diet high in maize), because of a malabsorption syndrome, or due to certain medications (e.g., some TB medications). The "4 D's" can occur with advanced pellagra and usually appear in this order:

- Diarrhea
- Dermatitis
- Dementia
- Death

Patients may experience weakness; may have a typically symmetric, erythematous rash in sun-exposed areas; and may be irritable or short-tempered before dementia becomes evident. Treatment involves replacing the niacin orally and eating foods rich in niacin and tryptophan (e.g., turkey, tuna, chicken, beef, peanuts, brewer's yeast). Correct malabsorption issues (e.g., alcoholism). Carcinoid tumors or gastric tumors may cause obstruction that prevents absorption of niacin, and should be surgically removed if possible. Niacin is metabolized and stored in the liver and excreted in the urine. Niacin toxicity can occur (e.g., flushing, pruritus, nausea/vomiting, hepatotoxicity).

VITAMIN B6 AND B6 DEFICIENCY

Vitamin B6 is a water-soluble vitamin that is important in **protein metabolism, hemoglobin synthesis, antibody synthesis, and proper nerve function**. A deficiency can be caused by a primary deficiency (inadequate intake) or a secondary deficiency (malabsorption, alcoholism, drugs that inactivate pyridoxine). A B6 deficiency results in peripheral neuropathy, anemia, seborrheic dermatitis, cheilosis, glossitis, a pellagra-like syndrome (characterized by diarrhea, dermatitis, and dementia), and possibly seizures. Treatment involves supplements and eating B6-rich foods, including liver, meat, fish, seeds, chickpeas, and bananas. Correct malabsorption issues and give patients on isoniazid concomitant pyridoxine. Vitamin B6 is metabolized and mostly stored in the liver (also stored in muscle and brain) and excreted in the urine. Megadoses can lead to B6 toxicity, which manifests as peripheral neuropathy, impaired vibratory sensation, impaired proprioception (sense of your body's position), and ataxia.

VITAMIN B12 AND B12 DEFICIENCY

Vitamin B12, or cobalamin, is a water-soluble vitamin that is important for **DNA synthesis, RBC production, proper nerve function, and cell metabolism**. Vitamin B12 works with folate in several chemical processes, including RBC production and maturation. Vitamin B12, like folate, must be ingested, since it cannot be produced by the body. It is only found in animal products; therefore, strict vegans are at an increased risk of a primary B12 deficiency. Vitamin B12 deficiency may also be caused by impaired absorption due to age, decreased gastric acid production, lack of intrinsic factor (i.e., pernicious anemia—often seen in the elderly), or intestinal disorders. Vitamin B12 deficiency can result in megaloblastic anemia, peripheral neuropathy, weight loss, glossitis, ataxia, and confusion or dementia. Diagnose with CBC with blood smear (hypersegmented neutrophils) and serum vitamin B12 and folate levels; the Schilling test (which tests for intrinsic factor) is not used as often as it once was. Treat with oral or IM vitamin B12, depending on the severity of the deficiency. Foods rich in vitamin B12 include clams, fish, meat, eggs, milk, and fortified cereals. Vitamin B12 is stored in the liver in large quantities and excreted in the urine. There appears to be no risk of toxicity.

> **Review Video: Pernicious Anemia**
> Visit mometrix.com/academy and enter code: 353419

FOLATE (FOLIC ACID) AND FOLATE DEFICIENCY

Folate, or vitamin B9, is a water-soluble vitamin that is needed for **DNA synthesis, mitosis, RBC production, and proper fetal development**. This vitamin cannot be synthesized by the body, so it must be ingested through foods and supplements. Folate supplements are especially important in pregnancy for prevention of neural tube defects. It is recommended to take folic acid 600–800 µg/day while pregnant and 500–800 µg/day while breastfeeding. Folate supplements must be accompanied by vitamin B12 supplements. This is because both folate and B12 deficiencies result in a megaloblastic anemia. Therefore, if a patient is treated with folate, the anemia will appear to be correcting while the nerve damage caused by a concomitant vitamin B12 deficiency continues. This can result in permanent nerve damage. Folate deficiency can be due to inadequate intake, increased age, malabsorption (e.g., chronic alcohol use, IBD), and certain medications (e.g., antacids, methotrexate). Folate deficiency can result in megaloblastic anemia, glossitis, diarrhea, confusion, and neural tube defects in pregnancy.

Diagnose with a CBC with blood smear, with serum folate or RBC folate levels, and serum vitamin B12 levels. Treat with oral folate and concomitant vitamin B12 if deficient. Foods rich in folate include dark green leafy vegetables, fruit, organ meats, and dairy products. Unlike vitamin B12, folate is not stored in large amounts in the body. Folate is metabolized in the liver and excreted in the urine. There appears to be no risk of toxicity.

VITAMIN A (RETINOL) AND VITAMIN A DEFICIENCY

Vitamin A is a fat-soluble vitamin that is an **antioxidant**, is helpful in **boosting the immune system, maintains epithelial and bone/teeth integrity, keeps the eyes healthy, and is required for night/low-light vision**. The antioxidant effects of vitamin A (β-carotene) may help prevent some forms of cancer. Vitamin A comes from animal sources (retinol, or preformed vitamin A) and vegetable sources (carotenoids; β-carotene converts to vitamin A). A primary vitamin A deficiency can be due to malnutrition, but this is rare in developed countries. Secondary vitamin A deficiency can be due to malabsorption, including malabsorption of fats (which decreases the absorption of vitamin A), impaired vitamin A transport, or liver disease. Deficiency can lead to diarrhea, increased infections, respiratory disorders, dry/brittle hair and nails, decreased growth rate, night blindness, and eventually complete blindness. **Xerophthalmia**, or pathologic dry eyes, leads to keratinization, Bitot spots, and eventually corneal ulcerations and blindness. Although rare in the US, this blindness is especially seen in malnourished children in developing countries.

Deficiency is diagnosed clinically, and serum retinol levels can be measured. Treat by giving supplements and eating foods rich in vitamin A (e.g., liver, fish oils, egg yolk, sweet potatoes, dark leafy greens like spinach, and carrots). Treat malabsorption disorders if possible. Vitamin A is stored in the liver (typical reserves last about 1 year) and metabolized in the cell, and toxicity can develop. Toxicity causes birth defects, nausea/vomiting, headache, increased intracranial pressure (ICP), dry/rough skin, and liver damage. **Carotenemia**, or **carotenoderma**, is harmless and causes yellowing of the skin due to increased ingestion of β-carotene.

VITAMIN C AND VITAMIN C DEFICIENCY

Vitamin C, or **ascorbic acid**, is a water-soluble vitamin that acts as an **antioxidant** and is vital for **immune health, wound healing, collagen formation, and proper function of blood vessels, and it aids in the**

absorption of iron in the intestines. Vitamin C must be ingested, since the body cannot manufacture it. Those at an increased risk of a vitamin C deficiency include alcoholics, smokers, the elderly, and those with poor nutrition. A deficiency in vitamin C causes an illness known as **scurvy**. Historically, this was seen in those who were at sea for extended periods of time and did not have access to foods rich in vitamin C. Scurvy causes weakness, bruising, bleeding gums/gingivitis, hemorrhages, hair and tooth loss, arthralgias, rash (e.g., perifollicular hyperkeratosis/perifollicular hemorrhage), and poor wound healing. In children, this can appear as impaired bone growth and growth delay. Treatment of a vitamin C deficiency requires supplementation and dietary changes that increase the consumption of foods rich in vitamin C, such as citrus fruit, strawberries, potatoes, broccoli, and red/green peppers. Vitamin C is metabolized in the liver and excreted in the urine, and is not thought to be toxic, but may cause diarrhea if taken in high doses.

VITAMIN D AND VITAMIN D DEFICIENCY

Vitamin D is a fat-soluble vitamin that plays a vital role in **calcium absorption** into bones to provide healthy, strong **teeth and bones**. Vitamin D is known as the "sunshine vitamin"; it is produced within the skin after exposure to sunlight, and 5–30 minutes/day (depending on skin type, location, and time of the year) of sun exposure can help increase a person's vitamin D level. It then undergoes two hydroxylations in the liver and kidney to become the hormone, 1α,25-dihydroxyvitamin D (calcitriol), which is the biologically active form of vitamin D. A deficiency of vitamin D leads to a condition called rickets in children and osteomalacia in adults. **Rickets** will produce a bowing of the legs of children because of bone softening due to decreased bone mineralization. Bone growth will also be stifled without vitamin D. **Osteomalacia** in adults causes periosteal bone pain, muscle aches, weakness, and decreased bone mineralization or "soft bones," which places these individuals at higher risk of compression fractures.

Diagnose with serum 25(OH)D levels, which will be low (while PTH levels may be elevated), and radiographs. Treat with vitamin D supplements (e.g., ergocalciferol) and by increasing intake of dairy products, fortified foods, and saltwater fish. Correct any concurrent calcium or phosphate deficiencies. Vitamin D is stored in the liver and adipose tissue and metabolized in the liver and kidney. Toxicity can occur from megadoses of supplements. Toxicity results in hypercalcemia, causing bone pain, nausea/vomiting, poor appetite, constipation or diarrhea, kidney stones, and kidney failure.

VITAMIN E AND VITAMIN E DEFICIENCY

Vitamin E is a fat-soluble vitamin that acts as a vital **antioxidant**, which is important for protecting **lipids**, in the cell membrane and throughout the body, from **free radicals**. It is also important for immune function, nerve function, metabolic processes, RBC formation, and blood vessel health. There are 8 isoforms, but only α-**tocopherol**, which is the body's preference, can correct vitamin E deficiency. A deficiency can be due to a primary lack in the diet or a secondary cause (e.g., fat malabsorption). Vitamin E deficiency results in hemolytic anemia, muscle weakness/pain, ataxia, and nystagmus. The late effects of severe deficiency can result in cardiac arrhythmias, blindness, and dementia. Diagnose with a serum α-tocopherol level. Treat with vitamin E supplements (tocopherol) and by eating foods high in vitamin E, like vegetable oils, seeds, nuts, spinach, broccoli, and fortified foods. Vitamin E is stored in adipose tissue and metabolized in the liver, and toxicity can develop. Toxicity results in weakness, headache, nausea, abdominal cramps, and diarrhea, and it can cause blood clotting issues (easy bruising/bleeding). Vitamin E interacts with anticoagulant/antiplatelet medications, and it interferes with the action of vitamin K, and therefore can increase the risk of bleeding.

VITAMIN K AND VITAMIN K DEFICIENCY

Vitamin K is a fat-soluble vitamin that acts as a coenzyme and plays a vital role in the **clotting cascade** to prevent excessive bleeding. It is involved in the formation of factors II (prothrombin), VII, IX, and X. It also helps maintain bone and tissue health. Vitamin K comes in three forms: **Vitamin K1** (from plants), **Vitamin K2** (produced by bacteria in the intestines), and **Vitamin K3** (synthetic). A deficiency in vitamin K is very rare, but it can be seen in those individuals with a malabsorption syndrome that prevents the absorption of fats from the GI tract, leading to a decreased amount of vitamin K absorbed from foods. The blood-thinning drug warfarin (Coumadin) blocks the function of vitamin K in the clotting cascade, which promotes bleeding and an increased clotting time.

For treatment, a vitamin K deficiency can be reversed with injectable vitamin K1 (preferred method is SC or IM; oral also available). Also, this is given to infants IM shortly after birth (within 6 hours) to help prevent excessive bleeding. Diet is the main source of vitamin K, and it is found in abundant supply in green, leafy vegetables. Malabsorption issues that prevent absorption of fats from the GI tract should be treated, if possible. Vitamin K has low stores in the body, and is metabolized in the liver and excreted in the feces and urine. Toxicity can occur with vitamin K3. This causes jaundice in newborns and hemolytic anemia, and therefore is no longer used to treat vitamin K deficiencies.

METABOLIC DISORDERS

PHENYLKETONURIA

Phenylketonuria, or **PKU**, is a disorder in which an infant is not able to digest **phenylalanine**, a protein found in most foods. This causes phenylalanine to accumulate in the bloodstream and leads to severe brain damage and intellectual disabilities. Screening is done nationwide at birth to identify infants suffering from this condition. Patients who do have PKU may have lighter skin and hair because phenylalanine helps to produce melanin in the body. These children will be developmentally delayed and show signs of intellectual disabilities. They are more likely to suffer from a seizure disorder, jerky movements, and hyperactivity. PKU is diagnosed by an elevated serum phenylalanine, or by identifying PAH mutations by molecular analysis for prenatal diagnosis. PKU can be treated, but early identification is necessary. All children should be tested at birth for the presence of PKU. If PKU is diagnosed, a diet very low in phenylalanine should be strictly followed. If this is adhered to, intellectual disabilities can be mild and there may be minimal impairment in function. If this diet is not closely followed, intellectual disabilities will result. Pegvaliase is a new option for adults and is the first enzyme substitute to be released by the FDA (in 2018).

Genitourinary System

GENITOURINARY TRACT DISORDERS

NEPHROLITHIASIS AND UROLITHIASIS

Nephrolithiasis (kidney stones or calculi) and urolithiasis (calculi anywhere in the urinary tract) are common in the US. There are 4 main types: **calcium** (~75%; calcium oxalate and calcium phosphate), **struvite** (15%; infection), **uric acid** (6%), and **cystine** (~2%) stones. Nephrolithiasis affects men more often than women, and there is a genetic predisposition to forming stones. However, struvite stones (due to UTI) affect women more often than men. Other risk factors include a high-salt or high-protein diet, hypercalciuria, hyperparathyroidism, renal tubular acidosis, and cystinuria. Symptoms may include intense, sometimes radiating, intermittent flank pain causing the patient to constantly move around; diaphoresis; nausea/vomiting; urinary urgency/frequency; and hematuria.

Diagnosis is made clinically and with a noncontrast helical CT. A UA (urinalysis) with culture, urine creatinine, and stone identification is also helpful. Usually stones <5 mm pass on their own and may be treated with rehydration, analgesics, and medical expulsive therapy like α-receptor blockers (e.g., tamsulosin). If not able to pass in 4–6 weeks or with stones ≥10 mm (that cannot pass on their own), removal is required using various techniques (e.g., extracorporeal shockwave lithotripsy, ureteroscopy, percutaneous nephrostolithotomy). Stents may be placed in the ureter to help relieve symptoms while awaiting surgery. Treat infections with appropriate antibiotics, and alkalinizing the urine (e.g., with potassium citrate) can help dissolve uric acid or cystine stones. Complications of nephrolithiasis include UTI, scarring and stenosis of ureter, renal outflow obstruction, infective hydronephrosis, and loss of renal function.

BENIGN PROSTATIC HYPERPLASIA

Benign prostatic hyperplasia (**BPH**) is a benign enlargement of the **prostate gland**. Incidence increases with age, and there is no definite known cause; however, it seems to be familial and related to hormone changes. The prostate gland is located at the base of the bladder, surrounds the urethra, and is responsible for producing seminal fluid. Whenever there is a change in the size of the prostate gland, a complete assessment should follow to rule out a malignancy. Patients may complain of urinary frequency or urgency, straining, decreased force of urination, incomplete emptying, dribbling, and nocturia. Patients may have recurrent urinary tract infections.

A combination of history, PE, and labs are used to make diagnosis. The prostate gland will feel smooth and enlarged on digital rectal exam. The prostate-specific antigen (PSA) may be mildly elevated. Order a UA with culture to rule out infection. It is important that other diagnoses be ruled out, especially carcinomas, bladder outlet obstruction, strictures, and overactive bladder. All men with BPH should be advised on the following behavioral modifications: reduce alcohol and caffeine; avoid antihistamines, decongestants, and opioids; avoid fluid before bedtime or certain activities; and practice double voiding to try to fully empty the bladder. α-adrenergic blockers (e.g., Cardura, Flomax, Hytrin) help relax the smooth muscles and can help with voiding issues. Medications that help slow the growth of the prostate—the 5α-reductase inhibitors—include Proscar and Avodart. If symptoms of upper urinary tract injury develop, surgery may be necessary to remove a portion of the prostate (e.g., TURP or laser ablation). Complications include urinary retention, hematuria, UTIs, bladder and kidney dysfunction, and bladder calculi.

CRYPTORCHIDISM AND TESTICULAR CANCER

Cryptorchidism occurs when one (most common) or both of the **testicles** fail to descend into the **scrotum**. This can be due to prematurity, low birth weight, or hormone imbalance. In most boys, the undescended testis will descend spontaneously within the first 3–4 months of life. Cryptorchidism resolves in most infants by the first birthday, but about 1% of infants don't resolve. Patients should be referred by 6 months of age if not descended by then to help reduce complications. The initial newborn exam includes palpating the scrotum to feel that both testes are there. They may be palpable a little further up the inguinal canal on one or both sides. Repeated checks should be done at follow-up visits to ensure the testes descend. Some testicles will descend and then temporarily retract again. This condition is not true cryptorchidism.

Diagnose by physical exam. Further testing is required if hypospadias or epispadias is also present to rule out a disorder of sex development. If the testicle is not descended by 6 months of age, surgical intervention (orchiopexy, in which the testicle is sutured or fixed to the scrotum) will be needed, as it is very unlikely to spontaneously descend after that time. Hormonal treatments are no longer recommended. Complications of untreated cryptorchidism include testicular torsion, infertility, testicular cancer, and inguinal hernia. **Testicular cancer** usually affects males between 15–35 years old and presents as a painless testicular mass that does not transilluminate. Therefore, it is important to encourage monthly self-exams, especially in young men.

PHIMOSIS AND PARAPHIMOSIS

Phimosis, or the inability to retract the **foreskin** in uncircumcised males, is physiologically normal in male children and usually resolves by 5 years old. If not, circumcision is the treatment of choice. **Paraphimosis** is a condition that occurs in uncircumcised or partially circumcised males and can develop into a medical emergency. It occurs when the **foreskin** of the penis becomes trapped behind the **glans**. The foreskin can normally be retracted manually and will slide back over the glans on its own or with little effort. With a paraphimosis, the foreskin and glans become red and edematous, and patients will complain of pain from the constriction. This can compromise the blood flow and may lead to gangrene if untreated.

Various techniques (e.g., lubricant, ice, osmotic agents) can be used to assist in manually sliding the foreskin over the glans to its normal position. More invasive techniques can also be used; these include the Dundee technique (a small-gauge needle is used to create punctures in the foreskin, and then the edematous fluid is compressed from the tissue so the foreskin can be slid down) or aspiration of the glans. If these procedures fail, surgery may be necessary to create a vertical slit in the foreskin to enable it to slide back to its normal position. A circumcision may be performed in these patients to prevent recurrence. Complications include recurrence, infection, necrosis, gangrene, and autoamputation.

HYDROCELE

A hydrocele is a painless collection of fluid in the **scrotum**, surrounding the testicles. In the US, this is most common in infant boys (6%) due to a patent processus vaginalis and usually resolves within the first year of life. Occasionally, the fluid does not reabsorb because it is not able to flow back into the abdomen. A hydrocele can also occur in adult males, usually over 40, due to an injury or infection. In the developing world, the most common cause of hydroceles is **filariasis**, caused by a parasitic roundworm that enters the lymphatic system. Patients do not usually have any pain in the scrotum when a hydrocele is present. Pain will be present if an infection is the cause, or if there has been an injury to the scrotum.

Diagnose per PE. To help differentiate a hydrocele from hernia, mass, or hematocele, be aware that the hydrocele will make the scrotal sac transilluminate due to the fluid, and also, this fluid will lie anterior and superior to the testis. Rule out an inguinal hernia, and an ultrasound can be used if further investigation is needed. Most of the time, a hydrocele will resolve spontaneously. Rarely, surgery may be necessary to remove the hydrocele from the scrotum. Aspirating the fluid is not recommended since it is not curative and may introduce infection. Complications are rare, but large hydroceles may cause ischemia and infertility. The main concerns are usually cosmetic issues.

VARICOCELE

A varicocele is an engorgement of the **veins of the pampiniform plexus**. This plexus is part of the **spermatic cord**, which travels through the inguinal canal, terminating in the testes. A varicocele is more likely to occur in the left testis (90%) because the veins from there run vertically into the renal vein, while the veins from the right testis empty into the inferior vena cava. A varicocele is usually idiopathic in nature but can be caused by compression preventing the veins from draining. This condition can occur as early as adolescence, but usually occurs in males ages 15–25. A malignant tumor (e.g., renal tumor) should be considered in patients who develop a varicocele after the age of 40. Patients may be asymptomatic or may complain of a heavy, aching fullness in the affected side. On exam, the scrotum may appear visibly enlarged with engorged veins, and when palpated, it may feel like a "bag of worms." The swelling may increase with a Valsalva maneuver and may decrease when the patient is recumbent. If asymptomatic and there are no fertility issues, watchful waiting is the usual approach. If mild, a scrotal support may be used to try to resolve the condition on its own. If this is not effective, embolization or surgery (e.g., ligation) may be necessary. Complications include infertility and atrophy.

TESTICULAR TORSION

Testicular torsion is a medical emergency that occurs when the testicle **rotates** and causes **strangulation of the blood vessels**. This can be seen in males who are 7–10 days old, since many times the testes haven't descended yet and therefore haven't attached to the tunica vaginalis. Also, the testicle is usually posteriorly held in place by the **tunica vaginalis**, which allows little movement. Some males have a congenital anomaly in which the tunica vaginalis is fixed too high, which allows the testicles to move easily and rotate horizontally on the spermatic cord. This leaves them susceptible to developing testicular torsion, in which a testicle can twist on the spermatic cord, causing obstruction of blood flow to the testicle. Peak incidence is between 12 and 18 years old, and it is infrequent over age 30. Patients will complain of sudden, severe testicular pain with nausea and vomiting. The affected testicle may appear swollen or discolored, or may appear elevated when compared to the other, and the cremasteric reflex is usually missing.

Diagnose per clinical exam and use a color Doppler ultrasound if the diagnosis is unclear. Treatment should be emergent (≤6 hours from initial symptoms) due to the risk of tissue death from decreased blood flow. The torsion may be resolved by manually manipulating the testicle—rotating it outwardly, back into a normal

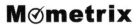

position—but emergent surgery may be necessary. With tissue death, an orchiectomy is performed. Complications include infertility, testicular infarction, and tissue death/loss of the testicle.

INFECTIOUS/INFLAMMATORY CONDITIONS

CYSTITIS AND URETHRITIS

Urinary tract infections (UTIs) are infections that can affect the bladder (**cystitis**) or the urethra (**urethritis**). Cystitis is more common in women because of an anatomically shorter urethra, but it can also occur in men. It is most common in women aged 20–40 during childbearing years, and in men over 50 because of enlargement of the prostate, obstructing urine flow. It is also more common with catheter use and in postmenopausal women. A UTI is caused by bacteria (usually *Escherichia coli*) that travel up the urethra to the bladder and multiply. Women are more susceptible to developing a UTI after frequent sexual intercourse because of bacterial exposure. Cystitis may be complicated (e.g., recent urinary surgery, comorbidities that increase the risk of infection, unusual pathogens, and structural or functional issues) or uncomplicated.

Signs and symptoms include dysuria, urgency, frequency, suprapubic pain, and hematuria. Patients may have a fever, but this is more likely with pyelonephritis. A clean-catch, midstream UA usually shows WBCs, RBCs, positive nitrite, and bacteria. Culture and sensitivity screening can be obtained to isolate the causative organism. For uncomplicated cystitis, the drugs of choice are nitrofurantoin, TMP-SMX, or fosfomycin, but local susceptibility patterns should be considered. For complicated cystitis, follow culture and sensitivity results and treat longer. Anesthetizing medications (e.g., phenazopyridine) can be given to reduce the pain. Symptoms should improve within 72 hours after antimicrobial therapy begins. Complications include recurrent infections, pyelonephritis, kidney damage if untreated, and sepsis.

PROSTATITIS

Prostatitis is inflammation or infection of the **prostate gland** and may be classified as: **acute or chronic bacterial prostatitis** (both usually caused by *E. coli*); **chronic prostatitis/chronic pelvic pain syndrome, CP/CPPS** (most common; 90–95%); or as **asymptomatic inflammatory prostatitis**. Chronic prostatitis/CPPS can be either noninflammatory or inflammatory and is possibly caused by blockage of urine flow or spasms of the urinary sphincters. Patients with acute or chronic bacterial prostatitis may complain of urinary urgency/frequency, decreased stream (and other obstructive symptoms), or lower abdominal/back or perineal pain; but a fever, systemic symptoms, and pain are much more pronounced with acute prostatitis. CP/CPPS is characterized by pain for ≥3 months and can involve pain on ejaculation as well as voiding symptoms. On exam, the prostate may feel boggy and enlarged, and is usually tender. Avoid prostatic massage with acute bacterial prostatitis.

Diagnose clinically, with UA (before and after prostate massage, unless contraindicated); urine culture and sensitivity and Gram stain can help guide therapy. For acute or chronic bacterial prostatitis, TMP-SMX or a fluoroquinolone are usually the drugs of choice, but check local susceptibility patterns; treat for 4–6 weeks, or longer if needed. Chronic prostatitis may benefit from α-blockers, muscle relaxants, and anti-inflammatory agents. Surgery is rarely needed. Complications include acute urinary retention (will need bladder drained by urethral or suprapubic catheter), recurrent UTIs, abscess, sepsis, infertility, and epididymitis.

EPIDIDYMITIS AND ORCHITIS

Epididymitis is inflammation of the **epididymis**, which is located on the posterior surface of each testicle and functions to store **sperm**. Epididymitis is most common in males under age 35 and is frequently due to a bacterial infection from an STD (e.g., chlamydia or gonorrhea). **Orchitis** is inflammation of the testes; when it occurs along with epididymitis, it is termed **epididymo-orchitis**. Orchitis is typically due to a bacterial STD or the mumps virus (orchitis will appear 4–7 days after parotitis). Symptoms are usually unilateral. Patients may complain of pain that begins on the back of the affected testicle and spreads. They may also have dysuria, urgency, and frequency, along with referred, lower abdominal pain. Fever and chills may also be present (high fever with mumps). On exam, the testicle may feel warm and swollen, with a palpable enlarged and tender epididymis. With orchitis, the testis is tender and enlarged, and the scrotum is swollen and erythematous.

Diagnose clinically and confirm with ultrasound. If the patient complains of acute testicular pain, it is important to rule out testicular torsion with a color Doppler ultrasound (because a positive Prehn sign is not as reliable for diagnosing epididymitis). If urethritis/STD is suspected, rule out an STD with NAA testing, and obtain a UA and urine culture. Supportive care includes analgesics, scrotal elevation, rest, and ice. Treat bacterial STDs (e.g., gonorrhea or chlamydia) with ceftriaxone plus doxycycline, OR if enteric organisms are suspected (e.g., *E. coli*), use levofloxacin or ofloxacin. Follow proper reporting protocol for patients who are positive for *C. trachomatis* or *N. gonorrhoeae*, evaluate partners, and counsel on condom use to prevent future STDs. Complications include a scrotal abscess, testicular atrophy (mumps), infertility, and (rarely) testicular infarction.

NEOPLASTIC DISEASES

PROSTATE CANCER

Prostate cancer is the third most common **cancer** diagnosed in the US, according to 2017 statistics. It is typically diagnosed in men ages 65–74, and is the second leading cause of **cancer death** in men. However, 5-year survival is close to 99%; and when caught early (localized or regional), it is 100%. Controversy surrounds the topic of screening. According to a 2017 draft by the United States Preventive Services Task Force, if the patient desires, and is expected to live for >10–15 years, screening for prostate cancer should occur at 55–69 years old with a PSA, and is usually accompanied with a digital rectal exam. There can be many false positives, since PSA may also be elevated with other disorders, like BPH. Screening should occur earlier, 40–45 years old, if at higher risk (e.g., African American, or first-degree relative diagnosed with prostate cancer).

Patients are usually asymptomatic, but symptoms may include difficulty urinating, urinary retention, blood in semen or urine, sexual dysfunction, and back pain. Urination difficulties can include difficulty starting or stopping the flow of urine, decreased force of urine stream, or dribbling. Bone pain in the lower back or pelvis may indicate metastasis. Use screening to guide workup: rectal exam reveals a palpable prostate that is enlarged and hardened, with a lumpy or uneven surface, and PSA blood levels may be elevated. Diagnose with a biopsy. Treatment varies according to the stage at diagnosis and includes surgery, radiation, and sometimes hormonal therapy for localized cancer or palliative therapy if it has moved outside the prostate. Complications include metastases, incontinence, urethral strictures (may need dilatation, stent, or surgery to correct), erectile dysfunction, and death.

RENAL CELL CARCINOMA

Renal cell carcinoma (**RCC**) is the most common **renal cancer** in the US and is more common in men than women. This cancer arises in the epithelium of the **proximal renal tubule**. Risk factors for developing RCC include obesity, smoking, exposure to chemicals, and some genetic disorders (e.g., von Hippel-Lindau syndrome, Birt-Hogg-Dube syndrome, hereditary papillary renal carcinoma). RCC may metastasize to the lungs (most common), bone, lymph nodes, liver, adrenal, and brain (least common). **Paraneoplastic syndromes** are common (20%) once it has metastasized.

The classic signs and symptoms are flank pain, a flank mass, and hematuria, but may include fever (often fever of unknown origin), weight loss, hypercalcemia, and hypertension. Since symptoms often don't appear until the disease is advanced, RCC is often diagnosed incidentally. Diagnosis is confirmed and staged with a contrast CT (procedure of choice) or MRI. Include a chest x-ray or CT to look for possible thoracic metastases. For localized disease, surgical resection is the treatment of choice. RCC is resistant to radiation and chemotherapy; therefore, if found early—before it has spread or metastasized—it can be treated by resection, otherwise the treatment is palliative (e.g., palliative surgery, immunotherapy, targeted therapy, experimental therapies). The primary complication is metastases, which brings with it a poor prognosis (8% 5-year survival, according to the ACS), along with paraneoplastic syndromes.

WILMS TUMOR

Wilms tumor, or **nephroblastoma**, is the most common **renal carcinoma** that affects children, usually ages 3–8. It is typically unilateral and affects males and females equally, except when bilateral, then it affects females more often. It is thought that Wilms tumors begin to form while in utero due to genetic mutations. The condition is usually diagnosed by age 1, though sometimes it may be as late as age 5. The prognosis is excellent, with a 5-year survival of 80–90%. Patients usually present with a painless abdominal mass. Wilms tumors can grow quite large before causing any symptoms in the child, so it may go undiagnosed until it becomes large enough to be palpable. Patients are usually asymptomatic but may experience abdominal pain/distension, hematuria, loss of appetite, nausea/vomiting, constipation, or SOB. Often a mass can be palpated in the abdomen and in the back over the affected kidney. Diagnosis is made with an abdominal ultrasound, CT, or MRI and confirmed with surgical examination and biopsies for staging. 90% of patients have favorable histology that shows no anaplasia. Treatment comprises surgery and chemotherapy; sometimes radiation is used if the patient presents with a higher-stage disease or has unfavorable histology. Complications include relapse, metastases, and treatment sequelae (e.g., CHF, renal insufficiency, liver damage, infertility, secondary neoplasms).

Hematologic System

ANEMIAS

IRON DEFICIENCY ANEMIA

Iron deficiency anemia is the most common form of anemia and causes a **microcytic, hypochromic anemia** due to a **lack of iron**. This can be caused by inadequate intake, impaired absorption, or bleeding. Iron is absorbed in the **duodenum and upper jejunum**, transported by **transferrin**, and stored as either **ferritin** (available for immediate use by the body) or **hemosiderin**. Iron requirements increase during times of growth (infancy through adolescence), during menstruation, and in pregnancy. Many patients are asymptomatic but may present with fatigue, weakness, cold intolerance, glossitis, cheilosis, koilonychia (concave nails), SOB, or signs of pica.

Diagnose with CBC, total iron-binding capacity (TIBC), serum iron and ferritin (reflects iron stores), reticulocyte count, and peripheral smear. These show reduced hemoglobin and hematocrit), reduced MCV, elevated RDW, elevated TIBC, reduced iron, reduced ferritin, and normal reticulocyte count; and as the anemia progresses, the smear shows hypochromic, microcytic RBCs with anisocytosis (unequal size) and poikilocytosis (shape variations). Treat with oral iron supplements; ferrous iron salts (e.g., ferrous sulfate, ferrous gluconate, ferrous fumarate) are best absorbed when taken on an empty stomach and with vitamin C, which increases absorption. The underlying cause should be determined and corrected, as well as any source of bleeding. Iron supplements are usually given during pregnancy. Complications include pregnancy issues, as well as hypoxemia resulting in irregular heart rate and CHF.

ANEMIA OF CHRONIC DISEASE (ANEMIA OF CHRONIC INFLAMMATION)

Anemia of chronic disease, or anemia of chronic inflammation, produces a microcytic or normocytic anemia due to an acute or chronic **activation of the immune system**. Causes include infections, cancer, autoimmune diseases (e.g., RA, SLE, DM, IBD), chronic kidney disease, or even severe trauma. The disease triggers the immune system, and in turn, several processes occur: The liver releases hepcidin, which decreases iron absorption in the duodenum and decreases the release of iron from macrophages. Old RBCs are degraded, and macrophages sequester and store more iron due to increased ferritin levels. Erythropoietin production in the kidneys is also decreased due to the inflammatory response. These processes all result in decreased iron availability and decreased RBC production, resulting in anemia. Patients may present with nonspecific signs and symptoms including fatigue, weakness, dizziness, cold intolerance, and pallor, as well as signs and symptoms of the disease triggering the anemia.

Diagnose with CBC with peripheral smear, serum iron, TIBC and ferritin, and reticulocyte count. These show reduced hemoglobin and hematocrit (moderately low), reduced TIBC, reduced iron, elevated ferritin, reduced reticulocyte count, and a normochromic or microcytic anemia on the smear. Treating the underlying disorder is the primary goal. In severe cases, erythropoiesis-stimulating agents (ESAs: epoetin alfa, darbepoetin alfa) may be used by hematologists or nephrologists (due to black box warnings), especially in those with chronic kidney disease (CKD) or patients undergoing chemotherapy for cancer; or blood transfusions may be necessary. Iron supplements are typically not used, but they may be if there is a concomitant iron deficiency anemia in patients with CKD if not on dialysis. Experimental therapies are under investigation. Complications include hypoxia, and increased mortality from cardiovascular disease and CKD.

THALASSEMIAS

Thalassemia is a group of **autosomal recessive disorders** that affects **hemoglobin (Hgb) formation**, causing a mild to severe **microcytic, hemolytic anemia**. This mostly affects those of African, Mediterranean, or South Asian descent. There are two main types: **α-thalassemia** and β-**thalassemia**. Both forms can produce a silent carrier state, a mild form called **thalassemia trait (thalassemia minor)** that is often diagnosed when a mild microcytic anemia does not respond to iron supplements, an intermediate form (Hgb H disease in α), and a severe form of the disease (**thalassemia major**: hydrops fetalis in α, Cooley's anemia in β). Symptoms usually start appearing after 6 months of life, when fetal hemoglobin starts being replaced by adult Hgb. Symptoms, if present, can include pallor, fatigue, jaundice, scleral icterus, and splenomegaly.

Diagnose with CBC, peripheral smear, and hemoglobin electrophoresis (usually normal in α-thalassemias, except Hgb H is elevated in Hgb H disease; elevated Hgb A2 and/or Hgb F in β-thalassemia trait; and elevated Hgb F in β-thalassemia major). Peripheral smear varies according to severity and ranges from a mild microcytic anemia, to Heinz bodies (Hgb H disease), or to target cells, nucleated RBCs, and basophilic stippling (β-thalassemia trait, β-thalassemia intermedia, β-thalassemia major). Treatment varies according to the severity of the disease. Patients who are carriers do not require treatment; those with the trait or intermediate disease may need blood transfusions; and those with Cooley's anemia depend on blood transfusions and iron chelation throughout their lifetime. Iron supplements are avoided. Splenectomy may be required, and a bone marrow transplant may be considered. Refer patients to genetic counseling. Complications include iron overload (rule out hemochromatosis), increased risk of infection, splenomegaly, bone deformities, heart failure, and (if severe thalassemia) death.

HEMOLYTIC ANEMIA

Hemolytic anemia results from destruction of **red blood cells (RBCs)**, and this is either inherited or acquired. It can be due to **intrinsic causes** (defect within the RBC itself) or **extrinsic causes** (from outside the RBC). Examples of intrinsic causes include sickle cell anemia, thalassemia, G6PD deficiency, thrombotic thrombocytopenic purpura (TTP), and hereditary spherocytosis. Extrinsic causes include drugs, toxins, autoimmune disorders (warm antibody hemolytic anemia or cold agglutinin disease), infections, hypersplenism, and prosthetic heart valves. Hemolysis can be acute, chronic, or sporadic; and it can occur intravascularly or extravascularly. Signs and symptoms depend on the underlying disorder causing the hemolysis, but may include pallor, fatigue, tachycardia, dyspnea, jaundice, ecchymosis, and dark urine from hemoglobinuria.

Diagnose with CBC with differential, peripheral smear, reticulocyte count, indirect bilirubin, haptoglobin, serum LDH (lactate dehydrogenase), and a direct Coombs test (i.e., direct antiglobulin test, DAT). The reticulocyte count is elevated in hemolysis and lower if the bone marrow is suppressed (e.g., aplastic anemia); the peripheral smear helps differentiate the cause (e.g., spherocytes, sickle cells, schistocytes); reduced haptoglobin, elevated indirect bilirubin, and elevated LDH are present in hemolysis; a positive DAT shows that antibodies or complement are present on RBC membranes, which indicates an immune-mediated cause (e.g., autoimmune, drugs, transfusion reaction). Treatment is directed at the underlying cause and may include steroids, blood transfusions, and a splenectomy or bone marrow transplant. Folic acid supplements are needed since folate is depleted during times of hemolysis; however, iron is usually not depleted during hemolysis, but is recycled, and therefore can be harmful if given. Avoid causative agents. Complications include bilirubin gallstones, heart failure, and death.

TRANSFUSION REACTION

Transfusion reaction is an adverse reaction after a **blood transfusion**. The reaction can be immune-mediated or non-immune-mediated and hemolytic or nonhemolytic. It can be acute or delayed (>24 hours to 2–3 weeks). Often the reactions are not serious and include febrile nonhemolytic reactions and allergic reactions. Hemolysis is serious and often fatal if due to ABO/Rh incompatibility. Patients with previous transfusions, and multiparous women, are at a higher risk of immune-mediated transfusion reactions due to the formation of alloantibodies. Transfusion-related acute lung injury (TRALI) is another possible serious complication of a transfusion.

Signs and symptoms of a transfusion reaction may include fever, chills, flushing, hypotension, dyspnea, wheezing, nausea/vomiting, anxiety, flank pain, and dark urine. Signs and symptoms of allergic reactions can include urticaria, pruritus, and wheezing. Blood typing and crossmatching before any transfusion helps decrease these reactions, but retype if a transfusion reaction occurs. Also use a DAT (direct antiglobulin test, also called direct Coombs test), which tests for antibodies directly attached to RBCs, to determine if the hemolysis is due to an immune-mediated process. The patient's plasma and centrifuged urine will appear pink or red if intravascular hemolysis/hemoglobinuria is present. Immediately discontinue the transfusion, give appropriate treatment (e.g., antihistamines, acetaminophen), and properly report if a transfusion reaction occurs. Complications include disseminated intravascular coagulation (DIC), TRALI, pulmonary edema, renal failure, volume overload, and anaphylaxis.

G6PD DEFICIENCY

Glucose-6-phosphate dehydrogenase (G6PD) deficiency is an X-linked **genetic disorder** in which the red blood cells undergo hemolysis, causing **hemolytic anemia**. This is due to an **enzyme deficiency** that affects RBC metabolism, and variants of the deficiency result in different levels of hemolysis. Many people will never experience symptoms or complications from the disorder. G6PD is the most common enzyme deficiency worldwide, and it is more common in males and in those of African, Mediterranean, or Asian descent. This condition is not constant but occurs during times of oxidative stress or certain triggers. Hemolysis may result from infection/fever, medication (e.g., acetaminophen, salicylates, sulfa drugs, Pyridium, chloroquine), or other triggers, like fava beans or mothballs. Hemolysis begins 24–48 hours after the oxidative stress and spontaneously resolves in 8–14 days. The patient may present with pale skin, jaundice, splenomegaly, dark urine, complaints of extreme fatigue, difficulty breathing, and an increased heart rate.

Diagnose the condition with a G6PD blood test (do not test during an episode of hemolysis due to high likelihood of false negatives). During hemolysis there is an elevated reticulocyte count, elevated LDH, and elevated indirect bilirubin. CBC shows anemia, and peripheral blood smear shows Heinz bodies and bite cells. Treatment is supportive during hemolysis since the episodes are self-limiting. Avoid triggers. Complications include chronic anemia and possible need of a transfusion (rare).

SICKLE CELL DISEASE/SICKLE CELL ANEMIA

Sickle cell disease (**SCD**) is an **autosomal recessive disorder of chromosome 11**, causing hemoglobin (Hgb) to be defective so that red blood cells (RBCs) are sickle-shaped and inflexible, resulting in their accumulating in small vessels and causing painful blockage (**sickle cell crisis**). While normal RBCs survive 120 days, sickled cells may survive only 10 to 20 days, stressing the bone marrow that cannot produce fast enough and resulting in **chronic hemolytic anemia**. There are variations of sickle cell disease, with homozygous Hgb S being the most common in the US (60–70%), affecting mostly African Americans. Sickle cell trait (Hgb A/S) occurs in 8–10%, is much less severe, and does not cause anemia. Different types of crises occur in SCD (aplastic, hemolytic, vaso-occlusive, and sequestration), and these can be brought on by stress, dehydration, and hypoxic states. Pain, pallor, jaundice, swelling in the extremities, weakness, and fatigue are common symptoms. Newborn screening is required in the US, and prenatal diagnosis is possible.

Diagnosis is per electrophoresis (Hgb S is present), PCR, or direct DNA testing. Hematology studies show: Hgb 5–9 g/dL, reduced Hct, elevated WBC, elevated reticulocyte count, and elevated platelets; and on peripheral smear: sickle cells, target cells, and possibly Howell-Jolly bodies. Treatment is supportive during a crisis (hydration, oxygen, analgesics); blood transfusions, iron chelation, and erythrocytapheresis may be necessary. Daily folate supplements (to prevent a megaloblastic anemia), penicillin prophylaxis (starting at 2 months until receiving all of their pneumococcal vaccines), and hydroxyurea therapy are also used. Stem cells transplantation is the only curative treatment and is about 85% effective. Complications of SCD include hemolytic anemia, aplastic crisis, avascular necrosis, organ damage, stroke, MI, acute chest syndrome, sequestration syndrome (spleen), chronic pain, increased risk of infection from encapsulated organisms, priapism, blindness, and pulmonary hypertension.

> **Review Video: Sickle Cell Disease**
> Visit mometrix.com/academy and enter code: 603869

PERNICIOUS ANEMIA (VITAMIN B12 DEFICIENCY) AND FOLATE DEFICIENCY ANEMIA

Pernicious anemia (or vitamin B12 deficiency) and folate deficiency both cause a **megaloblastic anemia**. Both B12 and folate must be ingested since they cannot be made by the body. **Pernicious anemia** is most often due to a lack of intrinsic factor in the stomach, which is necessary for the absorption of B12; it usually has an autoimmune etiology. Malabsorption of B12 can occur from gastritis, past surgeries to remove portions of the GI tract, and tapeworms. A deficiency of vitamin B12 can cause chronic fatigue; weakness; paresthesias; loss of appetite; weight loss; a sore, beefy red tongue; and mental changes, including confusion. **Folate deficiency** can be due to inadequate intake, increased age, malabsorption (e.g., celiac disease, alcoholism), or medications (e.g., metformin, methotrexate). Folate deficiency causes glossitis, diarrhea, confusion, and neural tube defects in pregnancy. This is difficult to clinically distinguish from pernicious anemia. Anemia may cause pallor, SOB, dyspnea, and tachypnea in either.

Diagnose with CBC with peripheral smear, and B12 and folate levels. CBC shows elevated MCV. Peripheral smear shows megaloblasts and hypersegmented neutrophils. Treatment consists of vitamin B12 replacement by IM injection or nasal spray, and begins with daily doses of vitamin B12 supplements, but then decreases to once monthly along with concomitant folic acid supplements. It is important to treat a vitamin B12 deficiency at the same time as giving folate, because folate will appear to be correcting the macrocytic anemia while the neurologic effects of a vitamin B12 deficiency continue to occur, resulting in permanent nerve damage. Complications include permanent neurologic damage if folate alone is used with a concomitant vitamin B12 deficiency.

APLASTIC ANEMIA

Aplastic anemia is a **pancytopenia** in which hematopoietic stem cells fail to make adequate **RBCs, WBCs, and platelets**. This is a rare but treatable condition. It can be genetic or acquired and can occur at any age; however, it is more common in the younger years and in the elderly. Genetic conditions that result in aplastic anemia include Fanconi anemia, familial aplastic anemia, and dyskeratosis congenita. Most cases of aplastic anemia are acquired; it can be caused by radiation, chemotherapy, toxins, medications, or viral infections, or it can be idiopathic (most common). The mechanism that causes aplastic anemia is thought to be either the direct damaging effects of an exposure or an immune-mediated response to various triggers (autoimmune).

The onset of signs and symptoms is insidious and may include pallor and fatigue, increased infections, and easy bleeding and bruising. Diagnose with a bone marrow biopsy. Treatment depends on the severity of the disease, and may be supportive or may include immunosuppressive agents (e.g., antithymocyte globulin, cyclosporine), blood transfusions, or hematopoietic stem cell transplants (HLA-matched sibling donors are preferred). Patients should be referred to a hematology expert. Complications include increased risk of infection and death.

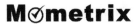

COAGULATION DISORDERS

CLOTTING DISORDERS

Factor VII deficiency can be genetic or acquired, and is due to a lack of factor VII (proconvertin). Factor VII is activated when combined with tissue factor, is necessary to complete the clotting cascade as an integral part of the extrinsic pathway, and is vitamin K-dependent. A prolonged PT and normal aPTT will be present. Treat with infusions of fresh frozen plasma (FFP) and recombinant factor VIIa.

Factor VIII deficiency (hemophilia A; classic hemophilia) is an X-linked recessive disorder causing a deficiency in factor VIII, which results in easy bruising and bleeding. It is typically genetic, but rarely may be acquired (autoantibodies). PT and platelets are normal, aPTT is prolonged, and there is reduced factor VIII; rule out Von Willebrand disease. Treat prophylactically before procedures and use replacement therapy with recombinant or concentrated factor VIII.

Factor IX deficiency (hemophilia B or Christmas disease) is an X-linked disorder, so it affects males more, and is less common than hemophilia A. Factor IX is vitamin K-dependent. A prolonged PTT, normal PT and platelets, and reduced factor IX assay will be present. Treat with infusions of factor IX (purified or recombinant).

Factor XI deficiency (hemophilia C or Rosenthal syndrome) is an autosomal disorder (males and females equally affected) and is more common in the Ashkenazi Jewish population. A prolonged PTT and normal PT are present. Infusions of fresh frozen plasma (FFP) are the primary treatment.

Von Willebrand disease is the most common bleeding disorder. It is usually autosomal dominant, and causes a deficiency of von Willebrand factor (VWF), resulting in platelet malfunction and low factor VIII. Labs show normal platelets and slightly prolonged aPTT. Diagnose with plasma VWF antigen, VWF ristocetin cofactor, and plasma factor VIII. Treatment may include desmopressin, recombinant VWF, and VWF/factor VIII concentrates.

HYPERCOAGULABLE STATES

Hypercoagulable states are a group of inherited or acquired disorders or conditions causing **increased coagulation**. They lead to an increased risk of **thromboembolic events** (venous or arterial). The risk of thrombosis has been described by **Virchow's triad**: hypercoagulability, endothelial injury, and stasis. The states of hypercoagulation include cancer, pregnancy, elevated estrogen (e.g., oral contraceptives, hormone replacement therapy), elevated or dysfunctional platelets, clotting disorders (e.g., factor V Leiden, prothrombin G20210A mutation, protein C or S deficiency, antithrombin deficiency), antiphospholipid antibodies, surgery or trauma, and blood stasis (e.g., immobilization, CHF, AFib). These increase the risk of venous thrombosis and pulmonary embolism (PE), which can be fatal.

Routine coagulation studies include: CBC with platelet count, PTT (intrinsic and common coagulation pathways), PT (extrinsic and common pathways), TT (thrombin time; only common pathway), and fibrinogen. A 1:1 mixing study helps determine whether the prolonged PT or PTT is due to a clotting factor disorder (clotting time corrects when mixed with normal pooled plasma) or due to the presence of inhibitors like heparin or autoantibodies (clotting time does not correct). Specific coagulation disorder studies include: factor V Leiden and prothrombin 20210 mutation tests, protein C or S activity tests, and antithrombin activity or antithrombin antigen tests. The presence of specific autoantibodies can be tested with a lupus anticoagulant, antiphospholipid antibody, or cardiolipin antibody test. A negative D-dimer, along with clinical judgment, helps rule out thrombosis.

IMMUNE (OR IDIOPATHIC) THROMBOCYTOPENIC PURPURA (ITP)

Immune (or idiopathic) thrombocytopenic purpura (ITP), also called **immune thrombocytopenia**, is a disorder causing bleeding and bruising due to a reduced number of **platelets** (thrombocytopenia). This is an autoimmune disorder (antiplatelet antibodies) that can be acute or chronic (>6 months), is seen in both

127

children and adults, and can be initiated by triggers including viruses, medication, or pregnancy. Children usually have acute ITP that is mild and self-limited, whereas adults usually have chronic cases of ITP. Consult a hematologist. Signs and symptoms include petechiae, purpura, bruising, and bleeding, but with a normal spleen size and no systemic symptoms.

This is a diagnosis of exclusion; rule out leukemia, myelodysplastic syndrome, SLE, and other secondary causes of thrombocytopenia (e.g., HIV, Hep C). Thrombocytopenia is defined as platelets $< 150,000/mm^3$, but bleeding is not usually seen until platelets are $< 50,000/mm^3$. Diagnose with CBC, platelets, and a peripheral smear; a bone marrow biopsy may be necessary to rule out other illnesses if the patient is unresponsive to treatment. Children with acute ITP usually do not require treatment. Treat with corticosteroids and possibly IV RhIG (e.g., RhoGAM) if Rh-positive, or IVIG (immune globulin IV) if Rh-negative. Other treatments include monoclonal antibodies (e.g., rituximab), other immunosuppressants, and thrombopoietin receptor agonists. Platelet transfusion may be necessary if there is severe bleeding, and a splenectomy may be necessary if the response to the initial treatment is inadequate. Avoid drugs that affect platelet function (e.g., NSAIDs). Complications include intracranial hemorrhages, GI bleeds, and recurrent disease.

THROMBOTIC THROMBOCYTOPENIC PURPURA (TTP)

Thrombotic thrombocytopenic purpura (TTP) is a rare **blood disorder** in which the formation of multiple thromboses (blood clots) in the small vessels results in a **low platelet count**. It is a medical emergency. It can be inherited or acquired (more common). The exact cause is unknown, but it can be triggered by drugs, pregnancy, or hemorrhagic E. coli; deficiency of the ADAMTS13 enzyme appears to be involved in some. Signs and symptoms can include microangiopathic hemolytic anemia, thrombocytopenia causing petechiae and purpura, fever, abnormal kidney function (however, not as severe as hemolytic uremic syndrome), and neurologic symptoms (e.g., altered mental status, paresthesias). Diagnosis consists of the following:

- CBC showing low platelets (20,000–50,000/μL) and low RBCs
- Blood smear showing broken and torn RBCs (schistocytes)
- Coagulation studies, negative DAT (Coombs), BUN, creatinine, elevated serum bilirubin, and elevated lactate dehydrogenase

The first line of treatment is plasma exchange, in which the patient's own plasma is removed and replaced with healthy plasma from a matching donor through transfusion. If the disease remains unresponsive to this treatment, immunosuppressive medications may be prescribed, and a splenectomy may be necessary. Complications include stroke, kidney impairment, and recurrence.

MALIGNANCIES, NEOPLASMS, AND MYELOPROLIFERATIVE DISORDERS
LEUKEMIA

Leukemia is a condition in which the proliferating malignant **hematopoietic cells** compete with and cause the suppression of normal **blood cell formation**. This results in several consequences, regardless of the type:

- Decrease in production of erythrocytes (RBCs), resulting in anemia
- Decrease in neutrophils, resulting in increased risk of infection
- Decrease in platelets, with subsequent decrease in clotting factors and increased bleeding
- Increased risk of physiological fractures because of invasion of bone marrow that weakens the periosteum
- Infiltration of liver, spleen, and lymph glands, resulting in enlargement and fibrosis
- Infiltration of the CNS, resulting in increased intracranial pressure, ventricular dilation, and meningeal irritation with headaches, vomiting, papilledema, nuchal rigidity, and coma, progressing to death
- Hypermetabolism that deprives cells of nutrients, resulting in anorexia, weight loss, muscle atrophy, and fatigue

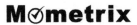

Leukemia occurs when one type of WBC proliferates with immature or inadequately functioning cells, with the defect occurring in the **hematopoietic stem cell**, either lymphoid (lympho-) or myeloid (myelo-). With **acute leukemia**, WBC count remains low because the cells are halted at the immature blast stage, and the disease progresses rapidly. **Chronic leukemia** progresses more slowly and most cells are mature, yet don't function properly. Risk factors include exposure to ionizing radiation or chemicals (e.g., benzene), previous chemotherapy, viruses, and chromosomal mutations.

> **Review Video: Leukemia**
> Visit mometrix.com/academy and enter code: 940024

ACUTE LYMPHOCYTIC LEUKEMIA AND CHRONIC LYMPHOCYTIC LEUKEMIA

Acute lymphocytic (lymphoblastic) leukemia (ALL) is the most common type of **pediatric cancer** in the US (may be seen in adults) and involves the proliferation of lymphoblasts (lymphoid precursors). Risk is increased with Down syndrome. Symptoms depend on whether there is primarily bone marrow involvement, or organs (e.g., spleen, liver, lymph nodes, thymus, CNS, gonads) have been infiltrated with blasts. Signs and symptoms include sudden onset of fever, fatigue, pallor, easy bleeding and bruising, petechiae, lymphadenopathy, and bone pain. Diagnosis is made with CBC (elevated WBCs) with peripheral smear and bone marrow biopsy (pancytopenia with >20% blasts). Refer to hematologist-oncologist. The cure rate is high in children.

Chronic lymphocytic leukemia (CLL) is the most common leukemia in **adults** (usually >60–70 years old) and involves the accumulation of mature but incompetent neoplastic lymphocytes (usually B cells). Incidence of CLL is increased in males. Risk factors include exposure to certain chemicals (e.g., Agent Orange) and a positive family history. CLL has an insidious onset, and patients may be asymptomatic when diagnosed (incidental finding). Signs and symptoms may include enlarged lymph nodes, hepatosplenomegaly, signs of anemia, and increased infections. Diagnose with CBC with peripheral smear (lymphocytosis, smudge cells), and bone marrow biopsy. Refer to hematologist-oncologist.

ACUTE MYELOGENOUS LEUKEMIA AND CHRONIC MYELOGENOUS LEUKEMIA

Acute myelogenous leukemia (AML) is a disease that originates in the **bone marrow** and involves the acute proliferation of **malignant myeloid precursor cells** (immature granulocytes and monocytes). AML is the most common **adult acute leukemia**. It may occur at any age but usually affects those >50 years old and affects men more than women. Risk is increased if the patient has myelodysplastic syndrome or previous chemotherapy/radiation. Signs and symptoms may include fatigue, fever, SOB, and gum issues (infiltrates, swelling, bleeding). Diagnose with CBC/peripheral smear and bone marrow biopsy (>20% myeloblasts; Auer rods). Refer to hematologist-oncologist.

Chronic myelogenous leukemia (CML) is a chronic disease that originates in the **bone marrow** and is almost always due to a **genetic mutation** (Philadelphia chromosome). CML involves the malignant production of granulocytes (neutrophils, eosinophils, basophils) and their precursors. It may occur at any age but is usually seen in adults. CML has an insidious onset and may present with general, nonspecific symptoms (e.g., fatigue, weight loss), splenomegaly (common), fever, night sweats, and signs of anemia. Diagnose with CBC, peripheral smear, and bone marrow biopsy (elevated WBCs; Philadelphia chromosome in bone marrow). Refer to hematologist-oncologist.

HODGKIN LYMPHOMA AND NON-HODGKIN LYMPHOMA

Lymphomas are cancers of the **lymphatic system**. The two primary types are Hodgkin and Non-Hodgkin lymphoma. **Hodgkin lymphoma** (previously, Hodgkin's disease) is a painless lymphoma usually in the cervical (most common), supraclavicular, mediastinal, or inguinal nodes. It is more common in males and in those 15–34 years old or >55 years old. Patients may present with fever, night sweats, weight loss (>10% body weight), dry cough, pruritus, splenomegaly, and palpable nodes. Some patients experience pain at the involved site when consuming alcohol. Diagnosis involves a biopsy and identifying Reed–Sternberg cells (a type of B cell). If caught in the early stages, most cases of Hodgkin lymphoma are curable. It spreads first to other nearby lymph nodes, and may sometimes eventually spread to the lungs, liver, or bone marrow. Treatment includes chemotherapy and/or radiation. Patients may desire to preserve fertility (egg or sperm banking).

Non-Hodgkin lymphoma is a group of **lymphocyte cancers**, is much more common than Hodgkin lymphoma (7th overall most common cancer), and can start in either T or B cell (more common) lymphocytes. It may occur anywhere in the lymphatic system and often spreads beyond (e.g., bone marrow, GI), even by the time of diagnosis. It is more common in males and is usually diagnosed in those ≥65 years old. Risk factors include environmental exposures, some viruses (e.g., Epstein-Barr virus), immunodeficiency conditions (e.g., HIV), and chronic inflammation. Signs and symptoms include painless peripheral lymphadenopathy that may cause compression symptoms; systemic symptoms are less common than in Hodgkin lymphoma. Biopsy enlarged nodes for diagnosis. Treatment involves chemotherapy, radiation, and monoclonal antibodies. Refer all lymphoma patients.

MULTIPLE MYELOMA AND MYELODYSPLASIA

Multiple myeloma is a cancer of the **plasma cells** and includes a range of diseases. The cancer cells invade the nearby **bone tissue** and destroy it. This affects men slightly more than women and is increased in African Americans, and incidence increases with age. Symptoms vary widely, and patients may be asymptomatic or may experience bone pain (especially in the back or ribs), osteoporosis, pathologic fractures, symptoms of anemia, and increased infections. Diagnose with CBC (elevated calcium), serum and urine protein electrophoresis, and x-rays; confirm with bone marrow biopsy. Treatment includes high-dose chemotherapy and autologous stem cell transplantation. The disease is progressive, and prognosis is poor.

Myelodysplasia (or myelodysplastic syndrome) is an abnormality in the development of **hematopoietic progenitor cells** and includes a wide range of **neoplastic disorders** depending on which cell line is affected. More dysplastic blasts are formed, and this causes a hypercellular (rarely it is hypocellular) bone marrow, but with peripheral cytopenia. This can be a precursor to acute myelogenous leukemia (AML). Risk factors include increasing age (>60 years), previous chemotherapy, radiation, and chemical exposure (e.g., benzene). Signs and symptoms depend on which cell line is affected. Decreased RBCs causes signs of anemia (pallor, fatigue, SOB), decreased neutrophils causes an increase in infections, and decreased platelets causes easy bleeding and bruising (e.g., bleeding gums). Diagnosis starts with CBC, peripheral blood smear, and bone marrow biopsy. Rule out other disorders causing a macrocytic anemia (e.g., vitamin B12 deficiency, folate deficiency). Refer to a hematologist-oncologist.

POLYCYTHEMIA VERA (PRIMARY POLYCYTHEMIA) AND THROMBOCYTHEMIA (THROMBOCYTOSIS)

Primary polycythemia (polycythemia vera) is a rare, chronic **myeloproliferative disorder** in which there is an increase in all three **myeloid cell lines** (RBCs, granulocyte WBCs, and platelets). This is due to a mutation (usually the JAK2 gene) in a **hematopoietic stem cell** and is usually diagnosed later in life (~50–70 years old). The blood volume expands and becomes hyperviscous due to the increased quantity of RBCs. Polycythemia vera places patients at an increased risk of thromboses and bleeding. Signs and symptoms include headache, vision issues, pruritus (often noted after a warm bath), reddish skin, fatigue, GI and gum bleeding, splenomegaly, hypertension, and SOB. Diagnosis is initially suspected with CBC findings (elevated Hct, Hgb, and RBCs). Secondary causes of elevated peripheral RBCs must be ruled out (e.g., disorders causing chronic hypoxemia, dehydration, tumors secreting erythropoietin). The primary treatment is phlebotomy. Consult with and/or refer to a hematologist.

Primary thrombocytosis is a chronic **myeloproliferative disorder** marked by an increase in **platelets**. This is more common in the elderly and is rare in pediatrics. The cause is unclear but seems to be due to mutations. Patients are at an increased risk of **thromboses and bleeding**. Patients are often asymptomatic, but signs and symptoms include headache, paresthesias, signs of thromboses, and bleeding or bruising. Diagnose initially with CBC (platelets > 600,000/mm^3) and peripheral smear; rule out other causes (secondary thrombocytosis may be caused by iron deficiency, infection, inflammation, neoplasms) since this is a diagnosis of exclusion. Treatment may include aspirin. Refer to a hematologist.

130

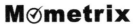

Infectious Diseases

BACTERIAL INFECTIONS

BOTULISM

Botulism is a potentially deadly disorder caused by the bacteria *Clostridium botulinum*. It causes symmetric, descending **paralysis** due to the toxin that blocks the release of **acetylcholine** from the neuromuscular junction. Symptoms usually begin 12–36 hours after ingesting the toxin from food (usually improperly canned food or infants ingesting honey) and begin with nausea/vomiting, diplopia, dry mouth, and dysphagia, progressing to respiratory failure. Treat with antitoxin and supportive care (airway). Wound botulism is also treated with penicillin. Spores can be destroyed at high heat when canning.

TETANUS

Tetanus (lockjaw) is a disease caused by the neurotoxin released by the bacteria *Clostridium tetani*, whose spores can be found in soil, dust, and animal feces. Spores thrive in anaerobic conditions and usually enter the body through a wound (especially puncture wounds, most often stepping on a nail). Symptoms usually start within 5–10 days of exposure and include headache, jaw stiffness or spasms, trismus (lockjaw), a fixed smile, dysphagia, and eventually generalized, painful muscle spasms, and even death. Treatment includes antitoxin, tetanus immune globulin (TIG), metronidazole (first-line) or penicillin, benzodiazepines for muscle rigidity, and airway support. Tetanus cases have decreased due to immunization (DTaP for pediatrics and Td or Tdap for adults). Postexposure prophylaxis includes TIG and a tetanus booster (if last tetanus vaccine ≥5 years).

CAMPYLOBACTER JEJUNI INFECTION, CHOLERA, ESCHERICHIA COLI, SALMONELLOSIS, AND SHIGELLOSIS

The following bacteria cause diarrhea (sometimes due to travel) and are confirmed with stool cultures:

- ***Campylobacter jejuni*** can cause crampy abdominal pain, watery and bloody diarrhea, and also systemic disease (e.g., fever). It is usually contracted by eating undercooked poultry; incubation is 2–5 days. It usually resolves spontaneously but may be treated with erythromycin or azithromycin.
- **Cholera** produces a profuse, watery diarrhea due to the saltwater-living bacteria, *Vibrio cholerae*. It is transmitted through the fecal-oral route (usually through ingesting contaminated water or food), and incubation is short, usually 1–3 days. Rehydration is the primary goal.
- ***Escherichia coli*** (*E. coli*) is a gram-negative rod normally found in the GI tract, yet certain strains cause diarrhea and even bloody diarrhea (O157:H7) due to toxins they produce. It is transmitted through water or food (ground beef). Symptoms start in 1–10 days with the O157:H7 strain and include severe cramping, bloody/watery diarrhea, and usually no fever; it can be complicated with hemolytic uremic syndrome (1–2 weeks after onset). Treatment involves supportive care (hydration).
- **Salmonellosis** is a disease caused by gram-negative bacteria from genus *Salmonella*. It can be spread via contaminated foods (poultry, eggs, beef) or animals (reptiles), and incubation is 6–72 hours. Symptoms include fever, abdominal pain, and watery diarrhea. Treatment is supportive. Sepsis can be a complication.
- **Shigellosis** (bacillary dysentery) is a disease caused by gram-negative bacteria, genus *Shigella*. It is spread through the fecal-oral route and incubation ranges from 12 hours to 4 days. Symptoms include high fever, nausea/vomiting, severe abdominal cramps, and a watery and bloody diarrhea. Treatment is supportive.

VIRAL INFECTIONS

CYTOMEGALOVIRUS (CMV)

Cytomegalovirus (**CMV**) is a **herpesvirus** (human herpesvirus 5). After the initial infection, CMV (like other herpes viruses) remains in the body in a latent phase. If contracted, CMV usually causes only mild disease and can even go unnoticed. CMV is one of the congenital **TORCH infections**, which can cause birth defects. More severe disease usually only affects the immunocompromised. It is spread through direct contact via **body fluids**, including by way of sexual contact, blood, and human milk. Those at increased risk of getting CMV

131

include health and childcare workers, pregnant women, transplant recipients, and those with HIV (immunocompromised). CMV can affect any organ system. Patients may be asymptomatic, or may present with mild flu-like symptoms or mononucleosis-type symptoms, with community-acquired pneumonia, or with fever of unknown origin; or if immunocompromised, may have severe disease, including retinitis, encephalitis, esophagitis, and colitis. Diagnosis is through serology tests, PCR, or viral cultures. Patients typically do not require treatment unless there is severe disease. Ganciclovir is the first-line treatment. Complications include birth defects, CMV relapse, hepatitis, Guillain-Barré syndrome, myocarditis, and anemia/cytopenias.

EPSTEIN-BARR INFECTION

Epstein-Barr virus (**EBV**) is a herpesvirus (human herpesvirus 4) and is responsible for causing **infectious mononucleosis**. After the initial infection, it remains latent in B cells and epithelial cells. It has been linked to certain epithelial and lymphatic neoplasms (e.g., nasopharyngeal carcinoma, Burkitt lymphoma, Hodgkin lymphoma). It is transmitted through **body fluids** like saliva, and hence is often referred to as the "kissing disease." It is most common in teenagers or college-age young adults, and incubation is typically 30–50 days. Symptoms of EBV infection range from being asymptomatic to having swollen painful lymph nodes, pharyngitis (can mimic strep pharyngitis), extreme fatigue, fever, and possibly hepatosplenomegaly. The WBC count is elevated (~10,000–20,000 cells/mL) with 10–30% atypical lymphocytes in the differential.

Confirm diagnosis with a mononucleosis spot test or EBV antibody serology tests. Treatment is supportive, and antibiotics are not helpful in treating this viral infection. Therefore, avoid unnecessary antibiotics in those with EBV, especially since administration of ampicillin or amoxicillin is often associated with a pruritic, maculopapular rash. Analgesics, warm saltwater gargles, increased fluid intake, and rest will help to relieve some of the symptoms. Symptoms may last for several weeks and fatigue may last even longer. Patients should avoid contact sports for up to 2 months. Complications include hepatitis, cytopenias (e.g., thrombocytopenia), Guillain-Barré syndrome, and splenic rupture.

HERPES SIMPLEX VIRUS INFECTIONS (HSV-1 AND HSV-2)

There are two types of the herpes simplex virus, human herpesvirus 1 (HSV-1) and human herpesvirus 2 (HSV-2). **HSV-1** usually causes a **gingivostomatitis** (often referred to as "cold sores" or "fever blisters") and is transmitted through **close contact**. **HSV-2** usually causes painful **genital lesions** through sexual contact. Either may be found in other areas of the body. Incubation time is ~2–12 days. The primary infection is usually more severe (causes systemic symptoms) than the reactivated infection, but it may be asymptomatic. After the primary infection, the virus remains dormant in the nerve ganglia, and can be reactivated especially during times of stress, illness, immunosuppression, or sun exposure. While patients are most contagious during times of active lesions, the disease may be spread while asymptomatic. The frequency of the outbreaks usually decreases over time. HSV lesions are grouped vesicles with an erythematous base. They are usually painful, and a prodrome of tingling, pain, or burning sensations may be felt hours to a couple days before the eruption. Lesions last for approximately 2–3 weeks in primary infection (up to 4 weeks with genital HSV), and 1–2 weeks in recurrent infections.

Diagnose clinically and confirm with a positive culture, PCR test, or HSV antibody tests (HSV-1 or HSV-2: IgM for active or recent infection; IgG for previous infection). Symptomatic treatment, proper wound care, and antivirals (acyclovir, valacyclovir, or famciclovir) may be given. Complications include perinatal infection, keratitis, herpetic whitlow, herpes gladiatorum, secondary infections, and encephalitis.

MEASLES

Measles (rubeola) virus is highly contagious, is spread through **respiratory secretions** (incubation is 7–14 days), and peaks in late winter to spring. It causes a prodrome of high fever (4–7 days), cough, congestion, and conjunctivitis; then Koplik spots (pathognomonic); and finally a maculopapular rash (spreads cephalocaudally). Report suspected cases immediately to the health department. Diagnose with a positive IgM antibody test (collected after 3 days of rash), viral culture, or PCR. Treatment is supportive.

MUMPS

Mumps (parotitis) is a viral infection that is spread via **saliva** (incubation is 12–24 days), and often occurs during winter and spring. It causes painful swelling of the salivary glands (parotid). Report to health department. Supportive treatment. Complications: orchitis (infertility), pancreatitis, meningitis.

RUBELLA

Rubella (German measles) is a virus that spreads via **respiratory droplets** (incubation is 2–3 weeks), and peaks in the spring. There is a mild prodrome (fever, aches, sore throat, conjunctivitis, swollen nodes [especially suboccipital, postauricular, and posterior cervical]), then a maculopapular rash (face first, then down). Report to health department. Confirm with rubella antibodies IgM or IgG. Symptomatic care.

ROSEOLA

Roseola is a herpesvirus (human herpesvirus 6 or 7) that is spread by **saliva** (incubation 5–15 days) and may occur any time of the year. It causes a high fever (3–5 days), then a fine pink/red maculopapular rash appears as the fever leaves (starts on trunk; lasts 2–3 days). Treat symptoms.

ERYTHEMA INFECTIOSUM

Erythema infectiosum, or "fifth disease," is caused by parvovirus B19, is spread via **respiratory secretions** (incubation is 4–21 days), and usually peaks in late winter to early spring. It causes a mild prodrome, then a "slapped cheek" appearance, then finally a lacy rash appears (patient is not contagious at this point). Treatment is supportive, as this is self-limited. Pregnant women should avoid contact with those with this virus (may cause stillbirth/hydrops fetalis).

HIV/AIDS

Human immunodeficiency virus (**HIV**) is a **retrovirus** that attacks the T lymphocytes (CD4+ cells), which weakens the immune system. There are two types: HIV-1 (most common in the US) and HIV-2. It is spread through blood, semen, genital/rectal fluids, and breast milk. The initial infection may go unnoticed, or 2–4 weeks after exposure, it may cause an **acute retroviral syndrome** (fever, fatigue, headache, lymphadenopathy, pharyngitis, rash, and myalgia/arthralgia), and during this time, **viral load** is high. Next there is an inactive or latent stage (length varies) and the viral load is lower. Screening (e.g., rapid HIV test) is recommended for those 13–64 years old and pregnant women.

Diagnose HIV through an antigen/antibody immunoassay, or a NAT (nucleic acid test) if it is indeterminate, and confirm with a second test that differentiates between HIV-1 and HIV-2. **Acquired immunodeficiency syndrome (AIDS)** is a progression of infection with HIV (average time is 11 years) that leads to opportunistic infections and neoplasms. Since patients may not immediately seek medical help, there is a wide range of presenting symptoms. AIDS is diagnosed when these criteria are met:

- HIV infection determined by lab
- CD4 count < 200 cells/mm^3
- AIDS-defining condition, such as opportunistic infections (cytomegalovirus, tuberculosis), wasting syndrome, neoplasms (Kaposi sarcoma), or AIDS dementia complex

It is important to review the following: CD4 counts to determine immune status, HIV RNA assay to determine the viral load; WBC and differential for signs of infection; cultures to help identify any infective agents; CBC to evaluate for signs of bleeding or thrombocytopenia; verify that vaccines are up to date; and repeat STD screens and TB tests periodically to determine if there is further exposure to diseases. Treatment aims to cure or manage opportunistic conditions and control underlying HIV infection through highly active antiretroviral therapy (HAART), ≥3 drugs used concurrently. Complications include opportunistic infections, dementia, neoplasms, wasting, and death. Refer appropriately.

INFECTIONS AND MALIGNANCIES ASSOCIATED WITH HIV/AIDS

The AIDS patient is highly susceptible to many bacterial, viral, fungal, and parasitic **infections**, as well as certain types of **cancers**, such as Kaposi sarcoma, central nervous system lymphoma, and non-Hodgkin lymphoma. **Bacterial infections** include *Streptococcus pneumoniae*; atypical mycobacterial disease (causes pulmonary infection), which includes *Mycobacterium avium-intracellulare* (MAI), also called the *Mycobacterium avium* complex (MAC); tuberculosis (TB); salmonellosis; syphilis; and bacillary angiomatosis. **Viral infections** include cytomegalovirus (CMV), viral hepatitis, herpes simplex virus (HSV), human papillomavirus (HPV), and progressive multifocal leukoencephalopathy (PML). **Fungal infections** include *Candida albicans*, *Histoplasma capsulatum*, cryptococcal meningitis, and *Pneumocystis jiroveci* pneumonia (PJP) (previously *Pneumocystis carinii* pneumonia, PCP), which is the most common opportunistic infection in those with HIV. **Parasitic infections** include toxoplasmosis and *Cryptosporidium*. The rate of contracting these types of infections in AIDS patients far exceeds the rates found within the general population. The AIDS-defining illnesses typically appear when the CD4 count is < 200 cells/mm^3.

INFLUENZA

Influenza (the flu) is a highly contagious viral infection that affects the entire **respiratory system** from the nose to the lungs. There are three types of influenza virus: **A** (causes epidemics), **B** (only in humans), and **C**. Types A and B are seen most often, and are the ones the annual flu vaccine is most effective against; type C is not as common and much less severe. Prevention is key, and annual, age-appropriate influenza vaccines should be given to those ≥6 months; two vaccines (separated by 28 days) are required in first-time vaccine patients if age 6 months through 8 years. Incubation is 1–4 days, and it is spread via respiratory droplets. Though symptoms can be very similar, the flu and the common cold differ in that the flu has a very sudden onset. Symptoms of influenza include a high fever (may last up to 5 days), headache, myalgias, dry cough, rhinorrhea, and fatigue. There may also be vomiting and diarrhea, although children are more prone to this.

Clinical judgment, community patterns, and rapid influenza tests (high specificity, but lower sensitivity) aid in diagnosis, but RT-PCR (reverse transcriptase-PCR) or viral culture definitively confirm the diagnosis; use pulse oximetry and chest x-ray as needed for pulmonary issues. Antibiotic treatment is not effective unless there is a secondary bacterial infection (e.g., pneumonia). Look for signs of secondary infections (e.g., dyspnea, cyanosis, fever that goes away and returns, confusion/lethargy). Treatment is supportive, with rest, fluids, and analgesics. Antivirals should be considered in those who are at high risk (<5 years old, elderly, pregnant, chronic conditions). These are most effective if initiated within 24–48 hours of symptom onset. The neuraminidase inhibitors (oseltamivir, zanamivir) treat type A, type B, and avian H5N1. There is extensive resistance to the adamantanes (amantadine, rimantadine), so they are rarely used. Complications include pneumonia, acute respiratory distress syndrome (ARDS), and death.

VARICELLA

Varicella (chicken pox) and herpes zoster (shingles) are both caused by a **herpes virus** (human herpesvirus 3), referred to as the **varicella-zoster virus**. Incubation is 10–21 days from initial exposure, and patients are contagious 2 days before the cutaneous eruption and until all lesions have crusted.

Varicella is the acute, initial infection with varicella-zoster virus and usually presents with a prodrome of fever, headache, and malaise, which is followed (in 2–3 days) by pruritic lesions that become vesicles with an erythematous base. Diagnosis is clinical and confirmed with a Tzanck smear or viral culture. Treatment is symptomatic; secondary infections are common. The first dose of the varicella vaccine is recommended at 12–15 months and the second at 4–6 years.

HERPES ZOSTER

Herpes zoster infection, or shingles, can be a very painful condition. It is caused by the same virus that causes chicken pox in children. The virus lies dormant in the **dorsal root ganglia** until increased stress or an immunocompromised state causes the virus to be reactivated, resulting in shingles. Patients may complain of burning pain and paresthesias 2–3 days before the lesions appear. Lesions most often erupt in the thoracic area, in a dermatomal pattern, though they can occur anywhere, including the face and eyes (trigeminal nerve; refer to optometrist). Vesicular lesions will open and eventually crust over. Patients may be left with chronic pain (**post-herpetic neuralgia**).

Diagnose per clinical evaluation, and a viral culture of vesicular fluid or polymerase chain reaction assay (PCR) can help confirm. Treating with antivirals within 48 hours of rash onset (e.g., acyclovir, valacyclovir, famciclovir) may reduce the length, severity, and complications. Topical analgesics or anesthetics (e.g., capsaicin or lidocaine patch) may help reduce the pain; anticonvulsants (gabapentin) and tricyclic antidepressants may help with the lasting pain of post-herpetic neuralgia. Immune globulin (VZIG) is given for post-exposure prophylaxis to those who are at high risk. Two doses of the shingles vaccine (Shingrix) 2–6 months apart are recommended for all those >50 years old, regardless of previous shingles or vaccination with Zostavax. Complications include disseminated infection (especially in immunocompromised) and visceral organ involvement (presents rapidly and includes encephalitis, hepatitis, and pneumonia).

FUNGAL INFECTIONS
CRYPTOCOCCOSIS
Cryptococcosis is an infection resulting from inhaling the **fungus** *Cryptococcus neoformans*, which is found worldwide in soil (can be associated with bird droppings), or *Cryptococcus gattii*, which is associated with certain trees in the Northwest. Cryptococcosis is most often due to *C. neoformans*, is found more often among those with compromised immune systems, and is an **AIDS-defining opportunistic infection**. Healthy patients may be asymptomatic, and the only finding may be pulmonary lesions on chest x-ray that resolve spontaneously. The fungus can disseminate and cause meningitis, encephalitis, and cutaneous lesions, and affect long bones and other tissues. Symptoms are based on the area of involvement. Patients may experience cough, pleuritic chest pain, weight loss, and fever if there is pulmonary involvement; headache, double vision, light sensitivity, nausea/vomiting, and confusion if CNS involvement; or cutaneous lesions (papules, pustules, nodules, ulcers) if the skin is involved.

Diagnosis includes microscopic analysis, culture (gold standard), or an antigen test (highly sensitive; good for detecting early infection) for *Cryptococcus* using cerebrospinal fluid (CSF), tissue, sputum, blood, or urine. Check CSF by India ink (limited sensitivity) or culture so meningitis can be ruled out. Confirm that no mass lesion is present by CT or MRI before LP is performed. Mild cases may only require monitoring to ensure that the infection does not spread. In more advanced cases, the infection is treated with different antifungal medications (e.g., fluconazole for pulmonary infections; amphotericin B, with or without flucytosine, for meningitis). The patient should also be monitored for CNS infection and medication side effects. AIDS patients may need lifelong antifungals. Complications include cryptococcal meningitis, neural deficits, optic nerve damage, and hydrocephalus.

HISTOPLASMOSIS
Histoplasmosis is an infection caused by inhalation of **spores** from the fungus *Histoplasma capsulatum*, which is found in soil and is associated with bird and bat droppings (e.g., in chicken coops, caves). Healthy patients are usually asymptomatic, and those with symptoms are typically immunocompromised or have had a heavy exposure to spores. The primary pulmonary infection occurs 3–17 days after exposure and can present with flu-like symptoms. It is typically self-limited but may become chronic. Histoplasmosis can also spread through the blood and can cause progressive disseminated disease in the immunocompromised (high mortality rate); this is an **AIDS-defining illness**. Diagnose through antigen tests (urine, serum), histopathology, or cultures; order a chest x-ray. Mild and even moderate acute pulmonary histoplasmosis may resolve on its own. If needed, treat mild to moderate infections with itraconazole, and severe illness with amphotericin B.

PNEUMOCYSTIS
Pneumocystis jiroveci is a **fungus** (previously known as *Pneumocystis carinii*) that causes **pneumonia** (PJP, previously PCP) in the immunocompromised. Most people have been exposed to this by the age of 3 or 4.

Symptoms of PJP include a dry nonproductive cough, fever, dyspnea, and weight loss. Chest x-ray may show diffuse bilateral infiltrates, or it may be normal; pulse oximetry may be low, especially on exertion.

Diagnosis is confirmed with sputum histopathology using sputum induction or bronchoalveolar lavage. Treat immediately with trimethoprim/sulfamethoxazole (TMP-SMX) for 21 days if HIV positive, and for 14 days in other cases. Steroids may be added for HIV patients with severe PJP. HIV/AIDS patients with CD4 counts <200/μL should receive PJP prophylaxis with TMP-SMX. Dapsone and pentamidine are alternatives. Complications include ARDS and death.

PARASITIC INFECTIONS
MALARIA

Malaria is a **blood-borne disease** caused by a **parasite** from the genus *Plasmodium* and found in tropical areas. There are four known to cause disease in humans (*P. malariae, P. vivax, P. ovale,* and *P. falciparum*). These protozoa are transmitted by the **female *Anopheles* mosquito**. They travel to the **liver**, where they multiply, are released, and then infect the RBCs, where they continue to multiply. Incubation time varies from 9 days to 1 month or even years based on the species of the infecting parasite. Signs and symptoms include headache, high fever with shaking chills and sweating (rigors; occurs when merozoites, an immature form of the parasite, are released from RBCs), jaundice, anemia, and hepatosplenomegaly. Take a thorough history, including recent travel.

Diagnose with 3 thin and thick blood smears (gold standard) stained with Giemsa (preferred) and obtained 12–24 hours apart. Labs typically show elevated LDH, thrombocytopenia, and atypical lymphocytes. Rapid antigen tests are also available, as well as PCR. Treat with chloroquine. If traveling, chemoprophylaxis depends on the area of travel due to species and resistance patterns, and may include chloroquine, primaquine, mefloquine, Malarone, or doxycycline. Report infections to your local or state health department. Complications include severe anemia and hemolysis, organ failure (liver, spleen, kidneys), cerebral malaria, ARDS, and death.

PINWORMS AND OTHER HELMINTH INFESTATIONS

Parasitic worms, or helminths, are broadly divided into **roundworms** (nematodes) and **flatworms**. Flatworms include tapeworms (which cause weight loss) and **flukes** (intestinal or liver). Roundworms include the genus *Ascaris*; hookworms, which cause anemia; **filariae**, which cause elephantiasis; and **pinworms**, which cause enterobiasis and are the most common helminth infestation. Pinworms are more prevalent in warmer areas of the country, and infestations occur more frequently in children. The worms lay eggs within the digestive tract and then travel to the anal area, where they are usually found. Pinworms are highly contagious. As a patient scratches the anal area where the eggs are located, the eggs cling to the fingers and can easily be transmitted to other people, either directly or through food or surfaces. The eggs can survive for 2–3 weeks on inanimate objects. Patients may be asymptomatic, or may have intense anal itching that is usually worse at night and can cause insomnia. Abdominal pain, nausea, and vomiting can also occur.

Diagnose with the "tape test," which involves pressing cellophane tape over the perianal area to pick up eggs or worms and examine under the microscope. Most other helminth infestations can be diagnosed with a stool sample for ova and parasites; filariasis requires a blood smear or antigen test. Anthelmintic medications (mebendazole, albendazole, or pyrantel pamoate) are given in a single dose and repeated in 2 weeks to kill the pinworms and their larvae. The entire family and close contacts should be treated simultaneously since pinworms are so contagious.

TOXOPLASMOSIS

Toxoplasmosis is an infection caused by the **parasite** *Toxoplasma gondii*, which is found in the soil. It is widespread and transmitted through cat feces; however, it also may be contracted by eating undercooked meat (especially pork, lamb, or venison) or poorly washed vegetables. Toxoplasmosis can cause serious disease and can affect various organs; the immunocompromised, and pregnant women and their unborn babies, are especially likely to have side effects of the disease (the "T" in congenital TORCH infections).

Healthy patients are usually asymptomatic; however, once the patient is infected, the parasite can remain latent until the patient becomes immunocompromised and the parasite is reactivated, causing symptoms. Toxoplasmosis can cause a flu-like illness with fever, myalgias, and lymphadenopathy. More serious effects include retinochoroiditis, brain lesions, and encephalitis. Congenital toxoplasmosis may cause retinochoroiditis, microcephaly, hydrocephalus, intellectual disabilities, and possibly miscarriage or stillbirth. Diagnose with serology for *Toxoplasma* antibodies IgM and IgG. Also, PCR may be used to test amniotic fluid, CSF, or tissue. Treat with pyrimethamine (preferred) plus folinic acid, or sulfadiazine plus folinic acid. Pregnant women should avoid high-risk practices like changing the cat litter and should avoid sandboxes.

SPIROCHETAL AND TICK-BORNE DISEASES

SYPHILIS

Syphilis is caused by the **spirochete** *Treponema pallidum* and is passed on through direct contact with a syphilitic sore by vaginal, oral, or anal sex, or through the placenta to an unborn baby. The disease has four phases, with an average incubation period of about 3 weeks (10–90 days):

- **Primary**: Chancre (painless) in areas of sexual contact, persisting 3 to 6 weeks.
- **Secondary**: General flu-like symptoms (sore throat, fever, headaches); red papular rash on trunk, flexor surfaces, palms, and soles; and lymphadenopathy. These occur about 3 to 6 weeks (up to 3 months) after end of primary phase, and eventually resolve.
- **Latent**: In the early latent phase (within 1 year of infection), the patient has a positive rapid plasma reagin (RPR), VDRL, or antibody test (FTA-ABS) and no symptoms, and is contagious; but in late latent phase (>1 year from infection) is not contagious, except to an unborn baby.
- **Tertiary**: Affects about 30% and includes CNS and cardiovascular symptoms 3 to 20 years after initial infection. Gummas (granulomatous lesions) may be widespread.

Neurosyphilis may occur at any stage of this disease. Early neurosyphilis occurs weeks to a few years after the exposure and presents as meningitis. Late neurosyphilis occurs 10–30 years after exposure and involves dementia, as well as nerve damage causing weakness and paralysis. Diagnosis is made by dark-field microscopy (primary or secondary) or serologic testing. An LP is needed in all patients with neurologic symptoms. Treatment for primary, secondary, and early latent is benzathine G penicillin 2.4 million units IM in 1 dose. For late latent or tertiary, treatment consists of benzathine G penicillin 2.4 million units IM weekly for 3 weeks (7.2 million units total). Complications include dementia, meningitis, neuropathy, hearing loss, ocular syphilis, thoracic aneurysm, aortic aneurysm, stroke, and cardiac valve disease. Report cases to the local health department.

LYME DISEASE

Lyme disease occurs from a bite from a **deer tick** (blacklegged tick) infected with the **spirochete bacterium** *Borrelia burgdorferi*. It is the most common tick-borne disease in the US and is more prevalent in heavily wooded areas. Adult ticks are more active during colder times, whereas the nymphs (<2 mm in size) are more active in the warm spring or summer months. Once the tick bites, it stays attached; however, it takes about 36–48 hours for nymphs and about 48–72 hours for adult ticks before the spirochete is transmitted to the person. Incubation is 3–30 days. There are 3 stages to this disease: 1) early localized, 2) early disseminated, and 3) chronic disseminated. In **stage 1**, 75% have the characteristic expanding red rash (erythema migrans; can be large, ~30 cm), which can progress to have central clearing (bull's-eye), headache, fever, chills, myalgias, and fatigue. **Stage 2** occurs weeks to months after initial infection and involves systemic symptoms (flu-like), neck stiffness, headaches, migrating pain in muscles and joints, rashes, paresthesias, Bell palsy, confusion, fatigue, myocarditis, and heart palpitations. **Stage 3** occurs months to years after initial infection and involves neurologic (e.g., encephalitis) and rheumatologic issues, especially arthritis of large joints (e.g., knee).

Diagnose using 2-tiered testing: antibodies (IgM, IgG), then Western blot. Antibiotic treatment for localized Lyme disease involves 2–3 weeks of doxycycline, amoxicillin, or cefuroxime axetil, and is started immediately after diagnosis. IV antibiotics may be needed for severe disease (e.g., IV ceftriaxone). Prevention is key: wearing clothes covering the skin, using tick repellents, showering soon after being outdoors in tick-prone areas, and thoroughly checking for ticks (especially in hard-to-see areas, by using a mirror). The Lyme vaccine is no longer available, and previous vaccine recipients are still at risk of contracting the disease, as protection decreases over time. Complications are prevalent with untreated Lyme disease; they include chronic arthritis, fatigue, chronic musculoskeletal issues, acrodermatitis chronica atrophicans, and memory and concentration issues. Report cases to the local health department.

ROCKY MOUNTAIN SPOTTED FEVER

Rocky Mountain spotted fever (**RMSF**) is a disease caused by a bite from a **tick** carrying the bacteria *Rickettsia rickettsii*. This can be found in all parts of the US and especially in eastern and central states. Of the tick-borne illnesses that can lead to death, RMSF is the most common. Prevention is key. Incubation is 3–12 days. Patients usually present with the sudden onset of fever, myalgias, headache, nausea/vomiting, abdominal pain, and a rash that usually appears within 2–4 days of the start of the fever (although the rash may appear later). A maculopapular pink rash usually begins on the wrists, forearms, palms, soles, and ankles and spreads centrally and to the extremities. Typically, the rash becomes darker red and petechial as the disease progresses; however, the rash is highly variable or can even be absent, leading to misdiagnosis. The disease can lead to severe illness, including encephalitis, myocarditis, uveitis, and gangrene.

Diagnosis can be difficult and is based on clinical findings and labs (e.g., thrombocytopenia, anemia, reduced sodium). RMSF can be confirmed with immunofluorescent antibody tests, but it may take weeks to confirm. It is vital to start empiric antibiotic treatment when RMSF is suspected since lab tests may be falsely negative in the first 7–10 days and since mortality is decreased if treatment is begun within the first 5 days of symptom onset. Treat with doxycycline. Hospitalization is often required. Complications include pulmonary edema, renal failure, shock, seizures, encephalopathy, hearing loss, DIC, and death. Report cases to the local health department.

PRENATAL INFECTIONS
TORCH

TORCH stands for:

- **T**oxoplasmosis (avoid contact with cat feces)
- **O**ther (syphilis, varicella-zoster, parvovirus B19 [erythema infectiosum], human immunodeficiency virus [HIV], Zika virus)
- **R**ubella
- **C**ytomegalovirus
- **H**erpes simplex virus type 2 (HSV-2)

These **congenital infections** are known to cause **sequelae** in unborn babies while usually only causing mild disease in the mother. The sequelae depend on the disease and include microcephaly, seizures, hearing loss, cataracts/blindness, neurologic deficits, intellectual disabilities, encephalitis, hydrocephalus, pneumonitis, prematurity, being small for gestational age/growth delay, jaundice, anemia, cardiac defects, miscarriage, and stillbirth. It is important to screen for and counsel pregnant women on prevention of these diseases.

ZIKA VIRUS

Zika virus is a **flavivirus** that is transmitted by the *Aedes* mosquito and through sexual contact. This virus can be passed on to an unborn baby, causing severe congenital defects, while causing mild or no disease in the mother. It is advised that all pregnant women avoid traveling to areas with the Zika virus (e.g., Central and South America, Mexico, Caribbean, Africa). Incubation period is 3–14 days and symptoms may last 4–7 days. The virus has been found to remain longer in semen than in other body fluids. If symptoms are present, they may include fever, headache, myalgias, arthralgias, a maculopapular rash, and conjunctivitis. Congenital defects include severe microcephaly, severe brain abnormalities, macular scarring, hearing loss, motor disabilities (e.g., hypertonia), and contractures. Women should be screened for Zika exposure at each prenatal visit.

Diagnostic testing is recommended for all asymptomatic pregnant women who have continued exposure to Zika, and for all symptomatic pregnant women who have possibly been exposed to the Zika virus. Testing includes RNA NAT testing on serum and urine, and serum IgM Zika antibody testing. Prenatal ultrasound helps determine if the effects of Zika are present. Report cases to the state health department; the CDC can be consulted. There is no treatment or cure for the Zika virus.

SEPSIS/SYSTEMIC INFLAMMATORY RESPONSE SYNDROME (SIRS)

SEPSIS

Sepsis is a systemic response by the body to **infection**; it can cause tissue damage, organ failure, and death. Mortality rates increase as the start time of treatment is delayed, and patient survival improves if treatment is started within 3 hours. Those at risk of sepsis include children <1 year old, the elderly (≥65 years old), those with chronic medical conditions, and the immunocompromised. Symptoms include fever (≥102 °F) or hypothermia, diaphoresis, SOB, tachycardia, altered mental status, pain/discomfort, and hypotension. A quick SOFA score (sequential organ failure assessment) can help identify those with sepsis. The three criteria are: respiratory rate ≥22 breaths/minute, systolic blood pressure ≤100 mmHg, and altered mental status. Patients with 2 out of these 3 criteria are likely to have sepsis.

Labs to help with diagnosis include a CBC with differential, BUN, creatinine (Cr), LFTs, and blood cultures/cultures from potential infection sites (e.g., wound or surgery site, CSF, urine) should be taken before antibiotics are started. If signs of septic shock, admit to the ICU and monitor ABGs, oxygen levels, renal function (urine output), blood glucose, lactate, and electrolytes. Treatment includes empiric antibiotics started immediately (follow local trends and antimicrobial resistance patterns when choosing antibiotics), reperfusion with IV fluids and vasopressors (if needed), oxygen, and other supportive measures. Complications include organ failure, septic shock, and death.

SYSTEMIC INFLAMMATORY RESPONSE SYNDROME (SIRS)

Systemic inflammatory response syndrome (**SIRS**) suggests that there is inflammation in the body. It is a way to assess for possible sepsis (assess risk of increased mortality due to sepsis).

SIRS is defined as meeting **2 or more** of the following criteria:

- Fever >100.4 °F or <96.8 °F
- Heart rate >90 bpm
- Respiratory rate >20 beats/minute or $PaCO_2$ <32 mmHg
- Abnormal WBC count (i.e., >12,000/μL or <4,000/μL or >10% immature bands)

However, SIRS is nonspecific. Processes other than sepsis (or infection) that can meet the SIRS criteria include trauma, surgery, burns, ischemia, MI, medications, malignancies, and pancreatitis. Workup includes CBC with differential, metabolic panel, and other studies based on the patient's history and physical exam (e.g., various cultures: blood, sputum, urine, CSF; cardiac enzymes; blood gases; lactate). Treatment varies greatly and is directed toward the cause. Since infection is the most common cause of SIRS, empiric antibiotic treatment should be directed at the source of infection and follow local resistance patterns. Complications of SIRS may include ARDS, renal failure, DVT, hyperglycemia, DIC, and death.

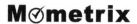

Musculoskeletal System

FRACTURES, DISLOCATIONS, AND SOFT TISSUE INJURIES

BOXER'S, COLLES, SMITH, AND SCAPHOID FRACTURES

A **boxer's fracture** occurs at the **distal end of the fifth metacarpal bone**. It earned its name because it is usually caused by the force of a fist hitting a hard surface, as with boxing. It usually heals within 3–4 weeks with splinting (ulnar gutter splint) and rest. Reduction and casting may or may not be necessary depending on the severity of the fracture.

A **Colles fracture** occurs at the **distal end of the radius with dorsal displacement** ("dinner fork" deformity) and is usually caused by breaking a fall with an outstretched (extended) hand. Depending on severity, surgery (open reduction) may be necessary, but often all that's needed is a closed reduction with a cast for 3–6 weeks until the fracture has healed.

A **Smith fracture** is a fracture of the **distal radius with volar displacement** (opposite of a Colles and not as common). This usually occurs from falling on a flexed wrist. Treatment involves open or closed reduction with a cast for 6 weeks. For both Colles and Smith fractures, assess for injury to the median nerve (palmar side of thumb, index, middle, and half of ring finger).

A **scaphoid fracture (navicular fracture)** occurs from a fall on an outstretched hand and is the most common carpal fracture. This will cause tenderness in the anatomic snuffbox at the base of the thumb in the wrist. With this fracture, there is risk of interrupted blood supply to this small bone, and osteonecrosis may occur. Treatment is with a thumb spica cast or splint, sometimes up to 6–8 weeks, and surgery may be necessary. Diagnose the above fractures with AP (anterior-posterior) and lateral x-rays. Add an oblique view for hand and carpal fractures. CT may be necessary; sometimes an MRI may be necessary with suspected scaphoid fractures. Care must be taken to note involvement of the epiphyseal disk (growth plate) in children since an open reduction and internal fixation (ORIF) may be required. Patients should be referred to an orthopedist.

NURSEMAID'S ELBOW

Nursemaid's elbow is a **subluxation of the radial head**. It usually occurs in children under 6 years old. A pulling mechanism on the arm, such as when swinging a child, causes the **radial head** to pull out of the **annular ligament** in which it sits. This results in partial dislocation, or subluxation, of the arm. The child may initially experience pain, but then usually acts normally while refusing to use the affected arm, and will hold it in a slightly flexed, adducted, and pronated position. There is no visible deformity, swelling, or bruising of the arm, but the child will guard the arm and prevent any movement of it to prevent pain.

Diagnosis is clinical; however, older children and adults may need an x-ray to rule out a fracture. A nursemaid's elbow is easily reduced using one of two techniques:

- The supination-flexion technique: The child's pronated arm is held at a 90° angle with pressure applied to the radial head. Next, the hand is supinated, and then the elbow flexed so the hand touches the shoulder.
- The hyperpronation technique: The child's pronated arm is held at a 90° angle with pressure applied to the radial head. Then the wrist is hyperpronated.

A pop or click is usually felt if it has been reduced, and typically the child immediately begins to use the arm (some take ~30 minutes). If this does not reduce the subluxation, the arm may be placed in a sling and orthopedic evaluation obtained. The parents should be advised to avoid swinging or pulling the child, especially by one arm, to help prevent this from recurring (recurs in about 30%).

GAMEKEEPER'S THUMB (SKIER'S THUMB)

Gamekeeper's thumb, or skier's thumb, is injury to the **ulnar collateral ligament** of the thumb. It is caused by a force that hyperextends the thumb away from the hand toward the body, as when falling on a ski pole. It earned its name from gamekeepers in Europe injuring the ligament while breaking rabbits' necks. It may also occur in sports (e.g., football, rugby), falls, and MVAs while bracing for impact. Patients will have significant pain with this injury, and depending upon severity, it can be disabling. The pain is greatly exacerbated when trying to grasp or pinch anything (e.g., holding car keys).

The area may be edematous, erythematous, or ecchymotic. Obtain AP, lateral, and oblique x-rays to rule out an avulsion fracture. Exam usually reveals ligament and first MCP (metacarpophalangeal) joint instability by using a lateral stress test (local anesthetic is needed, and this should not be performed if there is an avulsion fracture). Treatment consists of immobilization of the ligament with a thumb spica splint or cast for 4 weeks and NSAIDs. Surgery may be necessary if the ligament injury is not healing, and is required for a complete tear or rupture. Prognosis improves when the patient seeks medical attention shortly after the injury; if required, surgery should be performed within 3 weeks. Chronic instability is the primary complication.

DE QUERVAIN TENOSYNOVITIS

De Quervain tenosynovitis is a condition in which there is inflammation in the **abductor pollicis longus** and **extensor pollicis brevis tendons** in the thumb. They are held together in the thumb by the **extensor retinaculum**. If the tendons become inflamed and swollen, the retinaculum cannot expand to accommodate the inflammation, leading to tenosynovitis. This can be caused by overuse of the thumbs (e.g., carpenters; mothers or day care workers picking up infants), trauma, or arthritis, which can cause edema in the tendons, leading to this condition. Hormonal changes of pregnancy and water retention may lead to constriction and pain of the tendons. Patients complain of pain with motion of the thumb and wrist, and there is usually thickening and pain on palpation at the radial styloid (first dorsal compartment). Diagnose clinically and with the Finkelstein test (make a fist around the thumb and perform ulnar deviation; this elicits pain). Treatment consists of resting the thumb, splinting, and NSAIDs. If conservative treatments do not help, long-acting steroid injections into the sheath may reduce the inflammation. As a last resort, surgery can be done to release the extensor retinaculum.

CARPAL TUNNEL SYNDROME

Carpal tunnel syndrome occurs when there is irritation and pressure applied to the **median nerve** within the carpal tunnel of the wrist. In some cases, the cause is not known, but most patients have experienced some type of repetitive movement of the hands that caused irritation within the carpal tunnel. Signs and symptoms are gradually progressive and include numbness or tingling of the palmar side of the thumb, index, and middle fingers (median nerve distribution). Patients may describe grip strength weakness and frequent dropping of objects at home. Symptoms may be worse at night and may wake patients. Diagnose clinically and confirm with nerve conduction testing, EMG (electromyography), or ultrasound. Symptoms can be elicited by tapping on the volar surface of the wrist, over the carpal tunnel (Tinel sign). Wrist splints in a neutral or slightly extended position should be tried at night for 3–4 weeks to help relieve pressure on the nerve. Anti-inflammatory drugs and resting the hands and wrists may help. If conservative treatment does not work, corticosteroid injections may help. If it is severe or these other treatments are not effective, surgery to release the transverse ligament over the carpal tunnel usually resolves the condition.

LATERAL EPICONDYLITIS (TENNIS ELBOW)

Lateral epicondylitis, or tennis elbow, is common and occurs due to overuse of the **extensor muscles** in the forearm. These muscles attach to a tendon that attaches to the **lateral epicondyle** of the elbow. With overuse—such as with playing tennis (backhand), painting, or computer keyboard use—microtears and inflammation in the tendon at its insertion can occur. Patients may complain of pain and tenderness over the lateral epicondyle that can radiate to the forearm; this can be aggravated by extending the fingers and wrist. Symptoms will become worse while picking up an object or even shaking hands. Diagnose clinically. Testing involves having patients extend the wrist or fingers (especially the middle) against resistance, or supination

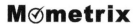

with resistance, which produces pain. Treatment includes rest of the elbow and forearm, ice, and NSAIDs, and a splint or a counterforce brace can be worn to help relieve pain. Stretching and exercises can also be done to help strengthen the extensor muscles of the forearm and decrease pain. Steroid injections can be performed around the tendon at the lateral epicondyle (not in the tendon because it will weaken and possibly rupture). Surgery may be needed if not improved in 9–12 months.

MEDIAL EPICONDYLITIS (GOLFER'S ELBOW)

Medial epicondylitis, or golfer's elbow, occurs due to overuse of the **flexor muscles** in the forearm. These muscles attach to a tendon that attaches to the medial epicondyle of the elbow. With overuse, such as with golfing, bowling, or typing, **microtears and inflammation** in the tendon insertion can occur. Patients will complain of pain and tenderness over the medial epicondyle, aggravated by flexing the fingers and wrist. Hand or wrist weakness may develop, and symptoms can become worse while grasping an object. Diagnose clinically. Testing involves having a patient extend the palm and attempt to flex the wrist toward the forearm against resistance or pronate against resistance, which should produce pain over the medial epicondyle. Use Tinel sign (tapping on the ulnar nerve at the medial epicondyle) to check for ulnar neuropathy. Treatment includes rest of the elbow and forearm, ice, and NSAIDs or acetaminophen; a cock-up wrist splint or counterforce brace can be worn to help relieve pain. Steroid injections can be performed around the tendon at the medial epicondyle. Once pain is better, exercises can be done to help strengthen the flexor muscles of the forearm. Surgery is rare, but may be needed if the patient is not improved in 9–12 months.

LOWER EXTREMITY

AVASCULAR NECROSIS

Avascular necrosis occurs when there is a **loss of blood supply** to the bone, and usually affects the **proximal femoral head** (Legg-Calvé-Perthes disease) but can occur in other bones as well (e.g., humeral head, carpal bones, metatarsal head, talus). This results in damage to the bone (osteonecrosis), causing pain and eventually **loss of joint function**. Avascular necrosis can be caused by trauma, stress fractures, chronic steroid use, radiation treatments to the area, chemotherapy, alcoholism, and chronic medical conditions, such as sickle cell anemia and SLE. Pain is the most common presenting symptom of avascular necrosis. Patients may have noticed a gradual progression of the pain, especially with weight bearing, or may develop a limp. X-rays will show the dead bone tissue once the condition is advanced. MRI is more sensitive in detecting early disease. Treatment focuses on treating the underlying cause and restoring blood supply to the bone. Bone grafting or joint replacement may be necessary. A core decompression procedure may help in early disease, and with pain, by drilling into the inner layer of bone to help regenerate blood vessels, thereby restoring blood supply. Complications include fracture, bone collapse, joint destruction, and osteoarthritis.

SLIPPED CAPITAL FEMORAL EPIPHYSIS

A slipped capital femoral epiphysis (**SCFE**) is a condition in which the **proximal femoral growth plate** becomes unstable; early diagnosis is crucial. This can occur due to trauma causing a Salter-Harris fracture, obesity, or abnormal growth of the bone and cartilage in the growth plate itself. It is most commonly detected in children (more common in boys) from 10–16 years of age. It usually occurs unilaterally, but may occur bilaterally, especially in children under the age of 10. Also, it may start unilaterally and progress to bilateral SCFE. Patients may complain of stiffness and a limp that becomes progressively worse. Pain may occur in the hip, groin, thigh, or knee. Internal rotation of the hip is typically painful and decreased. X-rays (AP and frog-leg lateral) will show widening of the epiphyseal plate or displacement of the femoral head. If the presentation is unusual, endocrinopathies and other disorders should be ruled out. Surgical repair is necessary to correct this condition. Internal fixation of the femoral head is performed to stabilize the joint. With severe disease, the child may end up with a discrepancy in the leg lengths, which can lead to chronic limp. Another complication is avascular necrosis.

OSGOOD-SCHLATTER DISEASE

Osgood-Schlatter disease is a condition in which **microavulsion fractures** develop around the **tibial tuberosity** at the knee, causing inflammation. It usually occurs during growth spurts with repeated stress on the **patellar tendon**, such as with running and kicking, which can cause the tendon to slightly pull away at its attachment to the tibial tuberosity. In severe cases, the tendon can completely tear at its attachment point. This is most common in active children involved in sports, usually in their preadolescent and early teen years. This resolves as the growth plate matures. Patients will complain of pain in the knee at the tibial tuberosity. The pain is aggravated with running, kicking, and squatting. There is pain with palpation at the tibial tuberosity and pain with resisted knee extension, and there may be swelling, redness, and decreased range of motion of the knee. Diagnose clinically; occasionally lateral x-rays are needed. Rest (avoiding aggravating movements), NSAIDs, and ice will usually resolve the condition. Occasionally short-term immobilization may be used. This condition can last for weeks to months, so it can be frustrating to the child to limit sports activities. Surgery is usually avoided in growing children for this condition.

KNEE INJURIES

The main knee injuries include anterior (ACL) and posterior cruciate ligament (PCL), collateral ligament, and meniscal injuries. All these are more common in athletes, especially in contact sports. **ACL injuries** involve **hyperextension of the knee**, usually when stopping quickly and changing directions. Patients usually report hearing or feeling a "pop," pain, and instability of the joint. The Lachman (most sensitive), anterior drawer, or pivot shift test helps diagnose, and an MRI confirms the diagnosis. Treatment involves conservative management and (if a candidate) surgical repair.

PCL injuries are less common since the PCL is the strongest ligament of the knee; they involve hyperflexion injuries, posterior force with hyperextension, or trauma to a bent knee (e.g., falling). Patients may report instability or pain when weight-bearing on a semi-flexed knee (e.g., walking down stairs). Diagnose clinically (posterior drawer test, posterior tibial sag sign). X-rays help rule out fractures; may confirm with an MRI. Treat conservatively (RICE and PT) or with surgical repair.

Collateral ligament injuries involve the **medial collateral ligament (MCL)** when outward (varus) force is placed on the knee while **lateral collateral ligament injury (LCL)** involves inner (valgus) force. This can involve complete or partial tears or sprains of the ligament. Patients may present with pain, swelling, stiffness, and instability (if severe). Diagnose clinically (varus and valgus stress tests); x-rays or an MRI may be ordered. Treat with RICE, NSAIDs, and if severe, surgical repair.

Meniscal injuries involve the C-shaped **cartilage between the femur and tibia**. This is usually due to rotational force injuries and the medial meniscus is injured more often. Symptoms include pain, edema, and knee locking or buckling. Diagnose clinically (McMurray and Apley test); x-rays and MRI as needed. Treat with RICE and surgical repair, if needed, and PT.

FOOT AND ANKLE INJURIES AND DISORDERS

Ankle **sprains** involve the overstretching or tearing of a **ligament**, which connects 2 bones together, whereas **strains** are the stretching or tearing of a tendon/muscle. Ankles are the most common sprain site in the body and are usually due to foot inversion and involve the anterior talofibular ligament. Assess stability, rule out fracture, treat with RICE (rest, ice, compression, elevation) and NSAIDs, protect with splints or braces (casting may be necessary in severe sprains, grade 3), and refer to orthopedist.

Grades of sprains:

- Grade 1: microscopic tearing only
- Grade 2: partial tearing and moderate loss of function
- Grade 3: complete rupture, inability to bear weight, and significant instability of the joint

Degrees of strains:

- 1st degree: microscopic tearing
- 2nd degree: partial tearing
- 3rd degree: complete tear or rupture

Plantar fasciitis is pain in the **plantar fascia**, which runs along the sole of the foot, providing support in the **arch**. This is common in runners. Pain is usually more pronounced at the origin site at the medial calcaneal tuberosity, worse in the morning and later in the day. Diagnose clinically and treat with ice, NSAIDs, rest, and arch/heel cushions; avoid high-impact activities. May need steroids/night splints.

Morton neuroma involves the irritation and thickening of the **interdigital nerve** at the ball of the foot, usually between the **3rd and 4th metatarsals**. It is more common in women. This causes progressive paresthesias and intermittent sharp, burning pain. Diagnose clinically; diagnosis may be confirmed with ultrasound or MRI. Treat by modifying footwear; or possibly steroid injections or surgery.

UPPER EXTREMITY

BICIPITAL TENDINITIS

Bicipital tendinitis (**biceps tendinitis**) is inflammation of the long head of the **biceps** as it runs along the **bicipital groove of the humerus**. The biceps both flexes and supinates the arm. This is a common overuse issue, especially in athletes (particularly with throwing) and those who lift heavy objects and objects overhead. This is often associated with a rotator cuff tear or a SLAP lesion (superior labrum anterior to posterior tear). Signs and symptoms include anterior shoulder pain over the bicipital groove, aggravated with flexion and supination; and, if unstable, it may cause a "snap" during range of motion (ROM) exercises.

Diagnose clinically (the Speed test: pain with shoulder flexion against resistance, with the elbow extended and arm supinated; Yergason test: pain with forearm supination against resistance, with the elbow flexed and shoulder adducted) and use x-rays, ultrasound, and MRI as needed. Treat initially with rest, ice (for 2 days), and NSAIDs for 3–4 weeks. Next, once pain free, PT may be used to stretch, then strengthen, the shoulder. Steroid injections may be used, with careful attention not to inject into the tendon itself, as that may cause atrophy and rupture of the tendon. Occasionally surgery may be necessary; refer to orthopedist. Complications include reinjury and biceps tendon rupture.

SHOULDER TENDINITIS

Shoulder tendinitis is inflammation of one of the **tendons** in the shoulder at its **insertion**. Common tendons affected by tendinitis include the **bicipital tendon** and **supraspinatus tendon**, which is often associated with an impingement issue since it runs under the acromion. Tendinitis typically occurs due to overuse from sports or work, especially with overhead and throwing motions. This results in pain (abduction and overhead motions), inflammation, and reduced ROM. Diagnose supraspinatus tendinitis clinically; pain at the greater tuberosity, Jobe test (pain or reduced strength when downward pressure, against resistance, is applied to an abducted and internally rotated arm), and Hawkins test (checks for impingement; pain with passive internal rotation of the shoulder, with both arm and shoulder flexed to 90°). X-rays help note bony changes (e.g., calcifications, sclerotic changes due to arthritis, and fracture); then obtain MRI for detailed information. Treat with rest, ice, and NSAIDs, and as it improves, use stretching and strengthening exercises. This should improve in 3–6 months.

SHOULDER BURSITIS

Shoulder bursitis is inflammation of a **bursa**, which is a fluid-filled sac that helps reduce friction between tendons/muscles and bones. The bursas in the shoulder are the **subacromial bursa** (most common site of bursitis), **subdeltoid bursa**, and **subcoracoid bursa**. Shoulder bursitis can be caused by overuse, trauma, inflammatory arthritis (e.g., gout, RA), or infection. Symptoms may include pain, swelling, erythema, and reduced ROM, especially with abduction. Diagnosis is usually clinical but may need an ultrasound or MRI.

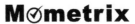

Aspirate bursa and study fluid if infection, inflammatory arthritis, or hemorrhage is suspected. Treat primarily with rest, ice, and NSAIDs; occasionally steroid injections around the bursa, or surgery, are needed.

ROTATOR CUFF TEAR

A rotator cuff tear involves an injury to one of the muscles that insert into the **shoulder (glenohumeral) joint** that help stabilize the humerus; it can be a partial or complete tear. The rotator cuff consists of the **supraspinatus** (most common tendon tear; used in abduction), **infraspinatus** (external rotation), **teres minor** (external rotation), and **subscapularis** (internal rotation) muscles. This may occur acutely or insidiously, or may be due to age (often affects those >40). Symptoms depend on the location of the tear and include pain (often at night), weakness, and reduced ROM. Diagnose clinically as follows. For supraspinatus and infraspinatus, use Jobe or Neer test; for teres minor, use Hornblower sign, which indicates a major rotator cuff tear; for subscapularis, use the lift-off test (patient places hand flat against back and tries to lift it away from back). MRI (best) and ultrasound may be used to evaluate the tear, and x-rays rule out changes in the bone (e.g., fracture, arthritis). Initially treat conservatively with rest, ice, and NSAIDs. Then work on restoring ROM with stretching and strengthening exercises. Steroid injections and surgery may be needed.

SHOULDER DISLOCATION

Shoulder dislocations occur when the **humeral head** separates from the **glenoid fossa**, usually anteriorly. This can occur due to a fall on an outstretched arm or other trauma. The acromion is prominent, and the patient does not want to move the arm. If anteriorly dislocated, the arm is held in slight abduction with external rotation. If posteriorly dislocated, the arm is held in an adducted and internally rotated position. Assess that nerves and blood vessels are intact. Order AP, axillary, and possibly Y-view x-rays. Treat with reduction, then immobilization (sling and swathed) for 1–3 weeks.

INFECTIOUS DISEASES

SEPTIC ARTHRITIS

Septic arthritis is an infection in a **joint**—most commonly the **knee**, though other joints may be affected. It is important to diagnose quickly since joint destruction can occur within 48 hours of the start of the infection. This is usually due to bacteria that have spread to the joint, but it can also be caused by a virus or fungus. The most common **bacterial causes** are *Staphylococcus aureus* (most common in ages <2 and >55) or *Neisseria gonorrhoeae* (most common in younger, sexually active adults). Patients at increased risk of developing septic arthritis include those with chronic illnesses (e.g., rheumatoid arthritis, DM), prosthetic joints, IV drug users, and those at risk of STDs. Patients will complain of acute onset of significant pain in the affected joint, fever, and reduced ROM, and the joint will appear red, swollen, hot, and very tender to the touch. Patients may or may not be aware of a recent bacterial infection elsewhere in their body.

Diagnose with arthrocentesis; consult orthopedist. Arthrocentesis with culture and sensitivity, blood cultures ×2, and STD testing should be performed before empiric antibiotics are started (follow local sensitivity patterns). Synovial fluid may show purulent discharge with elevated WBCs. Treatment is with IV antibiotics started at the time of diagnosis, followed by a course of oral antibiotics for a total of 2–4 weeks. Joint aspiration is usually necessary, and if the condition is severe, surgery may be needed (rarely) to drain and clean the joint. The primary complications are joint destruction and chronic arthritis.

OSTEOMYELITIS

Osteomyelitis is inflammation and destruction of the **bone** caused by an **infection** (usually bacterial). It may be acute or chronic. The most common **pathogen** is *Staphylococcus aureus*; the **lower extremities** are the most common site. Osteomyelitis may occur due to trauma (especially open wounds) or surgery, or may be blood-borne. Those at increased risk include those with DM or vascular insufficiency, or who are immunocompromised. Patients usually present with local pain, swelling, and erythema, and may have a fever. Diagnose clinically and confirm with x-rays (takes about 2 weeks to be visible on x-ray; periosteal thickening, soft tissue swelling, and bone loss may be noted), MRI, or bone scan. Blood cultures and bone biopsy with culture and sensitivity may be performed before antibiotics are begun. Treat with IV and oral antibiotics for 4–

145

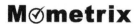

6 weeks following local empiric antibiotic susceptibility trends, and then (if necessary) change to follow culture and sensitivity results. Surgery may be performed to debride necrotic tissue and to remove areas of infection, including any fistulas or sinus tracts that may have formed in chronic cases.

DEGENERATIVE

OSTEOARTHRITIS

Osteoarthritis (**OA**) is a very common condition that occurs due to overuse of the joints. It is characterized by a wearing down of the cartilage and other structures within the joints and is a gradually progressive condition. It usually affects those >50 years old and commonly occurs in the hands (distal interphalangeal, proximal interphalangeal, and joint at base of thumb) and large weight-bearing joints, such as the hips and knees; but it can affect any joint in the body. Patients may note a gradual onset of a deep, aching pain in the affected joint, especially with activity, and may note joint stiffness in the morning or with inactivity that is relieved within 30 minutes with movement. There may be swelling in the joint, and osteophytes may be noted: Heberden nodes in the distal interphalangeal joints and Bouchard nodes in the proximal interphalangeal joints. On exam, crepitus can be felt with flexion and extension of the joint, and reduced ROM may be observed.

X-rays (gold standard) may show joint space narrowing due to worn-down cartilage, sclerosis, and marginal osteophytes. Treatment includes acetaminophen and rest of the affected joint, heat, or ice when it is painful; NSAIDs may be used if acetaminophen is not helpful. Exercise should still be performed, but not to the point that pain occurs. Physical therapy may help with muscle strengthening, and exercises that decrease the stress on joints, as well as weight loss, can be helpful. When OA is severe, surgery may be necessary to clean up or replace the joint.

RHEUMATOLOGIC DISORDERS

FIBROMYALGIA

Fibromyalgia is a chronic **neurosensory disorder** in which patients feel fatigued and have pain "all over," sleep disturbances, and memory difficulties. This condition affects the muscles and tendons. The cause of fibromyalgia is not fully understood, but it is believed to be a condition in which the body's **central nervous system** becomes hypersensitive to **peripheral stimuli**. This typically affects women more than men and appears in their 20s to 50s. Patients complain of chronic fatigue accompanied by tenderness or pain (must be continuous for >3 months) along with stiffness that is widespread. Signs of depression, difficulty sleeping, and concentration/memory problems may also be present. Many fibromyalgia patients also suffer from IBS and chronic headaches. Other disease processes like RA, SLE, hypothyroidism, and autoimmune disorders should be ruled out as the cause of the pain, but these diseases may be concomitant.

Patients may be diagnosed with fibromyalgia if the widespread pain index (WPI) is ≥7 and the symptom severity scale (SS scale) is ≥5 (or WPI 3–6 and SS scale ≥9), symptoms have been present for ≥3 months, and another disorder doesn't explain the pain. Tender points may be assessed during the PE. Treatment consists of non-opioid analgesics (e.g., tramadol, acetaminophen), tricyclic antidepressants, anti-anxiety drugs, and anticonvulsants. Currently, three drugs are approved for treating fibromyalgia: Lyrica (pregabalin), an anti-seizure medication; Cymbalta (duloxetine), a serotonin-norepinephrine reuptake inhibitor (SNRI); and Savella (milnacipran), an SNRI. Also, a healthy diet, exercise, stress management, sleep therapy, and psychotherapy can help.

GOUT AND PSEUDOGOUT

Gout occurs when there is increased **uric acid** in the blood, leading to urate crystals settling in a **joint**. Gout can be due to excess consumption of foods high in **purine** (e.g., asparagus, liver/kidneys, beer), reduced excretion by the kidneys, or elevated production of uric acid. It is more common in men and usually affects the big toe MTP joint but can occur in other joints. Patients complain of a sudden onset of severe pain, swelling, and erythema in the affected joint; even light pressure causes significant pain. Sometimes fever and chills are present. Diagnose clinically and with serum uric acid (>6.8 mg/dL) and synovial fluid analysis. Treat acute attacks with NSAIDs (indomethacin), colchicine (if tolerated), and steroids. Allopurinol can be taken regularly

146

for prevention of acute episodes and for chronic gout. Allopurinol reduces production of uric acid; the goal is a level <6 mg/dL. Patients should also be counseled on dietary changes to lower intake of purine-rich foods. Complications include gouty arthritis, tophi formation, and uric acid kidney stones.

Pseudogout is very similar to gout, except the causative agent is deposition of **calcium pyrophosphate dihydrate crystals (CPPD)** within a joint. It affects men and women equally, may be associated with OA, has a genetic component, and is self-limited (usually 10–14 days). The most common joints affected by pseudogout are the knees, but it can occur in other, often large, joints. Patients complain of an insidious onset of severe pain in the affected joint (takes days vs. hours), which appears red and swollen and is extremely tender on PE; fever may be present. Diagnose by examining the synovial fluid and x-rays. Treatment includes NSAIDs, colchicine (may cause several GI side effects; may not be well tolerated), and steroids. Maintenance therapy with colchicine may help reduce the number of acute attacks of pseudogout. Aspiration of the joint fluid can be performed to relieve pressure on the joint and help to reduce pain.

POLYARTERITIS NODOSA

Polyarteritis nodosa (PAN) is a systemic **vasculitis** in which necrotizing inflammation and damage occurs in the small and medium-sized **arteries**. This can occur anywhere within the body, but it most often affects the kidneys, intestines, skin, peripheral nerves, muscles, and joints; the lungs are usually not affected. It has no known definite cause, but it is often seen in patients who have been diagnosed with hepatitis B and sometimes hepatitis C. Patients may present acutely or may have an insidious onset, and it may affect one organ or many. Patients usually present with pain in the area that is affected by the arterial inflammation, fever, fatigue, weight loss, and weakness. If the damage is severe, there can be ischemia and infarcts of the bowel, kidney, or other affected organs. There can be asymmetric peripheral neuropathy if the peripheral nervous system is affected, hypertension if kidneys are affected, and if the skin is affected, ulcers, nodules, mottled skin, rashes, and purpura/cutaneous infarcts may be present. Diagnose with a tissue biopsy, which shows necrotizing vasculitis, and possibly with angiography. Treatment involves immunosuppression with corticosteroids (prednisone) and sometimes adding cyclophosphamide (not in hepatitis B cases). If patients have hepatitis B, appropriate therapy should be started to treat this condition. If polyarteritis nodosa is severe and tissue death has occurred, surgery is performed to remove the damaged tissue and make repairs. Refer these patients to general surgery.

OSTEOPOROSIS

Osteoporosis is a **metabolic bone disease** in which there is a decrease in the **bone mineral density (BMD)**. It may be classified as **primary** (postmenopausal, type I; or age-related/senile, type II) or **secondary osteoporosis** (e.g., due to cancer, hyperparathyroidism, steroid use). Type I involves mainly **trabecular bone loss** and type II involves mainly **cortical bone loss**. Osteoporosis is more common in Caucasians and more common in women than men; it is usually due to postmenopausal causes. **Estrogen** is thought to be bone-protective, and with the decrease in estrogen levels after menopause, the bones may begin to weaken. Other risk factors include smoking and alcohol use, medications (such as chronic steroid or heparin use), hormonal imbalance (such as hyperparathyroidism), reduced calcium intake, inactivity, and hypogonadal states. Patients may suffer an osteoporotic fracture, such as a compression fracture, as a result of little or no trauma.

Patients are asymptomatic until a fracture occurs; therefore, screening is vital. Screen all women ≥65 years old and all men ≥70 years old; screen earlier if risk factors are present. A DXA (dual-energy x-ray absorptiometry) bone mineral density scan of the hip or lumbar spine will show a bone density T-score of at least –2.5 standard deviations below the value of peak BMD. If a child, premenopausal, or a man <50 years old, then for diagnosis, use a Z-score ≤–2.0 standard deviations below the BMD that is expected for their age and sex. The FRAX tool can help identify those at increased risk of developing osteoporosis. Treatment includes weight-bearing exercise, modifying risk factors, and calcium and vitamin D supplementation. Also, bisphosphonates for up to 5 years (Fosamax, Boniva, Actonel; first-line) and calcitonin (which reduces bone reabsorption), or other newer medications (like denosumab) may be used for osteoporosis.

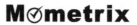

POLYMYALGIA RHEUMATICA

Polymyalgia rheumatica is a condition in which patients experience **proximal muscle stiffness** and severe pain, usually in the shoulders, hips, and neck. It is more common in adults over the age of 50 and two times more prevalent in women than men. The cause is unknown, but it may be an autoimmune disorder, it may have a trigger, and it is related to giant cell arteritis. It is self-limited but may last 3–5 years or more.

Polymyalgia rheumatica can have an insidious onset or occur very quickly. As the disease progresses, it will affect both sides equally, but may begin in a unilateral distribution. Patients typically complain of bilateral and symmetric muscle pain and stiffness in various proximal locations of the body (back, neck, shoulders, hips), especially first thing in the morning (may last ≥1 hour) and with inactivity. Patients may have bursitis and tenosynovitis. Patients may have a generalized feeling of malaise, fever, weight loss, and fatigue. Patients typically have normal muscle strength but a decreased ROM due to the pain. Diagnose clinically; ESR may be ≥40 mm/hr with elevated CRP, and anemia may be present on CBC; rule out other causes and rule out giant cell arteritis. Treatment is long-term corticosteroids, and patients may require 1–2 years of treatment; taper slowly. Patients should be closely monitored and counseled on the risks of long-term steroid use; refer to a rheumatologist.

POLYMYOSITIS

Polymyositis is an **inflammatory myopathy** in which chronic inflammation, degeneration, and weakness occurs in the **muscles**. It most commonly affects the muscles in the proximal large joints, such as shoulders and hips, and is gradually progressive. A definite cause is not known, but it may be due to an autoimmune reaction. This usually affects those >30 years old and is more common in women (2:1) and in the black population. Patients may complain of a slow progression of symmetric muscle weakness and sometimes pain. This is commonly present in the shoulders and arms, and patients will experience a sensation of fatigue after even light activity. Patients may have morning stiffness, arthralgias, progressive dysphagia, SOB, fever, and weight loss. Unlike dermatomyositis, polymyositis is not associated with a rash.

Diagnose with a muscle biopsy; creatine kinase is typically elevated. First-line treatment for polymyositis involves corticosteroids (prednisone), along with physical therapy. Medications that work by suppressing the immune system (e.g., azathioprine, methotrexate, and IVIG) can be used, especially in patients who don't respond to steroids. Complications of polymyositis include possible pneumonia due to decreased chest wall muscle expansion, and aspiration pneumonia due to dysphagia; it is also associated with malignancy.

RHEUMATOID ARTHRITIS

Rheumatoid arthritis (**RA**) is a chronic, progressive autoimmune disease that affects the **synovial linings of the joints**. The body's **white blood cells** attack this synovial lining and destroy it, leading to deformity and destruction of the joint. It is usually diagnosed in middle age and is more likely to occur in females than males. Patients typically start with fever, malaise, weakness, morning stiffness, and arthralgias, followed by a gradual progression of symmetric inflammation, erythema, and joint pain that generally starts in the small joints of the hands, wrists, and feet, which may eventually spread to include the larger joints of the body. Swan-neck and Boutonnière deformities of the fingers, as well as subcutaneous nodules (a later finding), may be present. There is decreased movement/ROM as the disease progresses.

Diagnose clinically (>6 weeks of typical symptoms; multiple joint involvement), with x-rays, elevated rheumatoid factor (RF), elevated anti-cyclic citrullinated peptide (anti-CCP), elevated ESR, and elevated CRP. There is no cure for rheumatoid arthritis, but the disease process can be slowed, and pain symptoms can be managed. Disease-modifying antirheumatic drugs (DMARDs) like methotrexate (first-line) or sulfasalazine are started at diagnosis to help slow the progress and damage caused by the disease. NSAIDs and steroids can help with pain relief as the patient waits for DMARDs to become effective. Some biologic DMARDs, such as the immunomodulator abatacept (Orencia) or the TNF-α inhibitor etanercept (Enbrel), can help reduce damage, control symptoms, and increase function. In severe cases, joint replacement surgery may be necessary.

JUVENILE IDIOPATHIC ARTHRITIS (JUVENILE RHEUMATOID ARTHRITIS)

Juvenile idiopathic arthritis (**JIA**), or juvenile rheumatoid arthritis, is a chronic arthritic disease affecting children <16 years old causing **joint inflammation and pain** for >6 weeks. JIA may be **pauciarticular** (≤4 joints), **polyarticular** (>4 joints), or **systemic** (spike fevers at predictable times, rash, hepatosplenomegaly). It may affect large or small joints and may be asymmetric or symmetric. JIA also may be associated with uveitis or psoriasis. The cause is unknown, but there is a **genetic and autoimmune component**. Patients typically present with a limp with either an abrupt or insidious onset. Other signs and symptoms may include morning stiffness, joint inflammation and warmth, guarding, pain, reduced ROM, and possibly systemic symptoms (e.g., fever, lymphadenopathy, rash).

Diagnosis is made with clinical criteria. X-rays or MRI, as well as RF (may be positive or negative), ANA (if positive, rule out SLE), anti-CCP (may be positive or negative), and CBC tests may be used to help confirm JIA and rule out other disorders. Be careful to rule out acute lymphocytic leukemia, septic arthritis, and postinfectious arthritis, as these may have similar presentations. Patients start treatment with an NSAID, which helps with the pain; intra-articular steroid injections also help treat the inflammation and pain in active disease. Disease-modifying antirheumatic drugs (DMARDs; e.g., methotrexate) may be added to slow the progression of the disease; the goal is complete remission. Patient care involves a team approach.

REACTIVE ARTHRITIS

Reactive arthritis (previously Reiter syndrome) is a collection of three conditions: **arthritis**, **conjunctivitis**, and **urinary tract symptoms** (urethritis); it is more common in young adult males. This condition is called reactive arthritis because it can occur in response to an **infection** (usually due to an STD or GI infection) somewhere in the body. The most common predisposing infection is *Chlamydia*; however, the bacteria *Salmonella*, *Shigella*, and *Campylobacter jejuni* may also cause reactive arthritis. Symptoms usually appear 1–4 weeks following the infection. Along with the triad of symptoms, patients may present with an acute onset of fever, fatigue, arthralgias, myalgias, or skin lesions or ulcers, and may have sausage-shaped fingers or toes. Arthritis primarily affects the large joints in the lower extremities and spine (low back pain). Sacroiliitis and spondylitis of the spine are common. Conjunctivitis and uveitis also may occur. Patients may have complaints of dysuria, urinary frequency, discharge, and (in men) prostatitis. Diagnose clinically. Treat symptoms. NSAIDs and corticosteroid injections can be helpful. If there is an active infection, appropriate antibiotics should be given. Refer to or consult a rheumatologist, an ophthalmologist if uveitis is present, and a cardiologist if the heart is affected. This becomes chronic in 30% of patients.

SJÖGREN SYNDROME

Sjögren syndrome is a chronic autoimmune disorder causing **dry eyes and mouth**. It is often seen with other types of connective tissue disorders (e.g., SLE, RA) and is much more common in women >50 years old. It is not known what causes Sjögren syndrome, though it is suspected that hereditary factors may play a part, and there may also be a link with viral infections being a trigger. Although the primary symptoms seen with Sjögren are dry eyes and a dry mouth, it may also affect almost any area of the body, including the lungs, kidneys, liver, joints, nervous system, and skin. Patients may complain of dry eyes, dry mouth, dry nasal passages, dry skin and pruritus, vaginal dryness, parotid enlargement, a dry cough, difficulty swallowing, and arthralgias. Since it is commonly seen in conjunction with other connective tissue disorders, symptoms of those accompanying diseases may also be present.

Diagnose clinically; may be supported with a positive ANA, a positive anti-SSA/Ro, a positive anti-SSB/La, or a positive RF. Topical gels and artificial tears can help with the dry eyes, and saliva production may be increased through chewing gum and/or using lozenges. Systemic medications to treat the symptoms include corticosteroids and immunosuppressants, especially if another connective tissue disorder is present. If dry eyes are severe, surgery can be performed to block small openings in the eyelids that drain tears from the eyes, thereby retaining moisture within the eyes. Complications include dental caries, eye infections, and an increased risk of lymphoma.

SYSTEMIC LUPUS ERYTHEMATOSUS (SLE)

Systemic lupus erythematosus (**SLE**), or lupus, is a **chronic inflammatory condition** with periods of remittance and flares in which the body's **immune system** turns against itself and begins attacking organs and tissues. It is primarily known to affect the skin, joints, kidneys, heart, nerves, and blood cells. This affects young women much more than men, and in the US appears more often in African Americans and Asians. There is no definite known cause of SLE, but genetic and environmental factors (e.g., sun exposure, medications) play a role in the development of this autoimmune disease. Patients may present with fever, fatigue, arthralgias, myalgias, a discoid rash, a photosensitive rash, or the typical malar rash (butterfly) across the nose and cheeks. Oral ulcers, serositis (e.g., pericarditis, pleuritis), Raynaud phenomenon, and renal (e.g., proteinuria) and neurologic disorders (e.g., depression) may also be present.

Diagnose clinically and by confirming the presence of autoantibodies and other lab criteria (e.g., positive ANA, anemia, proteinuria, positive renal biopsy for lupus nephritis). Patients must meet 4 of the 11 ACR criteria, or 4 of the 17 SLICC classification criteria, to be diagnosed with SLE. There is no known cure for SLE, but the symptoms can usually be controlled. Start the antimalarial hydroxychloroquine in patients with SLE to help decrease flares and mortality. NSAIDs and corticosteroids can help to decrease inflammation during an acute flare-up. Immunosuppressant medications (e.g., cyclophosphamide, azathioprine) may also be helpful in decreasing the symptoms in severe disease. Consult or refer patients to specialists as needed.

SYSTEMIC SCLEROSIS (SCLERODERMA)

Systemic sclerosis (scleroderma) is a chronic condition in which **fibrosis** (hardening) of the skin and connective tissues occurs due to excessive **collagen deposits**. This can be localized, limited (CREST syndrome), or diffuse and may become progressively worse and lead to involvement of the organs, like the GI tract, heart, lungs, and kidneys. There is no definite known cause of systemic sclerosis, but it is an **autoimmune connective tissue disorder**. It is more common in women and in those 20–60 years old. Risk of developing systemic sclerosis is increased in those with silica or solvent/chemical exposure. Patients may complain of whitish fingers or toes with exposure to cold (Raynaud's phenomenon), telangiectasias, puffy digits, and areas of tight, thickened, or hardened skin that will not go away, usually in the fingers, toes, or face. As the condition progresses, the skin becomes stiffer, range of motion (especially of the distal limbs/digits) decreases, and weakness develops. Scleroderma can even affect organs, such as the esophagus and stomach, leading to dysphagia and reduced gastric motility. If it affects the kidneys, it may result in renal failure.

Diagnose clinically and support with presence of autoantibodies (e.g., positive ANA, positive RF). Treatment is symptomatic; discontinue smoking. Topical medications and creams may help with the involved skin. NSAIDs and corticosteroids may help with pain as stiffness occurs. Medications to improve circulation (calcium channel blockers) can help, as can immunosuppressants, to decrease the symptoms and progression of this disease. Complications include contractures, distal ulcers, renal failure, and pulmonary hypertension.

SPINAL DISORDERS

ANKYLOSING SPONDYLITIS

Ankylosing spondylitis is a chronic systemic inflammatory form of **arthritis** involving the places where **ligaments and tendons** attach to bone (entheses), usually in the **vertebral column and the sacroiliac joints** (spondyloarthropathy). This inflammation causes **bony overgrowth**, especially in the spine, and may lead to fusion of the **vertebral bodies**. When it occurs at the joints of the ribs and spine, mobility of the rib cage can be affected, restricting respirations. Other systems that may be involved include the eyes, heart, lungs, kidneys, and GI tract. This has a genetic predisposition (HLA-B27) and is more common in men and in those in their late teens to 40 years old. Patients typically complain of fatigue and of pain and stiffness in the affected joints (usually back and SI joints) that's worse in the morning and with inactivity. The pain may occur at night and improves with exercise but not with rest. Ankylosing spondylitis may lead to kyphosis and possibly depressed respirations. Uveitis (or iritis) and inflammatory bowel disease may also be seen with this.

Diagnose clinically (pain ≥3 months and onset ≤40 years old) and by documenting SI joint involvement (sacroiliitis) on x-ray. X-rays may also show erosions with sclerosis, narrowing, or bony fusion ("bamboo spine") in the vertebral column. Blood testing includes CRP, ESR, and CBC, but these are nonspecific. Treatment includes anti-inflammatory drugs (NSAIDs are first-line), and steroid injections may be necessary to decrease inflammation. DMARDs and biologics are used second-line and may help to decrease symptoms. PT is helpful, and surgery may be needed to stabilize joints.

CAUDA EQUINA SYNDROME

Cauda equina syndrome is a condition in which there is severe compression of the **nerve roots** that exit the spinal cord below its termination at **L1** (which resemble a horse's tail). This can cause permanent **neurologic disabilities** and is a medical emergency. It is usually caused by an **acute herniated nucleus pulposus** (herniated disk); or it may be caused by compression from a **tumor**, or can occur due to **progressive degenerative changes** causing severe spinal stenosis in the lower lumbar spine. Patients usually have low back pain with pain radiating into one or both of the lower extremities. There will be saddle anesthesia present, along with bowel and bladder retention or incontinence (all red flags). The lower extremities are numb and/or weak and have depressed or absent reflexes. Diagnose with an MRI and refer immediately to neurosurgery. Treatment of cauda equina syndrome is urgent surgical intervention within 24–48 hours of severe symptom onset. If treated promptly, there is a chance that patients' symptoms will be reversed. The longer the symptoms are present, however, the less likely that patients will reach a full recovery. Steroids can be started to reduce the inflammation, but this is usually only until surgery is performed.

SPINAL STENOSIS

Spinal stenosis occurs when there is narrowing of the spinal canal or neural foramen, causing compression of the **spinal cord or nerve roots**. This most often affects the **cervical and lumbar spine**. Spinal stenosis is most often degenerative in nature (e.g., osteoarthritis, bone spurs) and therefore usually affects those >50 years old; however, there is an increased risk of developing this if there is congenital narrowing of the spinal column, and it may occur along with disk herniation or spondylolisthesis (slipping of the vertebrae). Patients typically complain of chronic pain in the affected portion of the spine and may have radiating pain, numbness, and/or weakness extending into the upper or lower extremities, depending on the stenosis location. With myelopathy (spinal cord injury), there will be profound weakness and hyperactive reflexes/spasticity.

Symptoms of neurogenic claudication (which is due to lumbar spinal stenosis) include pain that is aggravated with walking (especially downhill) and standing and is usually relieved with sitting and leaning forward. Severe lumbar spinal stenosis can cause cauda equina syndrome. Diagnose with an MRI (preferred) or CT/CT myelography, which shows narrowing of the canal. Symptoms may be slightly relieved with NSAIDs (first-line), pain relievers, antispasmodics, and epidural steroid injections, along with PT. Surgical correction in those with more severe symptoms (neurogenic claudication, radiculopathy, myelopathy) can be performed with a laminectomy or X-Stop procedure that relieves the pressure being applied to the spinal canal; refer to neurosurgery.

HERNIATED NUCLEUS PULPOSUS (HERNIATED DISK)

A herniated nucleus pulposus (herniated disk) occurs when the softer interior of the **intervertebral fibrocartilage** herniates through the outer fibrous material that surrounds the **nucleus pulposus**. This can occur anywhere in the spinal column but is most often seen in the **lumbar spine**. The disk can bulge in one direction or may be central. If this occurs above the level of L1, there is a risk of **spinal cord compression**. Herniated disks are seen more often in those with heavy-lifting jobs, and incidence increases with age. Patients may be asymptomatic or complain of pain at the level of the spine where the herniation occurs, along with radicular pain following the dermatome of the affected nerve. For example, if the herniation occurs at L5-S1, patients may complain of sciatic-type pain. Patients may develop numbness or tingling in the affected dermatome, along with weakness of the affected limb.

Assess strength and ROM, and thoroughly check for an intact neurologic system. Diagnose with MRI or CT. Patients may be managed conservatively with NSAIDs and pain relievers. Often, the symptoms will resolve with conservative treatment. Physical therapy to help with pain relief and stretching and strengthening can help. Steroids, either orally or per epidural injection, can help to reduce the inflammation. If neural deficits or signs of structural instability, refer to neurosurgery. Surgery may be performed with a microdiscectomy to remove the portion of the disk that has herniated.

LOW BACK SPRAINS AND STRAINS

Low back injuries and pain are a common presenting complaint of patients. A **sprain** is an injury to a **ligament** (connects bone to bone), and a **strain** is an injury to a **muscle or tendon** (connects muscle to bone). This often occurs due to sports and in those whose jobs require heavy lifting. The L4-L5 and L5-S1 are the most frequent locations of injury; however, injuries may occur anywhere along the back. **Back strains** are more common, and this is often caused by overuse or by a twisting motion while applying a force/muscle contraction (mechanical injuries).

Patients usually present with a history of the injury event, localized muscle/tendon/ligament pain on palpation, and increased pain with movement, and may have some radiating pain, muscle spasm, and reduced ROM. Red flags that may indicate other issues include fever or other systemic symptoms, midline vertebral pain, a positive straight leg raise test (may indicate sciatica/nerve root compression or a herniated nucleus pulposus), significant muscle weakness or paresthesias, sensory deficits, saddle anesthesia, bladder and bowel retention or incontinence, nocturnal pain, and a history of osteoporosis or cancer. Diagnose clinically and reserve imaging studies for those with red flags or if it is chronic (most patients heal within 6 weeks). Treat symptoms with rest and ice (for first 2 days), NSAIDs, and possibly muscle relaxants. After the acute phase, begin ROM and strengthening exercises. Educate patients in proper back safety and lifting techniques, and lumbosacral muscle corsets may be recommended.

SCOLIOSIS

Scoliosis is abnormal lateral curvature (≥10°) of the **spine** in an S or C shape. It can be classified as **infantile** (<3 years old), **juvenile** (3–10 years old), or **adolescent** (>10 years old). The cause is typically unknown, but it may have a genetic component and is more common in girls. It usually has an insidious onset in late childhood or early teen years when **growth spurts** are common. This is often first noted in a routine physical or by a school nurse during screening (Adams forward bend test), but asymmetry of the shoulders (right is usually higher), protruding scapula, uneven ribs, or ill-fitting clothes may be noted by a caregiver. Diagnose with AP and lateral x-rays showing a Cobb angle measurement ≥10°. If the Cobb angle is 10–19°, reevaluate every 6 months. Refer patients once it reaches ≥20°, and braces may be used at this point. Surgery is not usually used until >40°.

KYPHOSIS

Kyphosis is an abnormal forward curvature of the **thoracic spine** (≥50°) causing a "hunchback" appearance. Kyphosis has many possible causes but is most common in older women due to **osteoporosis** (compression fractures). **Scheuermann kyphosis** appears in adolescence and is slightly more common in boys. Patients may present with back pain; the curvature does not correct with hyperextension of the back, and patients may be cosmetically bothered by the curvature. Diagnose with posterior-anterior (PA) and lateral x-rays of the spine showing a Cobb angle ≥50°. Treat symptoms as needed (NSAIDs), treat underlying osteoporosis, and PT and bracing may be helpful. Surgery is usually reserved for more severe cases where curvature is >65–75° or if neurologic deficits are present.

NEOPLASMS

GANGLION CYST

Ganglion cysts, also referred to as **Bible cysts**, are soft-tissue cysts that are usually associated with **tendon sheaths and joint capsules**. This condition is more common in women (3:1) and is most often located on the **dorsal wrist**. It can also be found on the palmar (volar) side of the wrist, or in the finger, knee, ankle, or toe joints. It may appear gradually or rapidly and is most often accompanied by pain that worsens with joint use, and the lump may grow more prominent when the joint is engaged. The average size is 1 to 3 cm, which may fluctuate with time, and it is usually a solitary mass. The mass is soft and movable, and will transilluminate. Diagnose clinically. Ultrasound can also be useful in determining the makeup of the cyst. If not painful or interfering with function, no treatment is necessary, as the cyst may resolve on its own. Thick, clear fluid can be aspirated from the cyst to help relieve symptoms. If the cyst is problematic, surgical excision may be needed for some, but recurrence is common.

OSTEOSARCOMA

Osteosarcoma is a type of **bone cancer** that usually occurs in the **metaphyseal region of long bones** as they are growing. It is most often found at the distal femur, proximal tibia, and proximal humerus. It commonly affects children and young adults 10–20 years of age. Some hereditary diseases, such as hereditary retinoblastoma and bone dysplasia, may cause children to be more susceptible to developing osteosarcoma; and exposure of bone to high doses of radiation can also increase the risk of this disease. However, osteosarcoma will often occur without any known cause. Patients typically complain of bone pain that may have been present for months; they may have nocturnal pain, there is usually swelling at the site of the cancer, and muscle atrophy may be present. This condition may be mistaken for an injury or growing pains.

Systemic symptoms like fever and fatigue are uncommon. X-rays may show Codman triangle (a triangular area caused by the periosteum being lifted away), a sunburst lesion, or lytic lesions. This is followed by an MRI for staging and is then diagnosed with a bone biopsy. Treatment for osteosarcoma is surgery to remove the affected portion of the bone and chemotherapy (may also be given before surgery). In some cases, the cancer spreads to other organs of the body, especially the lungs. Refer to an orthopedic surgeon.

Neurologic System

CRANIAL NERVES

There are 12 pairs of cranial nerves that should be evaluated during a neurologic exam:

Nerve	Name	Function	PE Test
I	Olfactory	Smell	Test olfaction
II	Optic	Visual acuity	Snellen eye chart; accommodation
III	Oculomotor	Eye movement/pupil	Pupillary reflex; eye/eyelid motion
IV	Trochlear	Eye movement	Eye moves down & out
V	Trigeminal	Facial motor/sensory	Corneal reflex; facial sensation; mastication
VI	Abducens	Eye movement	Lateral eye motion
VII	Facial	Facial expression; taste	Moves forehead, closes eyes, smile/frown, puffs cheeks; taste
VIII	Vestibulocochlear (acoustic)	Hearing; balance	Hearing (Weber/Rinne tests); nystagmus
IX	Glossopharyngeal	Pharynx motor/sensory	Gag reflex; soft palate elevation
X	Vagus	Visceral sensory, motor	Gag, swallow, cough
XI	Accessory	Sternocleidomastoid & trapezius (motor)	Turns head & shrugs shoulders against resistance
XII	Hypoglossal	Tongue movement	Sticks out tongue

CLOSED HEAD INJURIES

CONCUSSION AND POST-CONCUSSION SYNDROME

Concussion is a mild **traumatic brain injury** that causes a disturbance in brain function. This commonly results from **sports injuries**. Signs and symptoms may include headache, dizziness, visual disturbances, light and noise sensitivities, confusion, amnesia (retrograde or antegrade), issues with concentration, loss of consciousness (only present in about 10%), emotional changes, nausea/vomiting, and balance or coordination issues. Persistent vomiting may be a sign of increased intracranial pressure and should be investigated further. Athletes should be immediately removed from play and should not return until cleared medically. Diagnose clinically, and possibly use imaging to rule out other injuries. Order a CT if loss of consciousness, a focal neurologic deficit, signs or symptoms of ICP, or Glasgow coma scale <15.

Post-concussion syndrome involves continued symptoms from the **concussion** and may persist for days, weeks, or months after the injury. This usually resolves but may become permanent. Signs and symptoms include chronic headaches, continued light and noise sensitivities, sleep disturbances, fatigue, personality changes (being more emotional or irritable), concentration issues, and short-term memory deficits. Diagnose clinically and treat with supportive care. Patients with repeated concussions (especially boxers and football players) are at an increased risk of developing **chronic traumatic encephalopathy**, which may not present until years after the last concussion. This causes progressive degenerative changes in the brain, which may manifest as mood/behavior issues, dementia, and motor dysfunction.

TRAUMATIC BRAIN INJURY AND INTRACRANIAL HEMORRHAGE

Traumatic brain injury (**TBI**) is an injury caused by external forces that may cause temporary or permanent **brain impairment**. TBI may occur from a variety of causes, including falls, motor vehicle accidents (MVAs) or other crashes, sports injuries, or gunshots/assaults. Helmet wearing, seatbelts, and child safety seats have helped reduce the incidence of TBI, but this continues to be a common cause of morbidity and mortality. This may be an open or closed head injury. Those with moderate and severe injuries may present with seizures or dilated pupils, and may be unresponsive. Increased intracranial pressure can cause what is known as the **Cushing triad**: hypertension, bradycardia, and irregular respirations.

Basilar skull fractures should be suspected if rhinorrhea (possible CSF), the Battle sign (postauricular ecchymosis), raccoon eyes (orbital ecchymosis), or hemotympanum. **Subdural hematomas** result from a venous bleed and may have symptoms that rapidly progress, or may have a more insidious onset, especially if chronic. **Epidural hematoma** patients often have loss of consciousness, then a period of lucidity, then rapid deterioration. **Subarachnoid hemorrhages** usually present with a severe "thunderclap" headache with nausea/vomiting and altered consciousness. Assess Glasgow coma scale within 48 hours of the injury: eye opening (1–4 points); verbal response (1–5 points); motor response (1–6 points). Mild TBI: 13–15; moderate TBI: 9–12; severe TBI: 3–8. Evaluation and treatment involve ABC management to stabilize the patient, a Glasgow coma scale, and obtaining a head CT. Mannitol may be used to help reduce ICP. Admit and refer to neurology or neurosurgery as needed.

HEADACHES

CLUSTER HEADACHES

Cluster headaches are a type of **trigeminal-autonomic cephalgia** (TAC) that are characterized by periods of severe unilateral orbital/periorbital or temporal pain with ipsilateral autonomic symptoms (e.g., lacrimation or conjunctival injection, rhinorrhea, miosis, ptosis) that occur frequently, perhaps for a few days or months, and then go into remission without headaches for a period of time. They can be classified as **episodic** (last 7 days to 1 year, with pain-free periods lasting ≥3 months) or **chronic** (last ≥1 year, without remissions or with remissions <3 months). There is no definite known cause of cluster headaches, though dysfunction of the **hypothalamus** may play a role. They are more common in males over 30 years old who are heavy drinkers and smokers. Cluster headache triggers may also include nitroglycerine, temperature extremes, and histamine.

These headaches last for 15–180 minutes and may recur from 8 times a day to every other day. Patients will not have an aura before the headache. Cluster headaches are extremely severe, described as a stabbing or sharp pain, and are more likely to occur at night or in the early morning. Patients are restless and prefer to pace rather than lie still. Patients may describe nasal congestion at the time of the headache, possibly with swelling around the eyes. Diagnose clinically. Abortive first-line treatment includes 100% oxygen, triptans (Imitrex, injection or nasal spray), or ergot alkaloids (e.g., dihydroergotamine). Some patients respond well to lidocaine administered nasally. Also, short-term use of corticosteroids and occipital nerve injections may help with episodes. Preventative first-line treatment includes the calcium channel blocker verapamil and the mood stabilizer lithium. Anticonvulsants (e.g., Depakote) may also help with prevention.

TENSION-TYPE HEADACHES

Tension headaches, now referred to as tension-type headaches (**TTH**), are the most common type of headache and are described as a **generalized, mild to moderate headache** that does not become worse with regular physical activity. It can be classified as **episodic** (frequent or infrequent) or **chronic**. It was previously thought to be mostly due to muscle contractions, but now is believed to result from many factors. Stress and poor sleep may affect these headaches. Patients will describe bilateral head pain that usually feels like a band squeezing around the skull, and may report difficulty concentrating. The pain typically starts toward the frontal or occipital regions and then spreads to the whole head. There can be muscular tightness and pain in the neck or upper back. There is no prodrome and no nausea/vomiting or light/sound sensitivity.

Diagnose clinically. The neurologic exam will be normal. NSAIDs (ibuprofen is usually the first choice) and other pain relievers may help, as well as relaxation techniques. Decreasing stress, sufficient sleep, and other lifestyle changes (like avoiding alcohol and caffeine and quitting smoking) may help control chronic TTH. Excessive use of NSAIDs can contribute to medication overuse headaches (rebound headaches) and GI bleeds. Other complications include dependence on narcotic medications or those containing caffeine; and patients with tension-type headaches are 4 times more likely to be diagnosed with epilepsy.

MIGRAINE HEADACHES

Migraine headaches are **moderate to severe, usually unilateral and throbbing headaches** with nausea, photophobia, and phonophobia that recur and become worse with regular physical activity. They can be classified as **migraines without aura** (previously common migraine), **migraines with aura** (previously classic migraine), or **chronic migraines**. These are fairly common, have a genetic component, and occur much more frequently in women. Several factors may trigger a migraine: changes in hormone levels during the menstrual cycle, stress, sleep disturbances, weather changes, smoking, red wine, MSG, and caffeine. Patients may describe a prodrome hours or 1–2 days before the migraine begins (e.g., fatigue, irritability, nausea, yawning). About 25% of patients describe an aura, which usually starts before the migraine begins but may occur after it starts. The aura lasts from minutes to an hour and is usually visual (flashes of light, dark spots, scotomas, bright zigzag lines), but may include a tingling sensation or other sensory/motor symptoms. The headache is severe, usually unilateral, and throbbing, and may be accompanied by photophobia, phonophobia, or nausea/vomiting. Migraines typically last for 4–72 hours, and patients prefer being in a dark and quiet room. The postdrome (fatigue, mood changes) lasts about 24–48 hours after the migraine has resolved.

Diagnose clinically; neurologic exam is typically normal. Rule out other disorders that may mimic a migraine (e.g., ruptured brain aneurysm or subarachnoid hemorrhage if a "thunderclap" headache, dissecting carotid artery, cancer, meningitis, giant cell arteritis). Triptan medications at the first sign of a migraine can help to abort it or lower the pain intensity and help in moderate to severe cases. Pain relievers (e.g., NSAIDs, Tylenol, or aspirin if mild), ergot medications, and antiemetics can also help. Prophylactic medications, such as β-blockers and antiepileptics, can also help to lower the incidence of migraines. Complications include seizures and strokes.

COGNITIVE DISORDERS

Delirium is an acute, usually reversible **decline in mental function** due to a medical condition, substance, or withdrawal that causes disturbance in attention, awareness, and cognition. This state fluctuates during the day and can be due to multiple factors. This is common, especially in the elderly and in hospitalized and surgical patients, and is associated with increased mortality. This clinical diagnosis requires prompt attention since it may be due to an infection or medication.

The current (DSM-5) terms that refer to dementia are major and mild neurocognitive disorders. **Major** refers to a significant decline in mental function, and the patient loses their independence. **Mild** refers to a mild or modest decline in mental function, and the patient maintains their independence. Neurocognitive disorders listed in the DSM-5 include: Alzheimer's disease, frontotemporal disorder, Lewy body disease, vascular disease, traumatic brain injury, substance/medication induced, HIV associated, prion disease, Parkinson's disease, and Huntington's disease.

Dementia is a chronic, progressive, typically irreversible state of **decline in mental function**. Its onset of cognitive impairment is insidious, and symptoms do not change drastically over the course of the day. This can affect many areas, including cognition, attention, memory, motor and visual perception, language, judgment, personality, and behavior. Level of consciousness usually remains intact until the later stages but may be complicated by delirium. Short-term memory is often affected early on. Personality changes and depression are common. The patient may have difficulty finding words for familiar and common objects (anomia) or the inability to recognize familiar people or objects (agnosia), and may experience aphasia, a difficulty finding appropriate words and expressing thoughts clearly. Sleep and wake cycles become fragmented. This progressively affects activities of daily living and can lead to death. Diagnose clinically; use the Mini-Mental State Exam and other questionnaires.

INFECTIOUS DISORDERS

MENINGITIS

Meningitis is an infection of the **meninges**, which surround the **brain and spinal cord**. It is most often due to a **virus**, which is self-limited, but can be fatal if a **bacterium** is the cause. It may also be due to a fungus, parasite, amoeba, or noninfectious cause (e.g., cancer, medication). It is referred to as **aseptic meningitis** when a source cannot be found (usually due to a virus). According to the CDC, the most common bacterial cause is *Streptococcus pneumoniae*, which may especially affect the young and elderly. In newborns, group B

Streptococcus is a common cause in the first week of life. **Meningococcal meningitis** is caused by the bacteria *Neisseria meningitidis*; it most often affects people aged 16–23 years, and is known to cause outbreaks on college campuses. *H. influenzae* type b and *Listeria monocytogenes* may also cause meningitis. Common viral causes include non-polio enteroviruses (most common), measles, mumps, influenza, arboviruses (e.g., West Nile), and herpesviruses. The young, elderly, and immunocompromised are more at risk of developing meningitis.

Patients usually present with a severe headache, stiff neck (nuchal rigidity; may have a positive Kernig or Brudzinski sign), and fever. They may also have lethargy, photophobia, confusion, and possibly seizures. Rashes may be present in viral or meningococcal (petechiae and purpura) meningitis. Diagnose with a lumbar puncture and CSF analysis (bacterial: high opening pressure, elevated WBC, decreased glucose, elevated protein; viral: normal opening pressure, elevated WBC, normal or slightly decreased glucose, normal or slightly elevated protein) with Gram stain and culture and sensitivity. If focal deficits or signs of elevated ICP, perform a head CT before the LP. While awaiting lab results, immediately start empiric IV antibiotics: ceftriaxone OR cefotaxime in addition to vancomycin, AND if age >50, add ampicillin. If viral, supportive treatment is all that is necessary, and it usually resolves within 7–10 days. Prevention is important with available vaccines. Complications are more common with bacterial meningitis (e.g., seizures, hearing loss, blindness, cerebral edema, coma, and death).

ENCEPHALITIS

Encephalitis is inflammation of **brain tissue** and may be a primary infection or secondary (postinfectious). It is usually due to a **viral infection**; however, often the source cannot be identified. Viruses that cause encephalitis include enteroviruses (most common), herpes viruses (herpes simplex 1 & 2, Epstein-Barr, CMV, varicella-zoster, roseola), measles, mumps, rabies, and arboviruses (e.g., Eastern and Western equine encephalitis, West Nile encephalitis, Zika virus). Other causes are bacterial, fungal, parasitic, and autoimmune. The viral prodrome is followed by a few symptoms of encephalitis, or the disease may be severe. Patients may present with a fever, severe headache, neck stiffness, nausea/vomiting, photophobia, focal neurologic deficits, lethargy, personality changes, confusion, or altered mental status, and seizures may be present.

Diagnose with an LP/CSF analysis including viral titers and Gram stain, head CT or MRI, EEG, and blood cultures and viral cultures as needed (head CT before LP if focal deficits or signs of elevated ICP). Viral CSF results show: normal opening pressure or slightly elevated; elevated WBC; normal or slightly reduced glucose; normal or slightly elevated protein. Definitive diagnosis is with a brain biopsy. While waiting for lab results, immediately begin treatment with empiric IV acyclovir. If herpes simplex or varicella-zoster encephalitis is confirmed, continue acyclovir for 14–21 days. May also start patients on empiric antibiotics as needed. Otherwise, treatment is mainly supportive. Anticonvulsants (benzodiazepines) may be necessary if patients are having seizures. Complications include epilepsy, memory issues, personality changes, balance/movement issues, coma, and death.

NEOPLASMS
BENIGN AND MALIGNANT BRAIN/SPINAL CORD TUMORS

Brain tumors may be benign or malignant and primary or secondary (metastases). Even **benign tumors** cause problems since they compress adjacent tissues within the skull. **Primary brain tumors** are more common in children, while **metastases** are more common in adults. Most metastases come from lung cancer, but they also are often from breast cancer, malignant melanoma, colon cancer, and renal cancer. **Pituitary adenomas** are common and are almost always benign. Brain tumors are classified according to where they arise. The most common types of brain and spinal neoplasms are **gliomas** (from glial cells in the brain or spinal cord; includes astrocytomas, oligodendrogliomas, ependymomas, medulloblastomas), **metastases**, **meningiomas** (from the meninges, so they may appear anywhere along the brain or spinal cord; benign and usually in adults), **pituitary adenomas**, and **acoustic neuromas** (from Schwann cells). **Glioblastoma multiforme** is the most common and the most aggressive primary brain tumor. Tumors are classified from grade I (slowest growing and noninvasive) to grade III or IV (fastest growing).

Based on the type and location of the tumor, signs and symptoms may include: headache (most common), vision/hearing problems, speech issues, nausea/vomiting, weakness/motor issues, changes in personality/mood, difficulty concentrating, and seizures. Deficits caused by tumor location: frontal lobe—personality, memory, learning, speech, motor; temporal lobe—memory, hearing, understanding language; parietal lobe—spatial awareness; occipital lobe—vision; cerebellum/brainstem—coordination/voluntary movement, cranial nerve palsies. Look for signs/symptoms of elevated ICP: headache, nausea/vomiting, diminished mental status, diplopia, papilledema, abnormal pupillary light reflexes, and Cushing's triad (decreased respiratory rate, decreased pulse, and elevated blood pressure). Initial diagnosis is usually made with a head CT after a thorough neurologic exam. An MRI may be obtained. Refer to neurosurgery.

NEUROMUSCULAR AND MOVEMENT DISORDERS

IDIOPATHIC FACIAL NERVE PALSY (BELL'S PALSY)

Bell's palsy, now called idiopathic facial nerve palsy, is a condition in which the muscles supplied by the **7th cranial nerve** (CN VII; facial nerve) are unilaterally weakened or paralyzed. The etiology of the CN VII impairment is unknown, but risk factors include a current or recent viral infection (most often due to herpes simplex or varicella-zoster), pregnancy, and diabetes mellitus. CN VII is a mixed motor/sensory nerve that has motor fibers that innervate the muscles of **facial expression** (including the forehead) and **sensory fibers** to the anterior two-thirds of the tongue. Patients may notice a tingling and rather rapid onset of weakness on one side of the face, which may occur quite suddenly over a few hours to a couple days. Both upper and lower parts of the face will be unilaterally affected, and may cause difficulty closing the eye, blinking, smiling, frowning, and wrinkling the forehead; taste disturbances may be present. Some patients may experience posterior ear pain, which may occur a couple days before the palsy sets in.

Thoroughly test the cranial nerves and perform a thorough neurologic exam (motor and sensory; impaired motor, but sensory is intact). This is a clinical diagnosis that is made after other causes are ruled out (e.g., infection, autoimmune disorder, CNS disease). If the onset is gradual, rule out a tumor. If only the upper or lower half of the face is affected, rule out a CVA. Bell's palsy is almost always a self-limited condition that lasts from a week to a few months. Treatment involves giving corticosteroids early on (start within 72 hours of symptom onset), which helps improve the outcome. If a virus is suspected, antiviral medications may be used (if given with steroids); however, their effectiveness is still being studied. Lubricating eye drops and/or ointment and eye patches, especially at night or if there is a corneal erosion or abrasion, may help the affected dry eye. Refer to neurology or ophthalmology as needed.

CEREBRAL PALSY

Cerebral palsy is a **movement disorder** that develops due to permanent brain damage that occurs during **prenatal or postnatal neural development**, or during **birth**. It affects a child's motor development and may or may not be accompanied by intellectual disabilities or seizures. It is diagnosed before 2 years old and may be classified as **spastic** (movement difficulties/ stiffness; most common), **dyskinetic** (involuntary movements), or **ataxic** (balance issues). It can result from a variety of incidents, including prenatal/postnatal infections, prenatal/postnatal exposures to toxins, trauma/intracranial hemorrhage, prematurity, or anoxia during or after birth. Parents will notice their children are not reaching developmental milestones (like sitting up, crawling, speaking, or walking) as they should. Cerebral palsy affects **motor function** usually by causing the muscles to be flaccid and weak early on, and then rigid and spastic. The limbs will appear underdeveloped and flaccid—or, more commonly, stiff, rigid, and with contractures. The child will be uncoordinated and hyperreflexic, and primitive (newborn) reflexes may still be present.

Diagnosis is made clinically and confirmed with an MRI. Rule out possible metabolic or neurologic causes. There is no cure for cerebral palsy, but physical therapy and kinesiotherapy can help with stretching the muscles and preventing contractions due to rigidity. Botulinum toxin, baclofen, and other muscle relaxants can be given to help decrease spasticity. Braces and surgery may also be used. If there are learning impairments, special education should be utilized to maximize the child's learning potential.

Multiple Sclerosis

Multiple sclerosis (**MS**) is a chronic disorder of the **CNS** in which inflammation, demyelination, and damage to **axons** occurs. The cause is unknown, but there may be genetic factors, viral, or other triggers to this autoimmune disease. This affects women more than men, is more common in temperate climates, and is usually diagnosed at 20–40 years of age. The 4 types of MS are **relapsing-remitting** (most common, 85%), **primary progressive**, **secondary progressive**, and **progressive-relapsing**. While it may or may not eventually lead to a diagnosis of MS, an episode that presents with at least 24 hours of one of the symptoms of MS is called **clinically isolated syndrome**.

Common presenting symptoms may include optic neuritis (vision loss, blurred vision, scotomas, eye pain), diplopia, focal sensory loss/paresthesias/weakness (usually in arms, hands, legs, face), muscle spasms, balance issues, urinary incontinence, cognitive problems, and depression. Typically, these episodes last for days, weeks, or months, and are followed by periods of remission that may last for months or years. **Attacks** are defined as lasting at least 24 hours and must be 1 month from the last attack. Clinical findings and MRI are used to diagnose this condition and to follow the progress of the disease. To diagnose MS, the MRI needs to show plaques or damage in at least two different areas that occurred at different times (lesions separated in "time and space"), or in one area of damage plus oligoclonal bands in CSF. Treatment involves corticosteroids for attacks or exacerbations, as well as disease-modifying agents (e.g., interferon) for long-term treatment.

Myasthenia Gravis

Myasthenia gravis (**MG**) is an **autoimmune neurologic disorder** that causes **skeletal muscle fatigue** with activity. **Autoantibodies** are produced that block the **postsynaptic acetylcholine receptor sites** at the neuromuscular junction, leading to fewer nerve signals being sent to muscle cells, which results in weakness. There is no definite known cause of MG, but the **thymus gland** may play a role in producing the antibodies for the disease. It most commonly affects middle-aged men and women, but typically appears earlier in women (20–40 years old) than in men (>50 years old). There are two main forms: **ocular** and **generalized**. Patients usually present with ptosis, diplopia, and fluctuating skeletal muscle weakness that worsens with activity and improves with rest. This can include difficulty breathing, chewing, swallowing, talking, performing exertive motions, or controlling eye movements. In a **myasthenia crisis**, normal respirations are affected, causing difficulty breathing, and possibly requiring a respirator; but mortality due to a crisis has greatly decreased through the years. A **cholinergic crisis**, which presents similarly to a myasthenic crisis, may also occur in MG patients, but this is due to ingestion of too much acetylcholinesterase inhibitor (e.g., pyridostigmine).

Diagnose with an AChR-Ab (anti-acetylcholine receptor antibody) test. A MuSK-Ab (muscle-specific kinase) test may be used if the first is negative. Use a chest x-ray or chest CT to rule out a thymoma. In patients with ptosis, a bedside ice test may be used to see if symptoms improve (improves in MG). Treat symptoms with the acetylcholinesterase inhibitor pyridostigmine. Also, over time, most patients improve after a thymectomy even if a thymoma is not present. Steroids and other immunosuppressants, plasmapheresis, and IVIG may also help reduce symptoms. The primary complication is respiratory failure.

> **Review Video: Myasthenia Gravis**
> Visit mometrix.com/academy and enter code: 162510

Essential Tremor

Essential tremor is an **involuntary shaking disorder** that usually occurs in older adults and typically affects the hands, forearms, head, chin, or even the voice. This is the most common tremor; its prevalence increases with age, and it affects men and women equally. These tremors are not accompanied by any other symptoms, as seen with the tremor of Parkinson's disease, but can be debilitating if severe. Most patients have a family history of essential tremors (autosomal dominant), but it is not known what causes the tremors. Patients usually complain of gradually progressive tremors in the hands or other areas. The tremors occur when maintaining posture against gravity or during voluntary movements. Tremors are most pronounced when performing simple activities such as eating, drinking, and writing. The tremors usually stop when patients are

Mometrix

resting and not moving, but restart when performing activities. Tremors worsen during periods of stress and are absent when sleeping. In some cases, alcohol can temporarily decrease the amplitude of the tremor. Muscle tone is normal, and reflexes remain intact.

Diagnose clinically. Rule out other causes of tremors: medications, caffeine, alcohol withdrawal, vitamin B12 deficiency, hyperthyroidism, and Parkinson's. Treat with the β-blocker propranolol or the anticonvulsant primidone, which can help control the tremors in most patients. When the tremor is severe and not responding to medical management, a thalamotomy may be performed, or a deep brain stimulator can be surgically implanted to try to control the tremor.

Huntington Disease

Huntington disease is an **autosomal dominant disorder** of the neurologic system that causes **progressive destruction of brain cells**, resulting in chorea, cognitive issues, and neuropsychiatric issues. Since it is an autosomal dominant disorder, only one parent needs to carry the gene for a child to develop the disease (50% probability). The disease results from a mutation on chromosome 4, and this primarily affects the caudate nucleus. There is no cure for Huntington's disease; it usually manifests around 30–50 years old, and patients have a life expectancy of about 10–30 years after the onset of symptoms.

Early signs and symptoms include personality changes, irritability, impaired concentration or memory issues, restlessness or clumsiness, and depression. Physical signs include imbalance, uncontrollable facial expressions, lack of coordination, and sudden spasm-like movements (chorea). These symptoms and dementia gradually progress to the point where patients are incapacitated and cannot care for themselves. Diagnosis is confirmed with genetic testing. First-degree relatives should be offered genetic counseling and then genetic testing. Anticonvulsants, antipsychotics, and antidepressants can help with some of the symptoms. Physical therapy, occupational therapy, and kinesiotherapy can all help with range of motion, but will not be able to stop the progression of the disease.

Parkinson's Disease

Parkinson's disease is a **movement disorder** that involves progressive damage and destruction of neurons in the **substantia nigra** that produce dopamine. The **basal ganglia** and the neurotransmitter **dopamine** are responsible for allowing the body to move smoothly and without rigidity or jerkiness. Symptoms result from an imbalance between dopamine-activated and acetylcholine-activated neural pathways in the basal ganglia. The exact cause of Parkinson's is not clearly understood, but it is thought to be due to genetic and environmental factors, as there is an increased incidence in people with chronic exposure to herbicides, pesticides, and well water. This affects men more than women, and symptoms usually start after the age of 60 but may begin earlier.

The onset is insidious and usually starts with a unilateral resting tremor in the hand, wrist, or fingers ("pill rolling") that improves with intentional motion. Other symptoms include gait disturbances with decreased arm swing on the affected side, soft voice, flat affect, and sometimes dementia. Rigidity, "cogwheel" movements, bradykinesia, akinesia, poor posture, and lack of balance and coordination, cause increasing problems with mobility, talking, and swallowing. Some patients experience sleep disturbances, depression, and mood changes. Diagnose clinically; be sure to rule out drug-induced symptoms. Treat symptoms with levodopa (precursor to dopamine) and carbidopa. Other drugs like ropinirole, safinamide, bromocriptine, and amantadine may be used in specific situations (like early or late disease) or to help with medication side effects. A deep brain stimulator may be surgically implanted to help with the movement disorders associated with Parkinson's.

Tourette Syndrome

Tourette syndrome (**TS**) is a **neurologic disorder** that manifests as repetitive, involuntary, nonrhythmic movements and vocalizations, referred to as **tics**. This is more common in males than females and there seems to be a genetic as well as an environmental component to this disease. These symptoms first appear in the preschool or early elementary-school child, often become worse during puberty, and usually resolve gradually during adulthood. **Simple motor tics** might include eye movements, grimacing, shrugging, twitching, or jerking; **simple vocal tics** might include throat-clearing, coughing, grunting, or sniffing. **Complex tics** are created with combined, coordinated activities, full words, or phrases (e.g., kicking, jumping, animal sounds, yelling). **Coprolalia** (use of profanity or inappropriate words) and **copropraxia** (obscene gestures) only occur in a minority of patients.

Symptoms worsen with stress or times of excitement and do not go away during sleep. Comorbid conditions like ADHD, learning disabilities, OCD, and depression are often present. Diagnose clinically: rule out other causes; symptoms of both motor and vocal tics must be present for >1 year and must appear before 18 years old according to DSM-5 criteria. Treatment is not required unless the tics interfere with normal daily functioning. Dopamine-blocking neuroleptics and other medications (e.g., haloperidol, pimozide, clonidine, topiramate) may then be considered as a means of providing some control. Side effects of haloperidol and other neuroleptics include extrapyramidal symptoms (e.g., acute dystonic reactions, akathisia [feeling of restlessness], Parkinson-like symptoms, tardive dyskinesia), which may not be reversible with prolonged use of the medication(s).

PERIPHERAL NERVE AND PAIN DISORDERS
COMPLEX REGIONAL PAIN SYNDROME

Complex regional pain syndrome (**CRPS**) is a **chronic pain condition** that usually manifests after an injury. CRPS is the newer collective name for reflex sympathetic dystrophy and causalgia. CRPS includes **type I**, which is linked to an initial injury or insult, and **type II**, which is due to an injury to a nerve. CRPS commonly occurs after a fracture, crush injury, limb immobilization/cast, surgery, or MI, and the pain is disproportionate to the injury. CRPS involves autonomic dysfunction, as well as sensory and motor issues and changes to the skin and possibly bone. It is more common in women and usually affects those in their 40s, although it may occur at any age.

Patients usually describe a regional burning, aching, or throbbing pain that starts days to weeks after an injury (often to an extremity), with other signs including changes in: temperature (>1 °C), color, edema, thinning skin, sweating, hair or nail growth changes, sensitivities to touch, muscle and joint stiffness, and decreased ROM. CRPS is a clinical diagnosis and requires 2–4 signs and 3–4 symptoms to be diagnosed, as well as ruling out other causes. Sometimes x-rays are taken that may show osteopenia. Early treatment is important and involves a multidisciplinary approach, with pain management, PT/OT, and psychological support. More research is needed, but medical treatment may include NSAIDs, opioids, corticosteroids, calcitonin/bisphosphonates, tricyclic antidepressants, gabapentin, clonidine, IVIG, and sympathetic ganglion blocks. Refer to neurology as needed.

TRIGEMINAL NEURALGIA

Trigeminal neuralgia is a **chronic disorder** that creates extreme pain, often described as stabbing or electric-shock-like, along one side of the **face** (follows the sensory distribution of CN V, usually the maxillary and mandibular nerve branches). This condition is rare but usually affects women >50 years old. It is typically idiopathic. Underlying causes are more likely to be determined in patients younger than 40—generally multiple sclerosis or a swollen blood vessel or tumor providing pressure on the **trigeminal nerve**. The pain usually lasts seconds to 2 minutes, and is typically sporadic at first, but may increase in frequency and can be quite debilitating. The pain may cause a facial tic due to muscle spasms. Triggers of the pain may include sound, touch, vibration or stimulation of the area through brushing teeth, chewing, drinking, eating, or shaving. The neurologic exam is normal.

Diagnosis is clinical but testing often includes magnetic resonance imaging (MRI). Treatment may include anticonvulsant medications (carbamazepine is usually first-line), muscle relaxants (baclofen), or tricyclic antidepressants. More aggressive treatment entails referring to neurosurgery and cutting or destroying part of

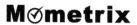

the trigeminal nerve (ablation), microcompression, tumor removal (if this secondary cause is found), or microvascular decompression.

GUILLAIN-BARRÉ SYNDROME

Guillain-Barré syndrome (**acute inflammatory polyneuropathy**) is an acute condition in which inflammation occurs in the **peripheral nerves** throughout the body, resulting in **progressive muscle weakness and decreased reflexes**. This typically begins in the lower extremities and ascends, which may cause respiratory depression requiring mechanical ventilation. There is no definite known cause of this disease, but over one-half of the people who suffer from Guillain-Barré have a history of a respiratory or gastrointestinal illness (usually *Campylobacter jejuni* or CMV) 2–4 weeks before they develop symptoms, so it may be due to an autoimmune disorder. Symptoms can progress rapidly from hours to days and usually peak within 2–4 weeks. Depending on the type (demyelinating or axonal injury) it may take weeks or months to recover, or even years. Patients develop symmetric paresthesias and weakness (usually affects proximal muscles more) in the extremities (usually lower first) that gradually spread up the limbs and may cause paralysis. This may be accompanied by pain, hypotension, and bladder/bowel incontinence.

Diagnose clinically and with nerve conduction studies, electromyography, and LP with CSF analysis (elevated protein but normal WBCs) to aid in the diagnosis process. Consult neurology, test for infectious cause, and rule out other causes. Admit patients with suspected Guillain-Barré syndrome, monitor closely, and intubate as needed. Treat with IVIG or plasmapheresis. The disorder generally begins to resolve after approximately 1 month. Most people make a full recovery from Guillain-Barré, with a small portion of patients having some degree of residual weakness. Complications include lasting sequelae, ARDS, and death.

SEIZURES

FOCAL SEIZURES

Seizures are broadly classified as focal, generalized, or having an unknown onset. **Focal seizures** (previously referred to as partial seizures) are misfirings of the electrical signals of the brain that are localized to a particular part of the brain. Focal seizures can be **simple** (conscious) or **complex** (impaired awareness). These may have motor, sensory (e.g., visual, auditory, olfactory, or taste), and autonomic (e.g., diaphoresis, flushed face) components, including an aura. Congenital defects, head trauma, disease, infection, or a stroke may increase the risk of developing a seizure disorder.

Epilepsy is the term used when >1 non-physiological seizure has occurred (e.g., it cannot be due to a fever). **Simple (aware) focal seizures** do not cause a loss of awareness, but rather a change in how things appear, taste, or smell, and can last for seconds to minutes. **Complex (impaired awareness) focal seizures** will cause a change in consciousness or loss of awareness (interruption in behavior or staring) with some motor changes, such as arm movements, lip smacking, repeated swallowing, or yelling out, and usually last for 1–1.5 minutes. Postictal confusion may last for a short time or for days. Diagnose clinically and with an EEG (electroencephalogram); rule out other causes. Treatment is with anticonvulsants (e.g., carbamazepine, divalproex sodium), but it may take several trials of drugs to find the most effective treatment for patients. Monotherapy at the lowest dose is the goal, but two or more medications may be required. Rarely, surgery is chosen if the seizures are unresponsive to medications.

GENERALIZED SEIZURES

Generalized seizures occur when **both hemispheres of the brain** are immediately affected by **abnormal electrical signals**, which results in a loss of consciousness. According to the 2017 International League Against Epilepsy, generalized seizures can be classified as motor or non-motor. These seizures include **tonic** (rigid), **clonic** (rhythmic jerking), **tonic-clonic** (grand mal), **myoclonic** (muscle group twitching or nonrhythmic jerking), **atonic** ("drop attacks"), and **absence** (petit mal; staring episodes usually lasting about 30 seconds). These generalized seizures all involve a loss of consciousness or loss of awareness and a postictal state of varying degrees. Head trauma, congenital malformation, infection, stroke, a tumor, and genetics may increase the chances of developing a seizure disorder.

Generalized seizures vary greatly. The mildest of these would be an absence seizure, or petit mal, in which patients stare blankly or have very subtle movements. The other end of the spectrum is a tonic-clonic seizure, or grand mal, in which there is loss of consciousness or loss of awareness with generalized jerking and possibly loss of bowel or bladder control. Diagnose clinically and with EEG and MRI; rule out causes (e.g., febrile seizures, infection). Treat with anticonvulsants (e.g., valproic acid, topiramate; ethosuximide or Depakote for absence), but it may take several trials of drugs to find the most effective treatment for patients, and sometimes multiple medications are necessary. Rarely, surgery is used if the seizure activity is unresponsive to anticonvulsants.

STATUS EPILEPTICUS

Status epilepticus is a condition in which the **seizure does not stop in 5 or more minutes** or in which there are repeated seizures (>2) where the patient remains **unconscious for 5 or more minutes**. It may be **generalized convulsive or nonconvulsive**. This is considered a medical emergency because of the physiological effects of sustained seizures, especially with the convulsive type (e.g., elevated heart rate, elevated temperature, elevated catecholamines, nerve cell death, pulmonary edema), and risk of asphyxiation or respiratory arrest during the seizure. Status epilepticus is most often due to patients not taking their **seizure medications** correctly or due to **changes in these medications**, but can also occur in acute illnesses such as meningitis, encephalitis, or very high fevers; or with decreased glucose levels, alcohol withdrawal, or head trauma. Patients exhibit signs of a tonic-clonic seizure persisting >5 minutes. There may be a known diagnosis of epilepsy or another illness.

Diagnose clinically and begin treatment before labs are back; obtain stat glucose, CBC, LFTs, BUN/Cr, ABG, anticonvulsant levels, and a toxicity screen. Check ABCs and give oxygen; the airway of patients should be protected; intubation may be necessary; and obtain an IV access. According to the 2016 guidelines from the American Epilepsy Society, the following is recommended: give a benzodiazepine as first-line treatment (e.g., IV lorazepam, IV diazepam, or IM midazolam); if the seizure persists >20 minutes, begin a second medication (e.g., IV fosphenytoin, IV valproic acid, or IV levetiracetam). More studies are necessary to determine the best way to handle seizures persisting longer than 40 minutes. If the cause of the seizure is not immediately known, an EEG and other testing should be done. If an acute illness is suspected, a lumbar puncture with CSF analysis and blood cultures should also be drawn to assess for sepsis. Complications include acidosis, rhabdomyolysis, hyperthermia, respiratory failure, and death.

VASCULAR DISORDERS

SYNCOPE

Syncope is an abrupt **loss of consciousness and muscle tone** ("fainting spell"); patients typically recover from the episode on their own. There are numerous causes of syncope, including a vasovagal response, hypoglycemia, dehydration, medications, orthostatic hypotension, arrhythmias, valvular or heart disease, MI, CVA/TIA, hyperventilation, breath-holding, and pregnancy. Anything that causes **decreased blood flow to the brain**, including decreased oxygen or glucose, may cause syncope. Those at increased risk include the elderly and those with cardiovascular disease. There may be presyncopal symptoms with a feeling of dizziness or light-headedness, weakness, sweating, blurry vision, or GI symptoms.

Red-flag symptoms include: palpitations, chest pain, syncope during exertion, syncope without a prodrome, severe headache or neurologic deficits, severe abdominal pain, and respiratory issues (especially if accompanied with lower-extremity edema or calf pain). Workup includes a thorough history and PE, orthostatic blood pressure (orthostatic hypotension is defined as: a sustained >20 mmHg decrease in systolic blood pressure and a 10 mmHg decrease in diastolic blood pressure within 3 minutes of standing from the supine position), and ECG. Also, a tilt table test, Valsalva maneuver, blood glucose, CBC, serum electrolytes, cardiac enzymes, and UA may be helpful in diagnosing. Treatment involves treating the underlying cause (e.g., vasovagal precautions/avoid triggers, orthostatic training/rise slowly, treat arrhythmias with medications or pacemaker, treat CHF with medications, stabilize blood glucose levels, rehydrate). If patient is at high risk, admit for observation and further workup.

TRANSIENT ISCHEMIC ATTACK

A transient ischemic attack (**TIA**) occurs when blood flow to an area of the brain, spinal cord, or retina is temporarily interrupted, causing **focal neurologic dysfunction**, but without causing tissue damage. This can occur due to atherosclerosis in an artery, arterial inflammation, emboli/thrombi, a hypercoagulable state, drugs (e.g., cocaine), or anything that causes a **temporary decrease in oxygen to a certain portion of the brain**. Risk factors for a TIA include a positive family history of TIA or CVA, African American or Hispanic descent, male, >55 years old, hypertension, DM, hypercholesterolemia, and smoking. About one-third of patients who have a TIA will eventually have a stroke, with most of those occurring in the next days or weeks post-TIA. Patients will have symptoms similar to a stroke, with possible hemiparesis, paresthesias, garbled speech, dizziness, cranial nerve dysfunction, and loss of vision in one eye. The difference between a stroke and a TIA is that, with a TIA, the symptoms will resolve spontaneously—within 24 hours, and often much less (minutes).

This is a clinical diagnosis with a thorough history and physical exam (thorough neurologic and cardiac exams, listen for carotid bruit), as there is no tissue damage to be seen on imaging. However, to rule out a cerebral infarct or hemorrhage, an MRI (diffusion weighted is most sensitive) or a CT must be obtained. Also rule out other causes (e.g., AFib, carotid stenosis) with appropriate labs, ECG, and imaging studies (e.g., carotid ultrasound, echo). After a hemorrhage has been ruled out, patients who have had a TIA should be started on daily antiplatelet medications (e.g., low-dose aspirin, clopidogrel, dipyridamole). Anticoagulants are started for cardiogenic TIAs (e.g., AFib). Lifestyle changes should be implemented, including eating foods lower in fat and cholesterol, quitting smoking, and losing weight, if necessary. The primary complication is a CVA.

STROKE

A stroke or **cerebrovascular accident (CVA)** occurs when **damage and death of brain cells** occurs from ischemia or a hemorrhage. It is a medical emergency. Neurons die within minutes without a blood supply, so early intervention is critical. According to the American Heart Association (AHA), most CVAs are caused by **arterial blockage causing ischemia** (87%), while bleeding of a vessel only accounts for about 13% of all CVAs. These two main types are termed ischemic and hemorrhagic strokes, respectively. **Ischemic strokes** can be due to a thrombus or embolus; a **hemorrhagic stroke** can be intracerebral or subarachnoid. Within the US, strokes are the fifth leading cause of death. The extent of the damage, presenting symptoms, and mortality are dependent upon the location and size of the vascular compromise.

Common symptoms include weakness, loss of voluntary movement (ataxia), paralysis, or a loss of sensation on one side of the body. The damage can result in problems with speech, swallowing, increased drooling, impaired balance, and vision or breathing issues; hemorrhagic patients typically appear sicker. If damage is extensive, unconsciousness or death may occur. Obtain a fingerstick glucose and diagnose initially with a noncontrast head CT: ischemic areas appear hypodense; hemorrhagic areas appear hyperdense. Remember, in an ischemic CVA, a head CT may appear normal early on (<12 hours) as the damage progresses. However, diffusion-weighted imaging can show damage within 15–30 minutes of the onset of an ischemic CVA. Angiography can be utilized for diagnosis and treatment. If signs of ICP or hemorrhage, refer immediately to neurosurgery. A hemorrhage must be ruled out in order to start thrombolytic therapy (start IV tPA [tissue plasminogen activator] within 3–4.5 hours of symptom onset for acute ischemic strokes). Complications include permanent neurologic deficits and death.

> **Review Video: Overview of Strokes**
> Visit mometrix.com/academy and enter code: 310572

SPONTANEOUS INTRACRANIAL HEMORRHAGE, CEREBRAL ANEURYSM, AND AV MALFORMATION (AVM)

A spontaneous intracranial hemorrhage occurs with sudden bleeding from a blood vessel in the brain. It is usually due to hypertension or occurs when vascular lesions in the brain leak/rupture. Examples include cerebral aneurysms and arteriovenous malformations.

A **cerebral aneurysm** is a dilatation in the wall of a cerebral artery that is usually asymptomatic until it leaks or ruptures. It may be saccular ("berry") or fusiform (spindle-like) in shape. About 5% of the population has this, and the risk of rupture is ~1%; however, mortality is >50% once it ruptures.

An **arteriovenous malformation (AVM)** is a tangle of vessels or malformed vessels that flow from arteries directly into veins. AVMs are rare (~1%), the rupture risk is ~3%, and mortality post-rupture is 12–66%.

Signs and symptoms vary depending on the area/size of the intracranial hemorrhage, but some include a severe headache (often with activity) described as "the worst of their life," speech and memory issues, confusion, visual deficits, nausea/vomiting, paresthesias or paralysis, other deficits, and loss of consciousness. AVMs may have less severe bleeding, and therefore less severe symptoms, or may even be asymptomatic. If non-emergent, these can be diagnosed with MRI, MRI angiography (preferred over CT angiography), or definitively through angiography. If it ruptures, follow emergency protocol (e.g., ABCs, fingerstick glucose, and noncontrast head CT) and immediately refer to neurosurgery. Complications from these include a subarachnoid hemorrhage (which is a medical emergency), chronic neurologic deficits, and death.

Psychiatry/Behavioral Science

ANXIETY DISORDERS

PANIC DISORDER

Panic disorder is a chronic condition in which people experience **unexpected panic attacks** that may become severe enough to affect their lives and level of functioning. Patients must experience >1 month of continued worry and behavioral changes (avoidance) regarding thoughts of a future panic attack in order to be diagnosed (DSM-5). These panic attacks may vary in intensity and frequency, and they are not caused by medications or other medical disorders. It is 2 to 3 times more likely to affect females, and it is more likely to start in late teens to early adulthood. It is likely to occur in families, and it is also commonly associated with other psychiatric disorders like major depression, OCD, and phobias. It may occur with other medical conditions like asthma, IBS, and migraines. The panic attacks experienced with panic disorder give patients a sense of extreme anxiety with rapid heart rate or palpitations, chest pain, paresthesias, chills or hot flashes, sweating, dyspnea, a choking feeling, shaking, dizziness, abdominal distress/nausea, derealization or depersonalization, and fear of dying or going crazy/losing control (must meet 4 of the 13 criteria). Patients may also have a fear of leaving their homes or encountering crowds of people (agoraphobia). Refer to a mental health professional.

Treatment includes cognitive behavior therapy (to correct thinking and "talk themselves down" from developing a panic attack), systematic desensitization therapy with small doses of exposure to the anxiety-provoking stimuli, and/or pharmacotherapy. First-line antidepressant monotherapy includes SSRIs (e.g., fluoxetine, paroxetine), SNRIs (e.g., venlafaxine), or tricyclic antidepressants (avoid tricyclics if patient has acute narrow-angle glaucoma or prostatic hypertrophy). Benzodiazepines may be used short-term while waiting for antidepressants to become effective, or may be used second-line in refractory cases.

GENERALIZED ANXIETY DISORDER

Generalized anxiety disorder (**GAD**) is a condition in which a person **worries** all the time about situations or conditions. This worry or stress is out of proportion with the general reaction of most people, and patients are unable to control the anxiety/worry. Also, it cannot be caused by medications or due to other medical conditions. This must be present for most days over a 6-month period over different situations or conditions. This is more common in females and often begins in childhood or adolescence. It is thought that an imbalance in the neurotransmitters **serotonin** and **norepinephrine** may play a role in the development of GAD.

GAD causes a generalized state of unrest or feeling keyed up, with muscle tension, irritability, fatigue, difficulty concentrating/mind going blank, and insomnia (must meet ≥3 criteria for diagnosis, DSM-5). On exam, patients may appear very restless, diaphoretic, with SOB and elevated heart rate, and they may complain of somatic symptoms such as nausea, diarrhea, difficulty swallowing, clammy hands, or headache. Treatment involves pharmacotherapy as well as psychotherapy. Psychotherapy helps GAD patients develop better coping skills and relaxation methods. First-line medical treatment includes SSRIs like fluoxetine or paroxetine, and SNRIs like venlafaxine. Sometimes benzodiazepines are started short-term while waiting for the antidepressants to take effect. SSRIs take 2–4 weeks to reach therapeutic levels. Medical treatment may involve several trials of different medications to find the treatment that works best for patients.

PHOBIAS: SPECIFIC AND SOCIAL (SOCIAL ANXIETY DISORDER)

Phobias can be specific or social. In both, the phobia cannot be caused by another medical condition or better defined by another mental disorder. In both, the fear and anxiety bring much distress, and patients greatly desire to avoid these objects or situations and will only endure them under immense distress. These fears must be present >6 months. They are more common in women. A **specific phobia** is a persistent, intense, disproportionate fear or anxiety regarding a certain **object or situation**, which causes immediate distress when the patient is exposed to it and interferes with how patients function as they try to avoid the object or situation. Some examples include fears of snakes, spiders, heights, water, weather, needles, medical procedures, and blood.

The primary treatment involves exposure therapy. Occasionally, short-term use of benzodiazepines is used in certain unavoidable situations. In **social phobias**, or **social anxiety disorder**, the object of the intense fear or anxiety is **public situations** where the patient may be scrutinized (e.g., speaking in public, performing, social interactions, eating, or using public restrooms). Patients worry that they will be looked down on, or that they will offend others with their actions. Treatment involves cognitive behavior therapy and pharmacotherapy. SSRIs are first-line; β-blockers may be added to help decrease the physical symptoms caused by performance anxiety.

> **Review Video: Anxiety Disorders**
> Visit mometrix.com/academy and enter code: 366760

TRAUMA AND STRESSOR-RELATED DISORDERS
ADJUSTMENT DISORDER

An adjustment disorder is a stress-related condition that occurs in response to some **change or stress** in a person's life. The behavioral and emotional symptoms begin within 3 months of the stressor and stop within 6 months after the stressor ends. The reaction to the stressor(s) is disproportionate to what is regularly expected and interferes with regular functioning. Therefore, this does not include normal bereavement/grief reactions that involve normal stages (e.g., denial, blame/anger, bargaining, sadness, acceptance). Examples of adjustment disorder stressors include relationship issues/divorce, work or money problems, becoming a parent, moving, illness, and natural disasters.

Signs and symptoms may include anxiety, depressed mood, sleep disturbances, sadness, irritability, withdrawing, feeling hopeless, or even thoughts of suicide. Patients may exhibit behavior changes and have conduct issues like abusing drugs or alcohol, getting into trouble, and destroying property. Children with adjustment disorder may have failing grades or may skip school. Treatment consists of psychotherapy to help work through the stress caused by the change in their lives and to develop healthy coping skills. Sometimes short-term antidepressants or benzodiazepines are added and may be helpful in relieving the symptoms of depression, anxiety, or insomnia.

POST-TRAUMATIC STRESS DISORDER

Post-traumatic stress disorder (**PTSD**) occurs following direct involvement in, witnessing, or indirectly learning a close friend or relative was exposed to an **extremely traumatic event** or the threat of such an event. This can include first responders or other professionals who repeatedly see or hear about traumatic events. But this does not include things only witnessed in photos, TV, or other electronic media. PTSD can occur after sexual or physical abuse or attacks, or from experiencing accidents, war, or a natural disaster.

Symptoms of PTSD usually begin within 3 months of the triggering event but may occur up to years later. Patients may have sudden, recurrent, unwanted, and disturbing memories or flashbacks of the trauma, nightmares, insomnia, irritability, difficulty concentrating, anger, guilt, and possibly self-destructive behavior. Small internal or external reminders of the trauma can send patients into an episode of severe distress, anger, fear, and intense physical reactions. There is avoidance of internal or external reminders, as well as an increased startle response, and there can be feelings of hopelessness and helplessness. Children <6 may experience different symptoms, including reenacting the trauma through play, regression, and delayed development.

For establishing a diagnosis, symptoms must last >1 month, including 1 or more "intrusion" symptoms, avoidance of triggers, 2 or more negative changes in "mood and cognitions," and 2 or more changes in "arousal and reactivity," and can't be due to a substance or other medical condition. Treatment involves psychotherapy and SSRIs (sertraline or paroxetine). Medical treatment can vary, depending on the predominant symptom a patient is experiencing (e.g., prazosin for insomnia).

BIPOLAR AND DEPRESSIVE DISORDERS
BIPOLAR DISORDERS

Bipolar disorders are chronic and characterized by **mood swings** that range from **major depression to mania**. The severity of the disorder varies among patients, but it usually greatly affects a person's life. The exact cause of bipolar disorders is unknown, but a positive family history, imbalances in the brain's neurotransmitters, and some environmental factors may play a role in its development. It can be classified as **bipolar I** (must have 1 manic episode with a hypomanic or major depressive episode), **bipolar II** (at least 1 hypomanic and 1 major depressive episode), or **cyclothymic disorder** (2 years of hypomanic and depressive "periods," not episodes). **Rapid cycling** refers to 4 or more mood episodes in a year; and bipolar I or II can have mixed features.

The "**low**" points of bipolar disorder cause the classic symptoms of major depression (must be present in the same 2-week period and have ≥5, with at least 1 of the first 2 symptoms, to be classified as a major depressive episode): anhedonia, depressed mood most of the day, fatigue, sleep disturbances, psychomotor retardation or agitation, decreased concentration/ability to think or indecisiveness, weight loss or gain, feelings of worthlessness or guilt, and suicidal ideation or an attempt. The "**high**" points occur during the manic phase (symptoms must be present for 1 week) and include (must have ≥3 to be classified as a manic episode): restlessness, racing thoughts, distractibility, lack of sleep, agitation or increase in goal-centered activities, pressured speech, inflated self-esteem (grandiosity), and increased involvement in high-risk activities. It is termed **hypomania** if ≥3 of the above manic symptoms last for 4 consecutive days. Medical treatment depends on the main symptoms and includes mood stabilizers (lithium is first-line), antipsychotics (haloperidol, risperidone), anti-anxiety (lorazepam, clonazepam), anticonvulsants (carbamazepine, valproate), and antidepressants (may heighten mania or suicide risk). Also include psychotherapy and ongoing monitoring.

MAJOR DEPRESSIVE DISORDER

Major depressive disorder (**MDD**) is a condition in which a depressed mood and/or anhedonia are present for most of the day for 2 weeks (usually lasts longer) and greatly affect a patient's ability to function. This affects women more than men and usually presents in adolescence or young adulthood. At least 5 of the following symptoms must be present in the same 2-week period, with at least 1 of the first 2 symptoms, to be classified as MDD: anhedonia, depressed mood most of the day, fatigue, sleep disturbances, psychomotor retardation or agitation, decreased concentration/ability to think or indecisiveness, weight loss or gain, feelings of worthlessness or guilt, and suicidal ideation or an attempt. Certain specifiers can be added to the diagnosis, including with anxious distress, mixed features, melancholic features, psychotic features, catatonic features, peripartum onset, and seasonal pattern.

DEPRESSIVE DISORDER WITH A SEASONAL PATTERN

Major depressive disorder with a seasonal pattern (also referred to as **seasonal affective disorder, SAD**) is form of major depressive disorder in which patients experience ≥5 of the above symptoms, which recur and remit during certain times of the year over a 2-year period. This typically presents in the winter and remits in the spring but may occur at other times of the year. Clinicians should screen for depression; there are multiple screening questionnaires, including the Beck Depression Inventory (BDI), Patient Health Questionnaire-9 (PHQ-9), and Zung Self-Rating Depression Scale. On PE, patients often have a normal appearance but may have poor grooming and hygiene as the symptoms worsen. Patients often have a flat affect, and speech may be slow or monotone. Rule out other causes of the symptoms, including drug-induced depression or other conditions. MDD is usually treated with both psychotherapy and medication. SSRIs are typically first-line, and other antidepressants include SNRIs, tricyclics, and MAOIs. If drugs are ineffective, ECT (electroconvulsive therapy) or phototherapy (for seasonal depression) may be used.

PERSISTENT DEPRESSIVE DISORDER (DYSTHYMIA)

Persistent depressive disorder (dysthymia) is a **DSM-5 diagnosis** that combines the previous DSM-IV diagnoses of **chronic major depressive disorder and dysthymia**. This usually has an insidious onset in childhood, adolescence, or young adulthood (referred to as "early onset" if diagnosed before 21 years old). The causes include a positive family history, imbalances in the neurotransmitters in the brain, and possibly environmental factors, such as tragedy in one's life. Patients are at an increased risk of personality disorders, anxiety disorders, and substance abuse.

Depression is a common illness, and most patients experience more than one major depressive episode in a lifetime. But patients with persistent depressive disorder have **continuous depressive symptoms** for ≥2 years (≥1 year in children/adolescents) for most of the day and for more days than not, along with ≥2 of the following symptoms: decreased appetite or overeating, insomnia or hypersomnia, decreased energy/fatigue, low self-esteem, decreased concentration or difficulty making decisions, and feeling hopeless. This is chronic, can be debilitating, and can be difficult to treat. Treatment includes a combination of psychotherapy and antidepressant medications (SSRIs). Inpatient treatment may be necessary in those contemplating suicide. It should be noted that suicide rates tend to be higher in patients as they are "coming out of" a major depressive episode, when their mood and outlook on life seem to be improving.

DISSOCIATIVE DISORDERS

Dissociative disorders are a group of disorders, according to the DSM-5, in which there is a disruption/discontinuity in the way people normally **integrate** consciousness, identity, memory or perception, their body representation, motor control, emotions, and their behavior. These usually appear due to **intense trauma** in a person's life. These disorders include: **dissociative identity disorder** (formerly multiple personality disorder; usually due to extreme trauma in childhood), **dissociative amnesia** (autobiographic memories are forgotten, usually surrounding a traumatic event), and **depersonalization/derealization disorder** (disordered perception, usually due to severe stress). All of these dissociative disorders may not be due to a substance, other medical condition (e.g., seizures), or other mental disorder that better describes the symptoms. These patients are at a high risk of self-harm and suicide. These are clinical diagnoses. Treatment involves psychotherapy (sometimes medications for symptoms), and it is important that patients feel safe.

EATING DISORDERS

ANOREXIA NERVOSA

Anorexia nervosa is an **eating disorder** in which patients have a considerably **below-normal body weight** due to food intake that is under the necessary requirements, an intense fear of weight gain/being fat, and misperceptions of their body weight and/or shape. Patients avoid eating, exercise a lot, and purge, and some even binge and then purge. This usually affects adolescent females. The cause is complex and not completely understood, but there is a genetic component. Those at higher risk include those with perfectionistic or obsessive tendencies, low self-esteem, a positive family history, conflict resolution difficulties, and a difficulty expressing negative emotions. Patients are at a higher risk of having OCD tendencies, bipolar disorder, depressive disorders, and anxiety disorders.

On PE, the patient may appear emaciated and have orthostatic hypotension, bradycardia, hypothermia, dry skin, and thinning or brittle hair and nails. Amenorrhea and osteopenia may be present, and cardiac dysrhythmias often develop, which increases mortality and the risk of sudden death. Lab results can show anemia, decreased WBC, decreased platelets, increased LFTs, hypoglycemia, hyponatremia, hypochloremia, hypokalemia, increased blood urea nitrogen (BUN), and either acidosis (from overusing laxatives) or alkalosis (from vomiting). Patients may need to be admitted to closely monitor while refeeding is slowly started; and treatment also includes various forms of psychotherapy to help patients develop a better self-image and learn healthy coping methods. Medication is typically only used for medical complications, but SSRIs may help with some of the anorexia symptoms. Close medical monitoring is necessary to detect any possible life-threatening effects of anorexia.

Bulimia Nervosa

Bulimia nervosa is an **eating disorder** characterized by episodes of **bingeing and purging**. Patients feel out of control and eat excessive amounts over a certain timeframe (2-hour period), then compensate through activities like inducing vomiting, over-exercising, or using laxatives/diuretics. The DSM-5 states that this must occur once a week for most weeks over a 3-month period to be diagnosed. This usually affects adolescent or young adult females. It is not entirely clear what causes bulimia, but a family history of eating disorders, along with a low self-esteem, anxiousness, depressive symptoms, and concerns over weight can contribute. Patients with bulimia are at an increased risk of having other mental disorders. Suicide risk is increased in both anorexia and bulimia nervosa.

Patients with bulimia usually appear normal in size to overweight and may have bilateral parotid gland enlargement. A positive Russell's sign (calluses or scarring on the knuckles from inducing vomiting), esophagitis, and dental caries or dental erosion (especially noted on the front teeth) can occur because of damage from stomach acids during vomiting. Dehydration, hypotension, electrolyte abnormalities (hypokalemia, hyponatremia, hypochloremia), metabolic alkalosis (due to vomiting), metabolic acidosis (due to laxative and diuretic abuse), and cardiac dysrhythmias may also occur and may be life-threatening. Treatment is usually on an outpatient basis and involves cognitive behavior therapy to develop an improved self-esteem and healthy coping methods; Prozac is also used. Prozac, which helps reduce bingeing, is the only medication indicated for treatment of bulimia. Close medical monitoring is necessary to detect any life-threatening effects of bulimia.

Neurodevelopment Disorders
Attention-Deficit/Hyperactivity Disorder

Attention-deficit/hyperactivity disorder (**ADHD**) is a **neurodevelopment disorder** that appears in early childhood and affects boys more often than girls. This must be properly diagnosed in order for prescribed medications to have the desired effect. Diagnosis is clinical and based on DSM-5 criteria. The following must not be typical for the patient's developmental level; they negatively affect the patient's interactions/activities, are present for >6 months, and include ≥6 of the following "inattention" criteria: doesn't pay attention to details and makes careless mistakes in school/other activities; difficulty keeping attention in tasks/play; does not appear to listen when directly spoken to; doesn't follow through on instructions/fails to finish tasks; difficulty organizing tasks/activities; avoids/dislikes/reluctant to engage in tasks that call for sustained mental effort; loses things needed for tasks/activities; easily distracted; often forgetful in daily activities. Hyperactivity and impulse-control symptoms include ≥6 of the following: often fidgets, taps hands or feet, squirms; often leaves seat in classroom/work; often runs/climbs where it is inappropriate; often not able to play/do leisure activities quietly; often on the go as if driven by a motor; often talks excessively; blurts out answers before question is finished; difficulty waiting turn; often interrupts/intrudes on others. For both categories, several must be present before 12 years old and must be present in ≥2 settings.

Treatment includes behavioral therapy and medication. Stimulants are first-line and include the following (extended-release and once-a-day dosing are usually preferred): methylphenidate (Ritalin), amphetamine-dextroamphetamine (Adderall), dexmethylphenidate (Focalin), dextroamphetamine (Dexedrine), and lisdexamfetamine (Vyvanse). In true ADHD, these drugs have a calming effect on the patient rather than a stimulating effect. Common side effects include reduced appetite, stomachache, headache, sleep disturbances, and depression.

AUTISM SPECTRUM DISORDER

Autism spectrum disorder is a **neurodevelopment disorder** in which there are **deficits in social interaction and communication** as well as **restricted or repetitive behaviors** that significantly affect how patients interact and function. This appears in early childhood and affects boys more than girls. The cause is unknown but may be affected by genetics, prenatal/obstetric complications (e.g., congenital rubella), and toxic exposure. DSM-5 diagnostic criteria include: persistent deficits in social-emotional reciprocity; deficits in nonverbal communication skills; deficits in developing/maintaining/understanding relationships; ≥2 of the following: stereotyped or repetitive movements, use of objects, or speech; insisting on regularity, having ritualized behavior/speech, or being inflexible to changing routines; highly restricted/fixated interests; under- or overreactions to sensory input. The severity of these 2 categories (social communication and restricted/repetitive behaviors) should be noted in the diagnosis. Treatment involves a multidisciplinary approach and may include intensive behavioral approaches, special education, speech and language therapy, PT and OT, nutrition, and medications. Early intervention appears to be key.

OBSESSIVE-COMPULSIVE DISORDERS

OBSESSIVE-COMPULSIVE DISORDER

Obsessive-compulsive disorder (**OCD**) is a condition, according to the DMS-5, in which a person has **intrusive and unwanted obsessions** (recurrent and persistent urges, thoughts, or images) and/or **compulsions** that compel them to perform repeated activities or mental acts (e.g., counting, praying) that must be rigidly followed, and completing them allows the person to lower anxiety and stress levels. These obsessions and compulsions cause distress (patients try to suppress or neutralize the obsession with a thought or action), are time-consuming (>1 hour/day), and interfere with their daily lives. Examples of obsessions include fear of contamination, desire for safety, forbidden or aggressive thoughts including harm to self or others, and needing symmetry or order.

The condition frequently begins during adolescence, affects males and females equally, and may be due to several factors, including environmental (e.g., abuse, traumatic events) and genetic; low serotonin levels may also play a role. Some research indicates there may be a link between group A streptococcal infections and OCD. Excessive stress can worsen OCD. Treatment is psychotherapy (e.g., cognitive behavior therapy) and SSRI antidepressants (e.g., Prozac, Paxil, Zoloft) or clomipramine (a tricyclic with serotonergic effects). These medications help to elevate serotonin levels in the brain. OCD patients are at an increased risk of suicide. Other OCD-related disorders include: body dysmorphic disorder, hoarding disorder, trichotillomania, and excoriation disorder.

> **Review Video: Obsessive-Compulsive Disorder (OCD)**
> Visit mometrix.com/academy and enter code: 499790

PERSONALITY DISORDERS

CLUSTER A PERSONALITY DISORDERS (ODD OR ECCENTRIC)

PARANOID PERSONALITY DISORDER

Paranoid personality disorder is characterized by **odd or eccentric behavior** that interferes with daily living due to a **pervasive distrust or suspicion of others**, leading the person to interpret others' motives as bad. There may be a genetic component to this disorder, and environmental factors—such as a history of child abuse or neglect—may also play a role in developing this disorder. Symptoms of paranoid personality disorder include 4 or more of the following: suspecting, without proper evidence, that others are out to harm, exploit, or deceive them; preoccupation with doubts that people are untrustworthy or disloyal; reluctance to confide in others due to fear that the information will be used against them; reading hidden meanings in innocuous comments or events; being unforgiving or bearing grudges; quickness to angrily react to perceived attacks on their character, and then counterattacking; and having recurring suspicions about the faithfulness of their spouse/partner.

This personality pattern begins by early adulthood, is chronic, goes against the social norm, and is present in all settings (social and work). These patients may find criticism in even the most innocent remark, have difficulty maintaining healthy relationships, and do not work well with others. Treatment of paranoid personality disorder is with psychotherapy (cognitive behavior therapy, group therapy), and sometimes medications (antidepressants, antianxiety, and antipsychotics) may be helpful in controlling some of the symptoms. Therapy can be difficult because of patients' inability to form trusting relationships with therapists.

SCHIZOID PERSONALITY DISORDER

Schizoid personality disorder is a condition in which people are **detached, withdraw from society, have difficulty expressing emotions, and avoid interaction with others**. This affects males slightly more than females; it usually appears before adolescence and definitely by young adulthood. They often find relationships too distressing and feel more comfortable when they are isolated. The cause is thought to be genetic. Symptoms of schizoid personality disorder include ≥4 of the following: doesn't enjoy or desire close relationships (e.g., being part of a family); prefers solitary activities; little to no interest in sexual activities with others; little to no pleasure in activities; lacks close friends (except maybe a first-degree relative); indifference to praise or criticism; emotionally cold, has a flat affect, shows very little emotion, or is detached. These patients may be poor students and seem to have no direction in life.

Psychotherapy is the mainstay of treatment with schizoid personality disorder. This is focused on developing social skills and helping patients find pleasure from interacting with others. Medications may be used to help treat some of the concomitant symptoms of depression or anxiety. This is difficult to treat since patients lack interest in others, and therefore have little desire to change.

SCHIZOTYPAL PERSONALITY DISORDER

Schizotypal personality disorder is a chronic condition in which people **isolate themselves from social situations** because of extreme anxiety when interacting with others due to **distortions in their perceptions and thinking**. The main risk factor is a family history of schizophrenia, and patients are at increased risk of major depressive disorder and substance abuse.

Symptoms of schizotypal personality disorder include ≥5 of the following: ideas of reference (interpreting ordinary events as having special meaning); odd beliefs, superstitions, magical thinking, or belief in special powers (e.g., mental telepathy); experiencing unusual perceptions; odd thinking and speech; suspicious or paranoid ideation; inappropriate and restricted facial expressions; odd/eccentric-appearing behavior; lacking close friends (except for first-degree relatives)/having problems relating with others; being anxious in social settings/social anxiety/having paranoid fears about the intentions of others. Stress can cause brief psychotic episodes but only last minutes to hours, and therefore does not meet diagnostic criteria for a psychotic disorder. Treatment is with a combination of psychotherapy (cognitive behavior therapy and skills training) and medications (atypical antipsychotics may help to relieve some of the symptoms of this condition, as well as antidepressants). Therapy can be difficult because of patients' inability to develop trusting relationships with therapists.

CLUSTER B PERSONALITY DISORDERS (DRAMATIC, EMOTIONAL, OR ERRATIC)

ANTISOCIAL PERSONALITY DISORDER

Antisocial personality disorder is a pervasive pattern of **disregard for the rights of others and society's rules**, so patients often repeatedly break the law, lie, cheat, steal, or harm others. The condition is often noticed during the teenage years, and symptoms tend to decrease as a person approaches middle age. It is much more common in males, has a genetic component, and may develop in those who suffer child abuse or neglect, especially if they already have conduct disorder. They are at an increased risk of other personality disorders (e.g., narcissistic, borderline), suicide, substance abuse, pathologic gambling, and becoming homicidal.

Symptoms include ≥3 of the following (symptoms must be present by age 15, but this cannot be diagnosed until 18): failing to conform to societal norms by repeatedly breaking the law; repeated deceitfulness/lying/conning others; impulsiveness/not planning ahead; being irritable and aggressive/often getting into fights/assaults; reckless disregard for the safety of self or others; being consistently irresponsible/can't keep jobs or meet financial responsibilities; lacking remorse. There must also be evidence of **conduct disorder** (e.g., bullying, being aggressive, threatening, beginning physical fights, having used a weapon, being physically cruel to people or animals, destroying property, stealing, breaking rules) before 15 years of age to meet the diagnostic criteria in DSM-5. These people don't like to be bored, are often poor parents, and are frequently imprisoned for their actions. Often, they people appear to be charming at first. Antisocial personality disorder is very hard to treat, and there is controversy about whether it is even a treatable condition. A combination of psychotherapy (cognitive behavior therapy) with antidepressants (SSRIs) or mood stabilizers (lithium, valproate) may help to control some of the symptoms (e.g., aggressiveness).

BORDERLINE PERSONALITY DISORDER

Borderline personality disorder (BPD) is a condition in which a person is **unstable in relationships, self-image, and mood**, and is **impulsive**. People with BPD are constantly in a **conflicting state** in which they cannot regulate their emotions. This condition is much more prevalent in women (75%), begins by young adult years, and is thought to occur due to a combination of genetics and environment (e.g., child abuse or neglect is common). They are at an increased risk of suicide and comorbid conditions like bipolar disorder, bulimia, substance abuse, and other personality disorders.

Symptoms of BPD must include ≥5 of the following (DSM-5): frantic efforts to avoid abandonment, either real or imagined; unstable and intense relationships that oscillate between idealizing a person and then devaluing them; unstable self-image; impulsiveness in at least 2 areas that can be harmful (e.g., substance abuse, overspending, reckless driving); recurrent suicidal or self-mutilating behaviors; reactive mood and affect; chronically feeling empty; difficulty controlling anger or angry outbursts; temporary paranoid ideation or dissociative symptoms that are related to stress. The roller coaster of mood swings makes relationships very difficult; they may be happy with their life situation one day and hate it the next, and they frequently change jobs. Treatment of BPD is with a combination of various forms of psychotherapy and medications. Mood stabilizers (lamotrigine, topiramate), atypical antipsychotics, and SSRIs may help control some of the symptoms. Do not use benzodiazepines in these patients since they are prone to substance abuse and overdose. Hospitalization is necessary if patients are at imminent risk of harming themselves.

HISTRIONIC PERSONALITY DISORDER

Histrionic personality disorder is a condition in which a person is **extremely emotional and attention seeking**. The condition seems to be equally or slightly more common in women than men, and the cause is not completely understood, though it may be due to a combination of genetic and environmental factors. It appears by early adulthood, and these people are at an increased risk of comorbid somatoform disorders and major depressive disorder. Symptoms of histrionic personality disorder are present in a variety of settings and include ≥5 of the following (DSM-5): being uncomfortable when not the center of attention; often acting provocatively toward others; rapidly changing and shallow emotions; using their appearance to draw attention to themselves; speech lacking details; expressing emotions in a dramatic, theatric, and over-the-top way; being suggestible and easily influenced by others or by their circumstances; considering relationships more intimate than they truly are. Treatment of histrionic personality disorder is usually with psychotherapy, but this can be difficult since patients may exaggerate symptoms and form inappropriate attachments to the therapist. Antidepressants and antianxiety medications may help with possible comorbid conditions.

Narcissistic Personality Disorder

Narcissistic personality disorder is a condition in which people **feel that they are superior to others, need to be admired, and have no regard for others**. It occurs more frequently in males than females, and symptoms often become evident in early adulthood. These people are at an increased risk of comorbid depressive disorders, substance abuse, and other personality disorders. Narcissistic personality disorder may be caused by multiple factors (neurobiological and environmental) but is not yet understood.

Symptoms occur in a variety of situations and must include ≥5 of the following (DSM-5): grandiose sense of self-importance; preoccupation with fantasies of unlimited success, power, influence, intellectual superiority, beauty, or ideal/perfect love; belief that they are special and can only truly be understood by those who are equally special (e.g., high-status); needing to be excessively admired; entitlement; exploiting others; lacking empathy for others; envying or thinking others envy him/her; having arrogant or haughty attitudes or actions. Criticism from others can be devastating, but these patients will often put down or counterattack those who do not praise them. They belittle others and have difficulty maintaining healthy relationships since take advantage of others to get what they want. The primary treatment for narcissistic personality disorder is psychotherapy. If there is underlying depression or anxiety, medications to treat these conditions may be helpful.

Cluster C Personality Disorders (Anxious or Fearful)

Avoidant Personality Disorder

Avoidant personality disorder is a condition in which a person feels **inadequate** and thus is very anxious or fearful of **social situations where they may be criticized**. The cause is not fully understood, but social, biological/genetic, temperamental (e.g., shy and fearful), and environmental factors may play a role in the development of this disorder. It occurs equally in males and females and begins by early adulthood, and patients have an increased risk of depressive, anxiety, bipolar, and dependent personality disorder. Symptoms must include ≥4 of the following (DSM-5): avoids work-related activities due to fears they will be criticized or rejected; avoids relationships with others unless they think they will be liked; is restrained in intimate relationships due to fear of being shamed or ridiculed; is preoccupied with thoughts of being criticized/rejected in social settings; is inhibited in new social situations due to feeling inadequate; has low self-esteem/feels inferior; doesn't want to be embarrassed and therefore is reluctant to take risks/be a part of new activities. Treat with a combination of psychotherapy and antidepressants or antianxiety medications.

Dependent Personality Disorder

Dependent personality disorder is a condition in which there is an **extreme need to be cared for**, which causes patients to be **submissive and overly clingy**. It may be slightly more common in women, it appears by early adulthood, and there is an increased risk for anxiety and adjustment disorder. ≥5 of the following must be present (DSM-5): can't make decisions on their own; need others to be responsible for most parts of their life; find it hard to disagree with others; have a hard time initiating things on their own; go to great lengths to get others' support; feel helpless and fearful of being alone since they don't think they can care for themselves; seek relationships with people who will care for them; are preoccupied with fears of being alone and unable to care for themselves. Treatment primarily involves psychotherapy (cognitive behavior therapy) and sometimes antidepressants (SSRIs). Therapists need to be careful not to encourage dependent attachments of the patient.

Obsessive-Compulsive Personality Disorder

Obsessive-compulsive personality disorder (as opposed to obsessive-compulsive disorder) is a condition in which people are preoccupied with being **orderly, perfect, and in control**, and so become **inflexible**. This is more common in men and appears by early adulthood, and these people are at an increased risk of depressive disorders and alcohol abuse. ≥4 of the following must be present (DSM-5): preoccupied with organization, lists, schedules, details, or rules; perfectionism that interferes with the task; overly devoted to work, neglecting leisure activities; inflexible in matters of morality, values, ethics; cannot get rid of old or worn-out things; reluctant to delegate unless the person follows exactly what they want; miserly in spending for both themselves and others; rigid and stubborn. Treatment involves psychotherapy (cognitive behavior therapy) and SSRIs.

OTHER SCHIZOPHRENIA SPECTRUM DISORDERS
DELUSIONAL DISORDER

Delusional disorder is a condition in which a person develops a very **strong, fixed belief** (delusion; must be present ≥1 month) in a specific situation that is **not true**, to the point that they alter their behaviors and life around this idea. However, there are no psychotic symptoms as in schizophrenia. This disorder may be caused by a combination of environmental or genetic factors, though no specific cause is understood. Delusional disorder can take different forms. Patients may have **delusions of grandeur** (grandiose type), believing that they are above everyone else and in a much higher standing than they really are. They may have **persecutory delusions** (persecutory type) that others are out to hurt, cheat, spy on, or conspire against them. They may believe **someone is in love with them** (erotomanic type) or that their **partner is unfaithful to them** (jealous type). They may also have delusions that **something is wrong with their body** (somatic type), like an odor, a sensation that bugs are crawling on them, or an infection, when there is nothing medically wrong.

Treatment can be challenging since many don't seek medical help, as they don't think anything is wrong; but it may include a combination of supportive psychotherapy and medications (antidepressants and antipsychotics may help to control the symptoms). Treatment can be difficult since patients firmly believe in their delusions, so the medical provider must work to develop an alliance with the patient.

SCHIZOPHRENIA AND SCHIZOAFFECTIVE DISORDER

Schizophrenia is a chronic disorder that includes the presence of ≥2 of the following, with at least 1 of the first 3 (most of the time in a 1-month period): delusions; hallucinations; disorganized speech; grossly disorganized/bizarre or catatonic behavior; negative symptoms like reduced expression of emotions. These psychotic symptoms (delusions and hallucinations) greatly affect how patients function. Signs of the disturbance are present for ≥6 months and can include certain stages of schizophrenia (prodrome, active phase, residual periods). This condition usually appears in late adolescence and affects males and females equally. Treatment includes antipsychotics: first-generation (e.g., haloperidol, chlorpromazine) cause extrapyramidal side effects; second-generation (e.g., clozapine) cause weight gain and glucose/lipid issues. Early treatment is key. Suicide risk is increased in this disorder.

Schizoaffective disorder is a combination of **schizophrenic symptoms** (≥2 schizophrenic symptoms) with **mood symptoms** (either major depressive or manic). These patients may have hallucinations and delusions with depression or mania; specify if patient is bipolar type or depressive type. The cause is unknown but may be due to imbalances of brain neurotransmitters. Symptoms may become severe enough that patients can be at risk for harming themselves or others. Treatment consists of a combination of psychotherapy and medications to control the symptoms: antidepressants (SSRIs) and antipsychotics in depressive types; mood stabilizers (e.g., lithium, carbamazepine, valproic acid) and antipsychotics in manic types. Hospitalization may be necessary for inpatient treatment, especially if patients are at risk of hurting themselves or others.

Pulmonary System

INFECTIOUS DISORDERS
ACUTE BRONCHITIS

Acute bronchitis is inflammation of the **bronchial tree**, usually caused by an **infection** (typically a virus). This irritation causes the bronchial structures to secrete more **mucus**, resulting in a cough. Patients with acute bronchitis usually describe recent history of a URI (e.g., congestion, rhinorrhea, occasionally a fever); complain of a cough, which may be productive; and may describe some wheezing or substernal discomfort when breathing or coughing. The color of the sputum does not indicate whether it is due to a virus or bacteria. Physical exam may reveal rhonchi and/or wheezing. Diagnose clinically; rule out other diagnoses like pneumonia or influenza. Treatment is supportive. Because acute bronchitis is usually caused by a virus, antibiotics don't help relieve symptoms unless there is a bacterial superinfection, which only occurs about 10% of the time. Using a humidifier at night to moisten the air, mucolytics, drinking plenty of fluids to thin the mucus secretions, and resting should help to relieve the symptoms within a week. The cough of bronchitis may linger for 2–3 weeks as the bronchial tubes heal.

ACUTE BRONCHIOLITIS/RESPIRATORY SYNCYTIAL VIRUS INFECTION (RSV)

Acute bronchiolitis is a disease of the **lower respiratory tract** that is caused by a virus, typically **respiratory syncytial virus (RSV)**. This most often affects infants and young children (<2 years old) because older children and adults have larger airways that can accommodate the inflammation, epithelial necrosis, and edema associated with it. Bronchiolitis peaks in the fall, winter, or early spring months. More severe disease is common in the youngest patients (1–6 months old) and may require hospitalization; bronchiolitis is the most common reason children <1 are admitted. Incubation is 2–8 days, with a prodrome of 1–3 days and symptoms that range from a common cold to severe respiratory issues. Patients may remain contagious up to 4 weeks from the onset. Parents of patients with acute bronchiolitis may describe their child wheezing and coughing frequently, appearing short of breath, being fussy and irritable, and feeding poorly. A low-grade fever is usually present. Coughing and wheezing may continue for 2–3 weeks, and rarely, severe respiratory symptoms can lead to respiratory arrest. Assess for wheezing, air exchange, respiratory rate, and retractions.

Diagnose clinically (a rapid antigen RSV test is available but not routinely required). Since the cause is viral, treatment is supportive, with nasal suctioning, antipyretics as needed, and plenty of fluids to prevent dehydration. Albuterol, racemic epinephrine, and steroids are no longer routinely recommended according to the AAP (American Academy of Pediatrics). A trial of nebulized albuterol may be used, but should not be continued if there is no improvement. If admitted, humidified oxygen and IV fluids are given. Premature infants born <29 weeks should receive palivizumab prophylaxis (a monoclonal antibody to RSV) during their first year of life.

ACUTE EPIGLOTTITIS

Acute epiglottitis is a medical emergency that may result in the **epiglottis blocking the trachea** if it is not treated immediately. It can be caused by the *H. influenzae* bacterium but is not seen as often due to the Hib immunization now available. Other causes are *H. parainfluenzae*, *Streptococcus pneumoniae*, and group A streptococci. Trauma to the throat can also cause inflammation of the epiglottis. Patients with epiglottitis usually have a muffled voice, throat pain, fever, difficulty swallowing, and possibly difficulty breathing. Patients lean forward in the classic tripod position to breathe and may even drool if swallowing is too difficult. If epiglottitis is suspected, one should NOT attempt to visualize the epiglottis directly with a tongue depressor during physical exam because this may cause more inflammation and could close the airway. Stridor, muffled voice, and a history of DM are indicators for the likelihood of airway intervention. Lateral neck x-rays will show an enlarged epiglottis (thumb sign). However, this is being replaced by nasopharyngoscopy/laryngoscopy in the operating room, which allows for direct visualization and thus a rapid, accurate diagnosis.

Treat with third-generation cephalosporins, like ceftriaxone (Rocephin), which are used due to the increasing resistance to ampicillin; amoxicillin/clavulanic acid is another option. If penicillin/cephalosporin allergic, chloramphenicol can be used. Patients should be kept calm and should avoid swallowing or talking, and intubation and cricothyrotomy equipment should be kept on hand in case of airway obstruction.

CROUP

Croup occurs because of inflammation around the **larynx and trachea** due to a **viral infection**. It occurs in children (especially ages 6 months to 3 years) and causes a **characteristic barking cough** that is seal-like and very distinguishable. It is most often caused by the parainfluenza virus (usually in the fall), though sometimes by adenovirus, RSV, or influenza. The barking cough associated with croup is usually worse at night and can wake a child from sleep. Patients typically present with recent history of URI symptoms and fever, a barking cough, inspiratory stridor, hoarseness, and some level of respiratory distress. More severe cases may have inspiratory and expiratory stridor at rest, retractions, and distress or agitation. Assess for hypoxia, tachypnea, and respiratory rate.

Diagnose clinically; AP/lateral neck and chest x-rays may be ordered if indicated. Symptoms typically last <1 week, and most cases can be treated at home with humidified air (cool mist vaporizer or sitting in the bathroom with steam from running a hot shower; however, there are no supporting research studies), keeping the child calm, cool drinks or popsicles to help ease the inflammation in the throat, staying hydrated, and antipyretics. Also, oral steroids may be prescribed for a few days, or a one-time dose of IM dexamethasone (especially helpful if given in the first 4–24 hours of the disease; effective within 6 hours). If racemic epinephrine (nebulizer) is given in the emergency department for moderate or severe distress, patients must be observed for 3–4 hours due to a possible rebound effect from the medication. Occasionally, hospitalization is necessary, with treatments including humidified oxygen, racemic epinephrine, steroids, or even intubation if very severe.

PNEUMONIAS
CAUSES

Pneumonia, which is an infection of the **lungs**, can be caused by bacteria, viruses, fungi, or parasites. Patients are at greater risk if they are >65 years old or <5 years old, are immunocompromised, have a chronic disease (e.g., CVD, DM, COPD, asthma), have had recent surgery, are asplenic, or smoke. Chest x-rays are helpful, but findings vary greatly, so they may not be used to diagnose a particular kind of pneumonia.

Bacterial pneumonia is most often caused by *Streptococcus pneumoniae* (most common), *H. influenzae*, and *Moraxella catarrhalis*. *Staphylococcus aureus* can cause severe pneumonia after having influenza, and the gram-negative organism *Klebsiella pneumoniae* is more common in alcoholics and produces a "currant jelly" sputum. *Mycoplasma pneumoniae* is an atypical bacterium that causes a milder disease (i.e., "walking pneumonia"). Other atypicals include *Legionella pneumophilia* and *Chlamydia psittaci* (carried by pet birds).

Viral pneumonia is commonly caused by influenza A or B. RSV (especially if less than 1 year old), parainfluenza, human metapneumovirus, and adenovirus are other common causes. Herpes virus pneumonias like herpes simplex, CMV, and varicella are rare in the immunocompetent patient.

Fungal pneumonia is usually caused by *Histoplasma capsulatum*, *Coccidioides immitis*, or *Blastomyces dermatitidis*. These may occur in healthy patients and are usually self-limited, but may cause illness. Serious disease usually doesn't occur unless patients are severely immunocompromised.

HIV-related pneumonia is most often caused by *Pneumocystis jiroveci*, though the immunocompromised patient is susceptible to contracting any type of pneumonia. Opportunistic fungal pneumonias like *Aspergillus*, parasites like *Toxoplasma gondii*, and herpes viruses like CMV, Epstein-Barr virus, and varicella-zoster are more common among HIV patients.

Community-acquired pneumonia (CAP) is most commonly caused by *Streptococcus pneumoniae*. Other typical pathogens of CAP include *H. influenzae*, *Moraxella catarrhalis*, atypical bacteria (e.g., *Legionella*, *Chlamydia pneumoniae,* and *Mycoplasma* species), and viruses. **Hospital-acquired pneumonia (HAP)** occurs after ≥48 hours of being in the hospital; it is most commonly caused by gram-negative bacteria (*Pseudomonas aeruginosa*) and *Staphylococcus aureus* (including MRSA) and is usually multi-drug resistant. Encourage influenza and pneumococcal vaccines for prevention.

SYMPTOMS AND TREATMENT

Patients with **bacterial pneumonia** typically present with a high fever, chills, a productive cough with purulent sputum, fatigue, pleuritic chest pain, SOB, dyspnea, elevated respiratory rate, and elevated heart rate, and appear quite ill. Patients may have crackles, reduced breath sounds, and a lung consolidation present on chest x-ray (PA and lateral). Blood and sputum cultures/Gram stain may be obtained if other organisms are suspected that would change treatment. Treat bacterial pneumonia with empiric antibiotics (if patient was previously healthy, use a macrolide; if comorbidities, antibiotics within the past 3 months, or inpatient but not in ICU, then use a respiratory fluoroquinolone OR β-lactam with a macrolide).

Viral pneumonia typically has a more gradual onset and presents with a low-grade fever, non-productive cough, viral prodrome, myalgias, and headache. Patients may be sick for several days before seeing a doctor. Chest x-ray is usually worse than the symptoms might suggest, and typically shows diffuse interstitial infiltrates with hilar adenopathy. Treat influenza with oseltamivir or zanamivir if started within 48 hours of symptom onset; acyclovir for varicella-zoster. Otherwise, treatment is symptomatic. Secondary bacterial infections are common with influenza.

Fungal pneumonias have similar symptoms but can also spread to become systemic. Treat with antifungals, depending on the infective organism.

HIV-related pneumonias have symptoms according to the type of pneumonia that's present; treatment depends upon the infective organism. Always follow local sensitivity patterns; patients should respond within 48–72 hours.

PERTUSSIS

Pertussis, or whooping cough, is a highly contagious **respiratory infection** caused by the gram-negative bacterium *Bordetella pertussis*. Pertussis is becoming more common now because immunity from the DTaP vaccine tends to wear off by adulthood, and because of a decrease in the number of people getting the vaccine. Incubation is 4–21 days. The symptoms come in 3 stages:

- The **catarrhal stage** begins gradually with symptoms of a cold such as runny nose, sneezing, lacrimation/red eyes, mild cough, and low-grade fever. This lasts 1–2 weeks.
- The **paroxysmal stage** is characterized by coughing spells that often leave the person breathless. These spells are followed by a loud inspiratory breath that makes a loud "whoop" sound. Post-tussive vomiting is common. This stage may last 1–6 weeks or longer.
- The **convalescent stage** lasts 2–6 weeks (sometimes months) as the chronic cough gradually fades.

Collect nasopharyngeal swab or nasal aspirates for PCR and culture before antibiotics are started. It is questionable whether antibiotics help to shorten the duration of symptoms, but they are given to reduce the spread of the disease. Treat with azithromycin for 5 days or erythromycin for 14 days. There are no proven effective treatments for the cough, but try not to agitate the child. Prophylaxis is given to close contacts (same as treatment). Report suspected cases to the local health department, which reports to the CDC.

TUBERCULOSIS

Tuberculosis (**TB**) is a disease caused by the aerobic bacillus *Mycobacterium tuberculosis*. It is spread through air droplets, and can cause either a **latent** TB infection (LTBI) or an **active** form. TB is more prevalent in those who are at a high risk, including those from countries with a high rate of TB, those in institutions/living in crowded conditions, the homeless, IV drug users, and those with weakened immune systems (HIV/AIDS). TB is seen more often in those frequently exposed to the disease, like close family contacts or medical professionals. TB typically causes pulmonary disease but may also occur at other sites (extrapulmonary TB; lymphadenopathy is most common). After the primary infection (which is usually asymptomatic), the body encases the bacteria and forms granulomas (LTBI); both the primary infection and the latent stage are not contagious. This latent phase can be reactivated and become active (contagious).

Symptoms of active TB may include night sweats, chronic cough, hemoptysis, dyspnea, low-grade fever, fatigue, loss of appetite, weight loss, and pleurisy. Those at high risk should receive a screening test of either a tuberculin skin test (purified protein derivative [PPD]) or an interferon-gamma release assay blood test (IGRA; use this if previous BCG vaccine, given in other countries). If either is positive (PPD [check for induration after 2–3 days]: ≥15 mm if no risk factors, ≥10 mm if some risk factors, ≥5 mm if HIV positive or high risk factors), order a chest x-ray and acid-fast bacilli (AFB) sputum smear and culture to confirm diagnosis. Chest x-ray (PA and lateral with apical lordotic view) may show cavitary lesions or multilobar opacities in apices and upper aspect of lower lobes. First-line treatment includes multiple antibiotics: isoniazid (INH), rifampin (RIF), pyrazinamide (PZA), and ethambutol for 2 months; then, if susceptible, continue INH and RIF for 4 more months; but if resistant, instead use RIF, PZA, and ethambutol for 4 more months. Once diagnosed, patients with active TB should be kept in isolation, and the local health department should be notified. Latent disease is usually treated prophylactically with INH for 9 months.

OBSTRUCTIVE PULMONARY DISEASES

ASTHMA

Asthma is a **chronic lung disease** in which the **airways** become inflamed and narrowed. In response to allergens or triggers, airways are constricted by edema, inflammation, and mucus, producing breathing difficulties and the classic "asthma attacks." Risk increases with a positive family history and exposure to tobacco smoke. It can be aggravated by allergen exposure, aspirin, cold air, exercise, infections, and stress. The symptoms of asthma include wheezing, difficulty breathing, and chest tightness; symptoms may be worse during the night. Coughing spasms can also occur as the airways constrict and the lungs attempt to expel the extra mucus that is produced. Diagnose clinically and confirm with pulmonary function test (PFT) if ≥5 years old to show obstruction and reversibility. Process is as follows:

- Spirometry before and after bronchodilator
- FEV1 is measured
  - Airway obstruction is when FEV1/FVC ratio is <70%
  - Reversibility should be ≥12% increase in FEV1 or for adults, a >200 mL increase in FEV1 from baseline
- Obtain chest x-ray and rule out other conditions

Asthma severity can be classified as **intermittent, mild persistent** (symptoms >2 days/week needing rescue medications), **moderate persistent** (symptoms every day needing rescue medications), and **severe persistent** (symptoms every day and night, needing rescue medications several times per day). The goal of treatment is prevention, which includes steps to reduce allergen exposure. Treatment can be divided between long-acting medicines and quick-acting "rescue" medications. The long-acting drugs include inhaled corticosteroids (ICS), long-acting β-2 agonists (e.g., salmeterol), leukotriene modifiers, theophylline, Cromolyn, and sometimes immunomodulators (e.g., omalizumab). The short-acting medications are used when patients are having an acute exacerbation and include short-acting β-2 agonists, ipratropium (Atrovent), and systemic corticosteroids. A stepwise approach to treatment is best; for intermittent asthma, use SA bronchodilators as needed; for persistent asthma, start with low-dose ICS and step up as needed (e.g., use medium-dose ICS or add an LA bronchodilator). The key is prevention by minimizing exposure to known allergens or triggers, using medications regularly, and not smoking.

CHRONIC BRONCHITIS

Chronic bronchitis is a type of chronic obstructive pulmonary disease (COPD) that occurs when the **bronchial tubes** are irritated and inflamed, causing hyperplasia of mucus glands, excess mucus secretion, and epithelial damage resulting in plugged airways and decreased oxygen flow. **Smoking** is the most common cause of chronic bronchitis; occasionally, chronic exposure to dust and other irritants can cause chronic bronchitis. Patients usually complain of a chronic, productive cough, shortness of breath, dyspnea on exertion, fatigue, chest discomfort, and wheezing. Physical exam may show rhonchi and wheezing. Patients have recurrent lung infections, and over time, signs of right-sided heart failure, cyanosis, and weight gain ("blue bloater").

Diagnosis is made by symptoms of a productive cough for at least 3 months during a 2-year period. Confirm with PFTs that show an increase residual volume, reduced FEV1, and FEV1/FVC ratio <70% that is not reversible with bronchodilators. Chest x-ray (PA and lateral) may show increased pulmonary markings and an enlarged heart; a chest CT may also be ordered. Treatment is symptomatic and usually includes bronchodilators (either short- or long-acting depending on the severity), inhaled anticholinergics (ipratropium bromide is short-acting; tiotropium is long-acting), inhaled steroids, and possibly systemic steroids or antibiotics during exacerbations. Patients may require supplemental oxygen at home if hypoxia is severe. Patients should quit smoking to help decrease irritation to the lungs and should stay up to date on vaccines.

EMPHYSEMA

Emphysema, another type of COPD, occurs with lung damage past the **terminal bronchiole**, causing alveoli that lose their elasticity, alveoli that incompletely empty air on expiration, and damage to the capillary bed. This causes **hyperinflation of the lungs** with difficulty drawing in the oxygen needed to take another breath. The most common cause of emphysema is **smoking**; a deficiency in α-1 antitrypsin protein can also lead to emphysema. Patients typically have a thin appearance with a barrel chest, are short of breath and easily fatigued, and may have a mild, usually non-productive cough. Patients often purse their lips when exhaling ("pink puffers"). On exam, patients may be tachypneic, hypoxic, and may have decreased breath sounds with a hyperresonant chest, but are not cyanotic. Over time, patients will develop fingernail clubbing and will increasingly use accessory muscles.

Diagnose clinically and confirm with PFTs, which show an increased residual volume, reduced FEV1, and reduced FEV1/FVC ratio; this is not reversible with bronchodilators. Chest x-ray shows hyperinflation, flattened diaphragms, increased retrosternal airspace, possibly bullae, and a small heart; a chest CT may also be ordered. Treatment consists of inhaled bronchodilators (short- or long-acting), inhaled anticholinergics, inhaled steroids, and possibly systemic steroids or antibiotics during exacerbations. Quitting smoking is the best treatment to help prevent progression of the disease. Patients may require supplemental oxygen at home. Rarely, surgery may be done to remove the damaged tissue (bullectomy).

CYSTIC FIBROSIS

Cystic fibrosis (**CF**) is an **autosomal recessive genetic disorder** affecting the **exocrine glands**, especially involving the lungs and GI tract. It causes **excessive mucus production** that leads to pulmonary obstruction, deficient pancreatic enzyme production, and infertility issues (especially in males). There is no cure for cystic fibrosis. The average life expectancy in the US is in the late 30s or early 40s; death usually occurs due to pulmonary complications or cor pulmonale. **Bronchiectasis** occurs; this is a condition of the bronchial tubes caused by chronic inflammation and infection, which causes dilatation and damage, resulting in increasingly purulent sputum. The lungs become chronically infected with, usually, *Staphylococcus aureus* early on, then *Pseudomonas aeruginosa* as the disease progresses.

Symptoms present early and may include recurrent lung/sinus infections with excessive congestion, bowel obstruction due to thickened feces (meconium ileus), and failure to thrive or poor nutrition because of decreased absorption of fat-soluble vitamins, fats, proteins, and carbohydrates. Check for clubbing, cyanosis, cough, increased AP chest diameter, hepatosplenomegaly, and abdominal distension. The newborn screen now tests for CF, and the diagnosis is confirmed with sweat-chloride testing and genetic testing. Still about 10% are diagnosed later on, but usually by teenage or young adult years. Refer to a specialist team. Postural drainage and chest physiotherapy can be performed regularly to promote drainage of lung secretions. Pancreatic enzymes and multivitamins are taken orally to aid in digestion and nutrition. Bronchodilators, inhaled antibiotics, and mucolytics are given to decrease secretions and irritation in the lungs. In severe cases, lung transplantation can be performed to improve quality of life, though this still does not cure the disease.

OBSTRUCTIVE SLEEP APNEA/OBESITY HYPOVENTILATION SYNDROME

Obstructive sleep apnea (**OSA**) is caused by partial or complete closure of the upper airway that leads to **apnea or hypoventilation** for >10 seconds during sleep. This may occur at any age and is more prevalent in men. In children, this is usually due to hypertrophy of the tonsils and adenoids, and in adults is often due to obesity, alcohol, or sedative use. Anatomical risk factors include a large neck, large tongue or uvula, and crowded oropharynx. OSA can lead to many consequences, including growth retardation, poor concentration and memory, poor performance at work or school, depression, weight loss or an increased BMI, hypertension, and

CHF. Signs and symptoms include snoring, difficulty staying asleep, fatigue, daytime sleepiness, and poor concentration/memory. Diagnose with an overnight polysomnogram (sleep study); OSA is indicated by ≥5 apnea/hypopnea episodes per hour with symptoms or ≥15 episodes per hour without symptoms. Treatment includes modifying risk factors, using appliances, CPAP, or occasionally surgery to correct anatomic issues that cause OSA.

Obesity hypoventilation syndrome (OHS; also called Pickwickian syndrome) is a **breathing disorder** due to obesity that causes **hypercapnia and hypoxia**. This may lead to pulmonary hypertension, cor pulmonale, erythrocytosis, and early death. This may or may not be associated with OSA.

NEOPLASMS
CARCINOID TUMORS

Carcinoid tumors occur in the **neuroendocrine system** and are most frequently found in the small intestine, rectum, or appendix, but may also be found in the lungs, bronchi, or pancreas. They may be **benign** but are often **malignant** (especially if found in the ileum or bronchus) and metastasize to the liver, brain, or lungs. They are slow-growing tumors and may not be diagnosed right away. They most often present in adults and are often not diagnosed until patients are 50–60 years old. Patients with carcinoid tumors may be asymptomatic, but they may secrete hormones like serotonin and produce symptoms of **carcinoid syndrome** (flushing, diarrhea, wheezing, weight loss, loss of appetite). Diagnose with an imaging study (e.g., CT, bronchoscopy), plasma or urinary 5-HIAA, and biopsy. Treatment of carcinoid tumors consists of surgical removal of the tumor. Chemotherapy, as well as radiation, may be given if the tumor has spread to other locations in the body. Interferon-α may be given to help decrease the growth of the tumor, especially if metastatic or unresectable.

LUNG CANCER

Lung cancer is the **most common cause of cancer death** for both men and women, and **smoking** is the most common risk factor (~85%). There are two main types: **small cell lung cancer (SCLC)** and **non-small cell lung cancer (NSCLC)**. SCLC has the worse prognosis, is aggressive, and often already presents with metastases when diagnosed. 85% of all cases of lung cancer are NSCLC, which can be adenocarcinoma, large cell, or squamous cell (bronchogenic). **Squamous cell** is typically found centrally, in the bronchi, while **adenocarcinoma and large cell** are usually found as a peripheral mass or nodule. Symptoms of **bronchogenic carcinoma** include a progressively worsening cough, dyspnea, and chest pain, with or without hemoptysis. Weight loss and fatigue may be present as the disease progresses. Patients may be asymptomatic for a while. As the cancer spreads, it may encroach on the laryngeal nerve, causing hoarseness, or may cause **superior vena cava syndrome** (SVCS; swelling in the face, neck, upper extremities, or trunk; cough; headache/head fullness) or may cause **Horner syndrome** (ptosis, miosis, anhidrosis). If metastases are present, patients may experience bone pain, abdominal pain, or confusion, depending on the location of the metastases. Some small cell tumors may serve as an ectopic source of hormone production, so symptoms that mimic an endocrine disorder may be evident.

Diagnose with chest x-ray, CT, sputum or fluid cytology, and biopsy (usually by bronchoscopy). Often, once diagnosed, prognosis is very poor with this disease. Treatment may involve surgery to resect (NSCLC) or to debulk a large tumor, or a lobectomy. This may be followed with radiation and/or chemotherapy depending on the location and type of cancer. New research shows promise with immunotherapy and targeted therapy for genetic mutations.

PULMONARY NODULES

Pulmonary nodules are **lesions** <3 cm, often found incidentally on chest x-ray or CT scan, that are surrounded by **aerated lung tissue**. If >3 cm, it is referred to as a mass. Pulmonary nodules may be benign (~90%) or cancerous. **Benign nodules** are slower growing and may have many causes, including infection (abscess, TB, fungal, parasite), granulomas from a previous infection, hemangioma, cyst, lymph node, lipoma, or fibroma. Risk for a **cancerous nodule** increases with age, smoking, previous history of cancer, and larger size of the nodule. High-risk patients >55 years old may be screened with a low-dose CT. Patients are usually asymptomatic but may have a cough. Diagnosis involves using imaging studies. Compare previous chest x-ray or CT scans. Evaluate the nodule using CT. It is more likely benign if the nodule has not grown or doubled in 2 years, is <1.5 cm, is solid, and has a smooth edge. PET scan may be used to check for malignancy. Biopsy the nodule if malignancy is suspected. Rule out an infectious cause. Treatment is based on the findings and may include observation or resection. Growing nodules and those suspected to be cancerous should be resected. If the nodule is <1 cm, reevaluate in 3 months, in 6 months, then annually for 2 years. If the nodule is confirmed to be benign, no further follow-up is necessary.

PLEURAL DISEASES

PLEURAL EFFUSION

A pleural effusion is an accumulation of fluid in the **pleural space**. It can have many causes, but is frequently caused by **infections** such as pneumonia, or by **chronic diseases** such as CHF or lung cancer. The effusion can be classified as a transudate (due to changes in hydrostatic and plasma osmotic pressure) or as an exudate (due to increased capillary permeability). **Transudates** are typically caused by CHF, cirrhosis, or nephrotic syndrome. **Exudates** are typically caused by pneumonia, PEs, TB, or malignancies. Patients may be asymptomatic or may complain of a cough, dyspnea, and pleuritic chest pain. On physical exam, there may be decreased breath sounds, pleural friction rub, reduced tactile fremitus, and dullness to percussion over the effusion. The effusion is evident on chest x-ray and may be better examined by CT imaging.

Treatment depends on the size and type of effusion. Small effusions may be watched, and diuretics may be used to decrease the effusion if it is due to CHF. For a new or unexplained effusion, a thoracentesis and pleural fluid analysis may be done to draw the fluid off the lungs and to diagnose the type of effusion; a thoracentesis is both diagnostic and therapeutic. Check fluid pH, glucose, protein, LDH, cell count with differential, and Gram stain and culture. Treat the underlying cause. If the effusion is chronic, treat with pleurodesis or drain with an indwelling catheter. Complications include empyema, scarring, and pneumothorax.

PRIMARY, SECONDARY, TRAUMATIC, AND TENSION PNEUMOTHORAX

A pneumothorax is when air gets into the **pleural space**, causing the lung to partially or completely **collapse**. Symptoms usually include sudden, sharp chest pain, dyspnea, and SOB. Physical exam findings may include reduced breath sounds, asymmetric expansion of the lungs, tachypnea, and possibly respiratory distress. The main types are spontaneous, traumatic, and tension pneumothorax. A **spontaneous pneumothorax** can be either primary or secondary.

A **primary pneumothorax** is not due to lung disease and usually occurs in young, tall males. This happens when a bleb ruptures on the lung, causing collapse of a portion of the lung. If small, it can be monitored with repeated chest x-rays and usually heals in 1–2 weeks. If large, hospitalization with a chest tube (tube thoracostomy) may be necessary.

A **secondary pneumothorax** is more serious than a primary, and occurs due to chronic lung disease, such as COPD, cystic fibrosis, or TB. It can potentially be life-threatening and may require hospitalization and a chest tube for treatment.

A **traumatic pneumothorax** occurs when there is trauma to the chest wall that results in air entering the chest cavity. This can result in a small pneumothorax that can be monitored, or it may be large enough to require a chest tube.

A **tension pneumothorax** is a medical emergency and can be fatal. It occurs when air becomes trapped in the pleural space and cannot escape (due to increased pressure within the pleural space compared to atmospheric pressure). This results in a worsening pneumothorax that will eventually cause hypotension, tachycardia, and hypoxia, and cause the structures in the cavity to shift. It is life-threatening and should be treated immediately with a needle decompression (at the second intercostal space and midclavicular line) before confirming with a chest x-ray. Follow this with a chest tube.

181

PULMONARY CIRCULATION

COR PULMONALE

Cor pulmonale is **right-sided heart failure**. This can occur because of **prolonged pulmonary hypertension** due to lung disease, which causes an increase in pressure within the **right ventricle**. Chronic lung disease, such as COPD or cystic fibrosis, can lead to cor pulmonale, or it may occur acutely due to a pulmonary embolus. Patients may complain of increasing shortness of breath and fatigue. They may have chest pain and dyspnea that is exacerbated with activity and not entirely relieved with rest as the disease progresses. On exam, patients may have jugular venous distension, hepatomegaly, ascites, or lower extremity edema.

Diagnose with chest x-ray and echocardiogram; a heart catheterization may be needed to confirm the diagnosis and assess the pressures. Treating the underlying cause is the focus of treatment with cor pulmonale. Patients may require anticoagulant therapy to prevent thromboembolism. Diuretics are sometimes used for chronic cor pulmonale, but should be used with caution since they may worsen symptoms. Calcium channel blockers and vasodilators may be given to help optimize cardiac function if the right-sided heart failure is due to primary pulmonary hypertension. Oxygen therapy may be given to patients for home use in order to improve oxygenation of the blood; this is especially helpful in COPD patients.

PULMONARY EMBOLISM

A pulmonary embolism (**PE**) occurs when a **thrombus** travels to the **lungs** and causes obstruction of the airway. PE can be caused by a **deep vein thrombosis** (usually from the lower extremity or pelvis) that travels to the lungs, by any conditions that cause the blood to be **hypercoagulable**, or by **cardiac dysrhythmias**. Factors that increase risk include immobility, increased age, cancer, heart failure, smoking, use of oral contraceptives, postpartum, and recent surgery or trauma. Patients with a PE may be asymptomatic, or may have gradual or sudden shortness of breath, and may complain of pleuritic chest pain, shoulder pain, sweating, cough, or hemoptysis. On exam, patients may be tachypneic and tachycardic, with hypotension, and there may be decreased breath sounds. Patients may become unconscious.

Check oxygen saturations with a pulse oximetry. Those suspected of having a PE should receive a chest x-ray and ECG. CT angiography is primarily used to confirm the presence of a PE. V/Q (ventilation-perfusion) scans are also used, but take longer; they are sensitive, but not as specific as CT angiography. Oxygen is given first to help patients. Anticoagulation is started, usually with heparin (typically SQ, fractionated LMWH) or fondaparinux, then switched to oral warfarin. Overlap with heparin therapy until therapeutic INR has been reached for 24 hours (2.0–3.0). Patients will need to stay on warfarin for 3 months or longer because of the risk of recurrent PE. "Clot buster" thrombolytic drugs may be given to break up large clots if the patient is hemodynamically unstable (e.g., hypotension). An inferior vena cava filter may be placed if anticoagulation is contraindicated or for recurrent DVTs/PEs. Complications include shock, cor pulmonale, and sudden death.

PULMONARY HYPERTENSION

Pulmonary hypertension is a **rise in pressure within the pulmonary artery** carrying blood to the lungs. Pulmonary hypertension is now classified in five groups. **Group 1** involves narrowing of the pulmonary arterioles and includes idiopathic pulmonary arterial hypertension (PAH), familial, drug or toxin-induced, and PAH associated with medical conditions like portal hypertension, sickle cell disease, scleroderma (connective tissue disorder), HIV, schistosomiasis, and congenital heart disease. It can be caused by left-sided heart failure (**group 2**; most common), especially as the ejection fraction decreases and left ventricular function decreases, or it may be due to lung disease, like COPD or hypoxia (**group 3**). **Group 4** includes cases due to chronic pulmonary thromboembolism; and **group 5** includes unclear, multifactorial causes. As resistance in the pulmonary vasculature increases, changes occur that can lead to **right-sided heart failure**.

The symptoms of pulmonary hypertension include SOB, dyspnea on exertion that becomes progressively worse, fatigue, and chest pain. Patients may also complain of a cough, sometimes with hemoptysis, and may even have syncopal episodes. Physical exam may show jugular venous distension, a right-sided heave, a split S2, and possibly an S3 in advanced cases. Diagnose with chest x-ray (enlarged pulmonary arteries), ECG (right-axis deviation), and echocardiography, and confirm with a right-sided heart catheterization. Management of pulmonary hypertension focuses on treating the underlying cause. Treatment may include oxygen therapy, diuretics (e.g., furosemide; avoid hypovolemia), digoxin, and anticoagulants, which may be useful in treating symptoms and in preventing complications from this condition. Other advanced treatment includes IV epoprostenol, prostacyclin agonists, or phosphodiesterase 5 inhibitors. Additional research is on going.

RESTRICTIVE PULMONARY DISEASES
PULMONARY FIBROSIS (IDIOPATHIC)

Pulmonary fibrosis (idiopathic) is a chronic and progressive condition in which the **alveoli** become damaged and are replaced by **fibrotic scar tissue**. This results in a thickening of the alveolar tissue, preventing the **transfer of oxygen**. The cause of pulmonary fibrosis is uncertain, but it is thought there is a genetic tendency for developing this disease. It is also thought that inhaled environmental agents, especially cigarette smoke, may increase the likelihood of developing pulmonary fibrosis.

Symptoms of idiopathic pulmonary fibrosis develop over time, and patients may complain of shortness of breath or dyspnea, especially during activity, and may have a dry, hacking cough and fatigue. Patients may also have a loss of appetite with significant weight loss. On exam, there may be fine inspiratory crackles (like Velcro) at both bases, clubbing, and a decrease in oxygen saturation on pulse oximetry. Diagnose with a high-resolution CT (diffuse subpleural and reticular opacities, subpleural honeycombing) and sometimes a biopsy. There is no cure for pulmonary fibrosis. Supplemental oxygen can be given to help with shortness of breath. Pirfenidone is a recently approved antifibrotic agent that may be used for treating idiopathic pulmonary fibrosis. In severe cases, a lung transplant may be performed. Complications include pulmonary hypertension, respiratory infections, and death.

PNEUMOCONIOSIS

Pneumoconiosis is an occupational lung disease that is due to **inhaling particulate matter**. It can be due to inhaling the dust from coal, asbestos, silica (rock and sand), beryllium, iron, talc, and other materials. The specific type of pneumoconiosis will vary depending upon the material inhaled. For example, asbestos workers can develop **asbestosis**, while those who work with silica develop **silicosis**. There is also **coal worker's pneumoconiosis (CWP)**, or black lung disease. There should be workplace safety monitoring in place to help protect workers. Patients are often asymptomatic for years, then typically complain of progressively worsening shortness of breath that is more pronounced during activities. They will also have a chronic cough that may be productive or nonproductive. On exam, there may be inspiratory crackles present.

Chest x-ray or CT may show consolidated areas where the inhaled dust has damaged the lung tissue. CWP shows round, nodular opacities and fibrosis; asbestosis shows reticular opacities, usually in the lower lobes, and pleural plaques; silicosis shows ground-glass opacities. There is no known treatment for the pneumoconiosis diseases. Supportive treatment with supplemental oxygen may be necessary. Patients should avoid any future contact with causative substances, and if they smoke, they should quit in order to prevent any further damage to the lung tissue that would further exacerbate the illness. In very severe cases, lung transplantation can be performed. There is an increased risk of developing **lung cancer** (mesothelioma) with asbestosis.

SARCOIDOSIS

Sarcoidosis is an inflammatory disease that usually appears in the **lungs or thoracic lymphatics**, but may affect any organ system in the body, causing **noncaseating granulomas** to form. It is often self-limited and resolves within a couple years, but in rare cases it may be fatal. It more commonly affects African Americans, 20- to 40-year-olds, and females. The cause of sarcoidosis is not known, but it is thought that it may be due to an immune response after exposure to a certain bacteria, virus, or toxin. Signs and symptoms vary depending on the organ system affected, and patients may be asymptomatic. With lung disease, patients may complain of shortness of breath with a chronic cough, and crackles may be heard. A skin rash, arthralgias, weight loss, fatigue, and red or watery eyes (uveitis) may also be present.

Diagnose with chest x-ray (shows bilateral hilar adenopathy) and biopsy. Bronchoscopy is performed for granuloma samples and for confirmation of the diagnosis. Lab tests may reveal an elevation in ACE and calcium, but this is not definitive for diagnosis. Treatment involves NSAIDs and corticosteroids, and may help to control some of the symptoms. Monitor with chest x-rays and pulmonary function tests every 6–12 months, and ECGs annually until resolved.

OTHER

ACUTE RESPIRATORY DISTRESS SYNDROME (ARDS)

Acute respiratory distress syndrome (ARDS) occurs when there is **acute inflammation and fluid accumulation within the lungs** that can quickly progress to **respiratory failure**. ARDS may be mild, moderate, or severe. ARDS can be caused by pneumonia, trauma, shock, aspiration, infection, sepsis, pancreatitis, chemical/gas inhalation, or burns/smoke inhalation. Damage occurs to the **alveoli and endothelium of the pulmonary capillaries**, which results in ARDS. The onset of this condition is usually 1–2 days following the triggering event.

Symptoms initially consist of dyspnea on exertion that progresses to dyspnea at rest and anxiety. Patients usually have rapid respiratory decline and multisystem organ failure to the point of becoming unconscious, and respiratory arrest can occur. On exam, crackles may be heard in the lungs because of fluid accumulation, and cyanosis is frequently present, along with tachypnea, tachycardia, and hypotension (cardiogenic shock). Diagnose with imaging tests (chest x-ray) and ABGs, which show pulmonary infiltrates and hypoxia; rule out a cardiac source for the pulmonary edema. ARDS is life-threatening, and patients are treated by specialists in the ICU with supportive therapy as the lungs heal. Maintaining proper oxygenation is the mainstay of treatment, and a prone position often helps with oxygenation. Patients are usually placed on ventilators until they can be weaned off and are able to breathe on their own. Treat the underlying cause; if an infection is present, appropriate antibiotics should be given. Diuretics may be given to decrease the fluid accumulation within the lungs. Mortality is about 30–45%.

ASPIRATION OF A FOREIGN BODY

Aspiration of a foreign body is commonly seen in children. Frequently, patients will initially experience **choking**, followed by a persistent **cough** and the feeling that something is stuck in their throat. Hoarseness, wheezing, or stridor may be heard, depending on the location of the blockage within the airway. If the condition is severe, the airway may be completely blocked, and this could cause patients to collapse and go into respiratory arrest. On exam, decreased breath sounds may be present on one side due to blockage of the main bronchus. Wheezing may also be heard in any portion of the lungs. Diagnose using an AP and lateral chest x-ray, and endoscopy may be used to diagnose and treat the condition. Treatment is focused on removing the object. In severe cases with complete airway blockage, the Heimlich maneuver should be given to forcefully expel the object from the airway. In emergency cases, an emergency tracheostomy may be performed to create a new airway below the level of the obstruction. In patients who are stable, bronchoscopy can be performed to physically remove the object.

> **Review Video: Aspiration of a Foreign Body**
> Visit mometrix.com/academy and enter code: 539288

HYALINE MEMBRANE DISEASE

Hyaline membrane disease affects **premature infants**. It occurs when infants are born before the lungs are producing adequate amounts of **surfactant** (usually <37 weeks gestation). Surfactant helps to prevent the lungs from collapsing. Adequate surfactant is usually present after week 35–36 of gestation, and amniotic fluid can be tested for adequate production of the substance. As the airways collapse, infants will struggle more and more to breathe, until they become **acidotic** and **multisystem organ failure** begins. The most common symptom of this condition is respiratory distress in the premature infant, with grunting, nasal flaring, and using accessory muscles to breathe. This starts soon after delivery. The baby can become cyanotic and become more dyspneic. Respiratory arrest can occur after the baby becomes exhausted.

Diagnose with chest x-ray (diffuse atelectasis) and ABGs (hypercapnia, hypoxemia). Rule out sepsis and transient tachypnea of the newborn (TTN). Treatment includes oxygen support with mechanical ventilation with positive pressure as needed. Artificial surfactant can be given through the endotracheal tube. Babies may suffer permanent respiratory illness because of hyaline membrane disease, but others make a full recovery and suffer no consequences. The best treatment is prevention by maintaining a healthy pregnancy to prevent premature birth. If premature delivery at 24–34 weeks is unavoidable, the mother is given betamethasone or dexamethasone 48 hours before delivery.

Renal System

RENAL DISORDERS
ACUTE KIDNEY INJURY

Acute kidney injury (**AKI**), the new term for acute renal failure (**ARF**), occurs when the **kidneys** acutely become unable to function; the damage is either reversible or irreversible. AKI can be due to three main causes: **prerenal** (decreased blood flow to the kidneys); **renal** (intrinsic inflammation or damage to the kidneys); or **postrenal** (urine blockage). Prerenal causes may include volume depletion (most common cause of AKI) due to hemorrhage, dehydration, or NSAIDs. Renal causes may include toxins such as some medications (e.g., aminoglycosides, methotrexate, imaging contrast), acute glomerulonephritis from infections or lupus, acute tubular necrosis, vascular diseases like malignant hypertension, and systemic diseases like sarcoidosis. Postrenal causes may include tubular obstruction and obstruction of the ureter or bladder. Signs and symptoms may include peripheral edema, muscle weakness, muscle cramps, nausea/vomiting, confusion, and possibly rashes or ecchymoses depending on the cause.

Diagnose with urine output, BUN, creatinine (Cr), UA, and renal ultrasound. There are various definitions of AKI, including the RIFLE and AKIN classifications. Most recently, the group Kidney Disease Improving Global Outcomes (KDIGO) defined AKI as: increase in serum creatinine by ≥0.3 mg/dL in 48 hours, or increase in creatinine ≥1.5 times the baseline within the last 7 days, or reduction in urine volume <0.5 mL/kg/hr for 6 hours. Treatment involves correcting the underlying issue (e.g., dehydration), diuretics for volume overload, and hemodialysis when K >6.0 mmol/L or when there are severe pH or electrolyte abnormalities that are unresponsive to treatment. Dietary treatment focuses on managing the patient with a low-sodium, low-potassium, low-phosphorus diet, fluid restriction, and providing adequate protein. As the disease progresses, it brings more pronounced complications in fluid and electrolyte balances, anemia, and uremia. Complications include SOB, chest pain, permanent renal damage, and death.

CHRONIC KIDNEY DISEASE

Chronic kidney disease (**CKD**), previously termed chronic renal failure, refers to long-standing renal disease that leads to renal damage and decreased renal function. CKD is defined as either renal damage or a reduced glomerular filtration rate (GFR) being present for ≥3 months. **Renal damage** means having one of the following: albuminuria (albumin-to-creatinine-ratio [ACR] >30 mg/g or albumin excretion rate [AER] ≥30 mg/24 hrs.); renal structure or histology abnormalities; urine sedimentation abnormalities; electrolyte or other abnormalities due to tubular disorders; or history of renal transplant. A **reduced GFR** is < 60 mL/min/1.73 m². The stages of CKD are predominantly categorized by GFR in units of mL/min/1.73 m²:

- **Stage 1:** Kidney damage with GFR >90
- **Stage 2:** GFR 60–89
- **Stage 3a:** GFR 45–59
- **Stage 3b:** GFR 30–44

- **Stage 4:** GFR 15–29
- **Stage 5:** GFR <15 or dialysis

Patients with stage 1–3 CKD are typically asymptomatic. Signs and symptoms appear as GFR decreases to < 30 mL/min/1.73 m² (stage 4–5) and include fatigue, muscle weakness, hypertension, edema, impaired cognitive function, restless leg syndrome, nocturia, nausea/vomiting, diarrhea, pruritus, and encephalopathy. Diagnose with labs using the above criteria: metabolic panel, CBC, UA with micro, and a lipid profile; and possibly a renal ultrasound. If possible, treat the underlying disease, and control hypertension, hypercholesterolemia, anemia, and DM. To protect the kidneys, avoid combining ACE inhibitors and ARBs, and adjust doses or avoid certain medications (e.g., NSAIDs, IV contrast) as GFR drops, especially if < 30 mL/min/1.73 m². Avoid nephrotoxic drugs. Complications include CV disease, hyperkalemia, metabolic acidosis, anemia, and end-stage renal disease requiring dialysis or transplant.

PYELONEPHRITIS

Pyelonephritis is a severe infection of the **kidneys** and can be life-threatening if not treated promptly. Chronic renal damage or scarring can occur, especially without treatment. Usually pyelonephritis is caused by *Escherichia coli* from a urinary tract infection (UTI) that spreads upward to the kidneys. It may also be caused by infection spreading through the bloodstream, and in cases of endocarditis or IV drug use, the causative pathogen is usually *Staphylococcus*. Pyelonephritis can be complicated by anatomical and functional abnormalities of the urinary tract (e.g., vesicoureteral reflux: diagnosed with voiding cystourethrogram (VCUG) and may require prophylactic antibiotics or surgery), immunity or metabolic issues (e.g., DM), antibiotic use, and recent urinary instrument use.

The classic symptoms of pyelonephritis are a fever (usually high), nausea/vomiting, and costovertebral angle tenderness. Also, similar to a UTI, patients may have urinary frequency, urgency, decreased stream, dysuria, lower abdominal pain, and foul-smelling urine. It is unusual for men to get UTIs/pyelonephritis, so if present, these should be considered complicated. Atypical presentations (e.g., failure to thrive, poor feeding, change in mental status) usually involve either young or elderly patients. Diagnose clinically and with clean-catch UA with micro, Gram stain, urine culture and sensitivity screen, and CBC. Blood cultures and imaging may be needed. Treat immediately with appropriate antibiotics, taking local resistance trends into consideration until susceptibility results are in. For outpatient cases, start empiric therapy with fluoroquinolones for 7 days (first-line). If severe or the patient has a complicated UTI, hospitalize and start treatment with IV fluoroquinolones for 24–48 hours (or until improving), switching to PO for a total of 10–14 days. Complications include recurrence, abscess, acute renal injury, chronic kidney disease, and urosepsis.

GLOMERULONEPHRITIS

Glomerulonephritis (**GN**) is inflammation of the **glomerular filters** within the kidneys. It is usually acute, but may be chronic, and can lead to permanent kidney damage if not treated promptly. There are many causes of GN, including **infections** (e.g., poststreptococcal infection, viral, bacterial endocarditis), **systemic disease** (e.g., SLE), **primary renal disease** (e.g., IgA nephropathy, membranoproliferative GN), and **vascular disorders**. As damage to the glomeruli occurs, the GFR decreases, which activates the renin-aldosterone system, causing water and salt retention—and, therefore, hypertension and edema. This causes **nephritic syndrome**, which is characterized by hematuria, proteinuria, oliguria, and hypertension. Patients may note oliguria; dark, tea-stained urine due to hematuria; foamy urine due to a high protein level; and edema (especially limbs and face) that can be quite profound. Blood pressure is elevated due to the increased fluid load.

Diagnosis is made clinically and with UA with micro, serum creatinine, BUN, ESR, and complement levels. The patient's age and history will help guide diagnostic tests and help disclose the most likely cause of GN. A renal biopsy may be needed to confirm the diagnosis. Treatment focuses on treating the underlying cause. If due to a recent streptococcal infection (antistreptolysin O is positive; peaks 3–5 weeks after strep) or bacterial endocarditis, appropriate antibiotic therapy should be prescribed. The condition will usually resolve on its own with management of the symptoms, such as ACE inhibitors to control hypertension and diuretics to reduce edema. Some patients may need dialysis during the acute episode. Complications include CHF, pulmonary edema, AKI, chronic kidney disease, and end-stage renal disease.

NEPHROTIC SYNDROME

Nephrotic syndrome (not to be confused with *nephritic* syndrome) is a condition that occurs due to damage to the **microvascular system** within the kidneys, leading to excess excretion of protein in the urine, resulting in **hypoalbuminemia**, which causes fluid to leak out of blood vessels (edema); high cholesterol is also part of this syndrome. There is an increased risk of developing blood clots and infections. Nephrotic syndrome can have primary and secondary causes. **Primary causes** include minimal-change nephropathy, focal segmental glomerulosclerosis, and membranous nephropathy. **Secondary causes** include diabetic nephropathy, SLE, viral infections, preeclampsia, amyloidosis, and drugs (e.g., NSAIDs, penicillamine, lithium). Nephrotic syndrome can cause a good deal of edema, especially in the extremities and face, and there may be noticeable weight gain or ascites due to this retained fluid. Patients may have a feeling of general malaise and note foamy urine due to proteinuria.

Diagnosis is made in the presence of proteinuria ≥3 g/day, hypoalbuminemia, and high cholesterol. Order a UA with micro (usually followed by a 24-hour urine protein study), serum albumin, and cholesterol. Depending on the patient's history and PE, other tests and a renal biopsy may be needed to confirm the diagnosis. Treatment focuses on treating the underlying cause and controlling the symptoms of nephrotic syndrome. Diuretics can reduce the edema, ACE inhibitors can be given to control hypertension, anticoagulants may be necessary to prevent blood clot formation, and steroids may be necessary for minimal change disease (most common in children). Complications include chronic kidney disease, infections, thrombi (renal vein thrombosis), emboli, hypercholesterolemia, CAD, and hypertension.

POLYCYSTIC KIDNEY DISEASE

Polycystic kidney disease (**PKD**) is a condition in which groups of fluid-filled **cysts** form within the **kidneys**. This can lead to **high blood pressure** and even **renal failure**. Polycystic disease is not limited to the kidneys and can affect the liver and pancreas as well; it is associated with an increased risk of colonic diverticulitis, brain aneurysms, and heart-valve abnormalities. This is a genetic condition that can be autosomal dominant or autosomal recessive (rare). Patients with the autosomal dominant version usually don't start having symptoms or get diagnosed until they are 30–50 years old, and typically don't progress to renal failure until 60–70 years old. However, patients with the recessive version are diagnosed early, usually in utero, and progress to renal failure very quickly. Patients with the autosomal dominant form may complain of abdominal or flank pain, gross hematuria, and an increasing abdominal girth. Hypertension is an early sign of PKD, and early signs of renal failure may be evident with elevated serum BUN and creatinine levels.

Diagnosis is suspected with a family history of PKD and confirmed with multiple cysts on ultrasound (sometimes a CT, MRI, or genetic testing). Treatment of PKD is focused on treating the symptoms and preventing renal failure by using antihypertensives (e.g., ACE inhibitors, ARBs), diuretics, and being on a low-salt diet. Close monitoring and control of blood pressure is crucial to slow the progression of the disease. Treat infections; contact sports should be avoided. If the cysts become large, they may need to be surgically drained. Dialysis and a kidney transplant may become necessary. Complications include hypertension, infection, preeclampsia, and end-stage renal disease.

FLUID AND ELECTROLYTE DISORDERS

HYPONATREMIA

Hyponatremia is defined as a **serum sodium (Na^+) <135 mEq/L** and is the most common **electrolyte disturbance** in hospitalized patients, affecting up to 30% of hospitalized patients. Serum sodium represents the extracellular Na^+ concentration, which is used as an estimation of total body sodium. Serum osmolality represents Na^+ concentration in the body's fluids. Both of these reflect the body's state of water balance, which in hyponatremia is usually a state of **water excess**. The most common form is hypotonic or hypoosmolar (<280 mOsm/kg) hyponatremia. Hyponatremia can be divided into three categories: **hypervolemic** (due to

CHF, or renal or liver failure); **euvolemic** (due to SIADH, hypothyroidism, or drugs); or **hypovolemic** (due to vomiting, diarrhea, diuretics, etc.). A pseudohyponatremia may be caused by hyperproteinemia, hyperlipidemia, or an increase in other osmoles like glucose (hyperglycemia).

Symptoms vary and depend largely on the rate of sodium loss. Patients may be asymptomatic or have nausea/vomiting, headache, malaise, lethargy, muscle weakness, and muscle pain. Severe hyponatremia (<125 mEq/L) causes changes in mental status, confusion, seizures, coma, and even death. Diagnose with serum Na^+, and determine the cause using serum and urine osmolality, and urine Na^+. If fluid overload (hypervolemia) is causing a dilutional hyponatremia, diurese and restrict fluid and salt intake. If SIADH is present or other euvolemic cause, treat the underlying disorder (e.g., treat cancer or infection, or discontinue causative drug) and restrict water intake. Treat hypovolemic causes with isotonic saline. If hyponatremia is severe or chronic (>48 hours), correct slowly with hypertonic saline IV fluids (3% NaCl). Complications include seizures, coma, and death.

HYPERNATREMIA

Hypernatremia is defined as **serum sodium (Na^+) >145 mEq/L**. This reflects the body's state of **water deficiency** and is rarely due to Na^+ excess. This is common in the elderly and hospitalized patient. Hypernatremia can be caused by water loss (most common), a decrease in fluid intake (e.g., elderly people who depend on others for water), an impairment in thirst, or not being able to concentrate urine as in diabetes insipidus (DI). Renal dysfunction can alter the excretion of Na^+ and result in higher levels within the bloodstream. Hypernatremia can be divided into three categories: **hypervolemic** (rare—due to increased Na^+ intake with limited access to water, salt water or tablet ingestion, hemodialysis, Cushing syndrome); **euvolemic** (DI, fever, hypodipsia, nephrotoxic medications like lithium and phenytoin, mechanical ventilation); and **hypovolemic** (most common—due to GI losses, enteral feeding, burns, loop diuretics, osmotic diuresis).

Signs and symptoms vary based on the cause of water loss; they include thirst, nausea/vomiting, diarrhea, fever, dry mouth, orthostatic blood pressure changes, polyuria, and dementia. Effects due to brain cell shrinkage include changes in mental status with irritability, somnolence, nystagmus, increased deep tendon reflexes, and seizures. Diagnose clinically and with serum Na^+. Treat the underlying cause (e.g., dehydration, DI), discontinue any causative medication, and replace free water deficit. How quickly water is replaced depends on whether it is acute or chronic. Free water deficit may be corrected quickly (over 24 hours) if hypernatremia has been present <24 hours, but slowly (0.5 mEq/L/hr) if present >48 hours, to avoid brain edema. Complications include cerebral edema, cerebral bleeding, coma, and death.

HYPOKALEMIA

Hypokalemia is defined as a **potassium (K^+) level <3.5 mEq/L**. Potassium is an essential **intracellular electrolyte** involved in the sodium-potassium exchange pump of the cells. K^+ losses can be due to increased excretion (most common; renal or GI), decreased intake, or a shift to inside the cells. Increased excretion of K^+ can occur with diuretics, renal tubular acidosis, increased mineralocorticoid (e.g., aldosterone, cortisol), hypomagnesemia, and dehydration from diarrhea and vomiting. Various medications can also cause hypokalemia (e.g., gentamicin, ampicillin, ephedrine, and bicarbonate). Intracellular shifts may be caused by insulin and albuterol. Inadequate intake may occur with dementia, eating disorders, and total parenteral nutrition (TPN). Hypokalemia can cause cardiac dysrhythmias, cardiac arrest, hypotension, muscle weakness and cramping, constipation, decreased respirations, reduced deep tendon reflex, and even paralysis. Severe hypokalemia (K^+ < 2.5 mEq/L) can occur in patients taking digoxin.

Diagnose with a serum K^+. ECG (very important) and a urinary K^+ and serum magnesium are helpful in determining the cause. ECG changes include flattened T waves, ST depression, QT prolongation, and U waves. Treatment consists of discontinuing any causative agents and treating the underlying cause of K^+ loss; give oral potassium (KCl) for mild hypokalemia. If severe hypokalemia, admit and use IV KCl with an infusion rate no greater than 10 mEq/hr. Patients must be closely monitored for signs and symptoms of hyperkalemia as potassium is replaced, especially cardiac effects. Other electrolyte levels (e.g., Na^+ and Mg^{2+}) should be closely monitored for abnormalities. Complications include digitalis toxicity, respiratory depression, rhabdomyolysis, paralysis, arrhythmias (VT, VF, torsades de pointes), and death.

HYPERKALEMIA

Hyperkalemia is defined as a **potassium (K^+) level >5.5 mEq/L**. This can be caused by decreased renal excretion (most common), increased K^+ intake, or a shift to outside the cells. K^+ is excreted through urine, so any dysfunction resulting in decreased urinary output can cause increased serum K^+ levels (e.g., AKI, CKD, tubular defects, reduced aldosterone, adrenal insufficiency, medications). Increased intake can occur with salt substitutes (KCl) or K^+ supplements; and any process that causes blood cell destruction, such as hemolytic anemia, can cause a rise in K^+ levels. Various medications (NSAIDs, heparin, ACE inhibitors, ARBs, K^+-sparing diuretics, penicillin VK) can also lead to hyperkalemia.

Symptoms range from patients who are asymptomatic to those with cardiac arrhythmias or paralysis. Symptoms usually start when $K^+ > 6.0$ to 6.5 mEq/L. The primary symptoms are neuromuscular and include weakness, lethargy, diminished reflexes, and paresthesias. Hyperkalemia can cause bradycardia, palpitations, and cardiac dysrhythmias (e.g., heart block, VF). GI symptoms of nausea, vomiting, and diarrhea may be present. Diagnose with serum K^+ and ECG. ECG changes are progressive and include peaked T waves, a long PR interval, wide QRS complex, loss of P waves, and eventually VF or asystole. If ECG changes or signs of cardiotoxicity, treat immediately with IV calcium gluconate or calcium chloride (cardioprotective). Also administer insulin with glucose, and albuterol, as these redistribute K^+ back into the cell. Calcium is not recommended if digoxin toxicity is present. Discontinue any causative agents. Kayexalate, given PO or rectally, binds with K^+ to increase excretion of K^+ through the GI tract. Hemodialysis may also be used in those with renal failure. Complications include paralysis and cardiac arrest ($K^+ > 8.5$ mEq/L).

HYPOCALCEMIA

Hypocalcemia is defined as a **total serum calcium (Ca^{2+}) level <8.8 mg/dL** (<2.2 mmol/L) or a **corrected total serum calcium level <8.5 mg/dL**. Correct calcium for changes in serum albumin (increase total serum Ca^{2+} by 0.8 mg/dL for every 1.0 g/dL albumin is below 4.0 g/dL). Hypocalcemia is frequent in hospitalized and chronically ill patients; Ca^{2+} is critical to the proper functioning of the body. This disorder can be caused by under-secretion of parathyroid hormone (PTH), resulting in more calcium remaining in the bones and less being circulated into the bloodstream. Calcium requires vitamin D to be absorbed in the GI tract, so a vitamin D deficiency can lead to hypocalcemia. It can also result from an alteration in renal function.

Symptoms range from asymptomatic patients to tetany. With hypocalcemia there is excitability of the nervous system, so patients may exhibit spasm of the facial muscles when tapped over the facial nerve (positive Chvostek sign), or a carpal spasm when a blood pressure cuff is inflated for 3 minutes (positive Trousseau sign). Other signs and symptoms include paresthesias, muscle cramps, bronchospasms, weakness, poor teeth, dry skin, coarse hair, brittle nails, altered mental status, irritability, hallucinations, and seizures. Patients may be hypotensive and have a prolonged QT interval on ECG. Diagnose with a total corrected serum or ionized Ca^{2+}; also check PTH, serum magnesium and phosphate, vitamin D levels, BUN, creatinine, and ECG. Treatment involves Ca^{2+} replacement (e.g., IV calcium gluconate or calcium chloride) if Ca^{2+} levels have dropped dangerously low (<7.0 mg/dL). Use oral Ca^{2+} replacement for mild hypocalcemia. Treat any underlying condition. Complications include seizures, respiratory arrest, and tetany.

HYPERCALCEMIA

Hypercalcemia is defined as a **total serum calcium (Ca^{2+}) level ≥10.5 mg/dL**. Calcium levels within the blood are controlled by many factors, but hypercalcemia is usually caused by **hyperparathyroidism** or **cancer**. Parathyroid hormone causes calcium to be reabsorbed by the bones if the Ca^{2+} level is too high, or causes Ca^{2+} to leave the bones and enter the blood if levels are too low. Tumors can cause paraneoplastic syndrome by elevating PTH levels, which results in elevated Ca^{2+} levels. Also, Ca^{2+} is excreted in the urine, so alterations in kidney function (e.g., CKD) can result in hypercalcemia.

Patients may be asymptomatic if mild or may have many symptoms. The signs and symptoms of hypercalcemia can be remembered with the mnemonic "bones, stones, groans, and moans:" bone pain; kidney stones; nausea/vomiting, anorexia, constipation, and abdominal pain; muscle weakness, fatigue, lethargy, depression, confusion, and coma. There may be hypotonia, a decrease in the reflexes, hypotension, bradycardia, arrhythmias, and a shortened QT interval on ECG, all due to nerve transmission malfunctions. Polyuria, nocturia, and decreased urinary output may occur due to kidney dysfunction. Diagnose with total corrected serum Ca^{2+} or ionized calcium. Use further labs to determine the cause (e.g., PTH, alkaline phosphatase, chest x-ray, ECG, serum phosphate, serum protein, BUN, Cr). Treatment depends on the severity and the cause, and may consist of adequate hydration (first-line in severe hypercalcemia), loop diuretics, decreased intake, prednisone, bisphosphonates, or calcitonin. Treat the underlying cause. Complications include osteoporosis, kidney failure, arrhythmias, dementia, coma, and death.

HYPOMAGNESEMIA

Hypomagnesemia is defined as a **serum magnesium (Mg^{2+}) level <1.8 mg/dL**; with this condition, serum levels do not adequately reflect total body stores (stored in bones, muscles, soft tissues). It is seen more often than hypermagnesemia and can cause many issues throughout the body, including cardiac issues. Magnesium is an important **intracellular electrolyte and coenzyme** that is involved in many critical processes (e.g., cellular metabolism, protein synthesis, cell replication, neurotransmitter release, muscle contraction). Hypomagnesemia can be caused by decreased intake, decreased GI absorption or GI loss, endocrine causes, excessive renal excretion, and some medications (e.g., gentamicin, ticarcillin, PPIs, cisplatin, loop or thiazide diuretics). It is often seen in patients who are alcoholics, hospitalized, or have DM.

Signs and symptoms include nausea/vomiting, muscle cramps, positive Chvostek and Trousseau signs, hyperreflexia, nystagmus, paresthesias, seizures, ECG changes (e.g., prolonged QT, PVCs), and mental status changes (e.g., irritability, depression). Diagnose with a serum Mg^{2+} level; and check serum Ca^{2+}, K^+, and phosphorus levels since this condition can be associated with hypocalcemia, hypokalemia, and hypophosphatemia. Treatment of hypomagnesemia depends on the severity and includes IV or IM magnesium sulfate if severe ($Mg^{2+} < 1.25$ mg/dL), and oral magnesium salts if the depletion is not as severe. Discontinue any causative agents; monitor often as Mg^{2+} is replenished and replace Ca^{2+} and K^+ as needed. Medications used to decrease the amount of Mg^{2+} excreted in the urine include potassium-sparing diuretics and triamterene. Complications include osteoporosis, arrhythmias, digitalis potentiation, VF, torsades de pointes, hypokalemia, and hypocalcemia.

HYPERMAGNESEMIA

Hypermagnesemia is defined as a **serum magnesium (Mg^{2+}) level >2.6 mg/dL**. It is not very common. When it does occur, it is most often caused by **renal failure** and **excessive intake** (e.g., antacids, laxatives, enemas, cathartics). Hypermagnesemia can cause nausea/vomiting, flushing, hyporeflexia, hypotension, muscle weakness, respiratory depression, and eventually cardiac arrest. Diagnose with serum Mg^{2+} levels. Also test for possible concurrent hypercalcemia and hyperkalemia. ECG may show a prolonged PR interval, widened QRS complex, and tall T wave. When severe (respiratory depression or cardiac changes), treat immediately with IV calcium gluconate, which will quickly reverse many of the symptoms. Also, discontinue any sources of magnesium. Other treatment options include furosemide (to promote Mg^{2+} excretion) and dialysis. Complications include respiratory depression, cardiac arrhythmias, neuromuscular paralysis, coma, and death.

ACID/BASE DISORDERS
METABOLIC ACIDOSIS

Metabolic acidosis is a condition in which there are excess **hydrogen ions** (H^+) within the system (due to elevated H^+ or reduced bicarbonate [HCO_3^-]), resulting in a **decreased serum pH level (arterial pH <7.35)**. The body will try to **compensate** by increasing the respiratory rate and depth of respirations in an effort to "blow off" some of the excess H^+ through carbon dioxide. The excess H^+ in the system can be due to excessive intake or production of acidic substances, decreased acid excretion by the kidneys, or by GI or renal loss of bicarbonate. These can result in a high anion gap metabolic acidosis or a normal anion gap acidosis. These can be remembered by the following mnemonics. **Increased anion gap:** GOLD MARK (Glycols, Oxoproline, L-lactate/lactic acidosis, D-lactate, Methanol, Aspirin, Renal failure/uremia, Ketoacidosis/DKA). **Normal anion gap** or hyperchloremic acidosis: USED CARP (Ureteroenterostomy, Small bowel fistula, Extra chloride, Diarrhea, Carbonic anhydrase inhibitors, Adrenal insufficiency, Renal tubular acidosis, Pancreatic fistula). Substances that increase acid include aspirin products, methanol, ethanol, and antifreeze. Symptoms usually reflect the cause of the acidosis (e.g., diarrhea, history of DM, lactic acidosis). Long, deep breaths (hyperpnea) are usually the first sign that is noted. With worsening acidosis, patients may experience nausea/vomiting, headache, and malaise; stupor, Kussmaul breathing, coma, or death may result without treatment. If chronic acidosis, bone demineralization can occur.

Diagnose with serum electrolytes and ABG, which reveal a reduced pH, reduced $PaCO_2$, and reduced HCO_3^-. Determine the anion gap and amount of respiratory compensation; use Winters' formula: expected $PaCO_2 = (1.5 \times HCO_3^-) + 8 \pm 2$. Treat the underlying cause and correct acidosis through bicarbonate (use with caution). Complications include coma and death.

METABOLIC ALKALOSIS

Metabolic alkalosis occurs when the **pH of the blood** becomes elevated (pH >7.45) due to too much **bicarbonate** (HCO_3^-) in the system. This can occur due to a decrease in hydrogen ions (H^+) or a direct increase in HCO_3^-. The means by which these two actions occur is usually through the **GI tract** or through the **renal tubule system**. With the loss of hydrochloric acid (HCl) in the stomach (e.g., vomiting or nasogastric tube suctioning), an alkalotic state can develop. Renal dysfunction or diuretic use can cause decreased secretion of HCO_3^-, which raises bicarbonate levels. Metabolic alkalosis can be divided into **chloride-responsive metabolic alkalosis** (e.g., GI loss, diuretic use; urine Cl^- <20 mEq/L) or **chloride-resistant metabolic alkalosis** (e.g., increased aldosterone effect/mineralocorticoid excess, hypokalemia, edema, hypertension; urine Cl^- <20 mEq/L).

Signs and symptoms can include hypoventilation (a compensatory mechanism), signs of hypocalcemia (positive Chvostek sign, neuromuscular excitability, headache, changes in mental status), signs of hypokalemia (weakness, myalgias, arrhythmias), hypervolemia or hypovolemia, and hypertension. Diagnose through serum electrolytes and ABGs. Urine Cl^- and aldosterone levels may be helpful. Lab studies show an elevated serum pH (7.45), elevated HCO_3^- levels, and possibly elevated aldosterone levels. Expected $PCO_2 = 0.7[HCO_3^-] + 20 \pm 5$. Treatment consists of correction of the underlying cause, and IV sodium chloride (isotonic saline solution, 0.9%) for chloride-responsive metabolic alkalosis. Chloride-resistant metabolic alkalosis involves treating the specific cause (e.g., removal of adrenal or pituitary tumors, K^+-sparing diuretics, dexamethasone). If edema is present, potassium chloride (KCl) should be used instead to balance electrolytes and reduce the edema. Complications include arrhythmias, tetany, seizures, and coma.

RESPIRATORY ACIDOSIS

Respiratory acidosis is due to a **depressed respiratory system** that prevents carbon dioxide (CO_2) from being "blown off," leading to **elevated acid levels** in the blood (pH <7.35). This can be acute or chronic. Blood pH is affected by the amount of CO_2 or carbonic acid (H_2CO_3) in the blood; the pH is controlled thorough the bicarbonate buffering system: $CO_2 + H_2O \leftrightarrow H_2CO_3 \leftrightarrow H^+ + HCO_3^-$. With chronic respiratory acidosis, the body will compensate by renal retention of bicarbonate (HCO_3^-) over a few days. Respiratory acidosis can be due to alveolar hypoventilation (most common), overproduction of CO_2 by the body, or an increased intake of CO_2. Some causes include COPD, asthma, sleep apnea, pneumonia, pulmonary edema, pleural effusion, pneumothorax, neuromuscular diseases (myasthenia gravis, Guillain-Barré), sedative drugs, and CNS depression. Patients may exhibit CO_2 narcosis: headache, confusion, somnolence, or stupor; but symptoms largely follow the underlying cause. If chronic, patients may appear asymptomatic or have subtle changes. Diagnose with serum electrolytes and ABGs, which reveal a pH <7.35 and $PaCO_2$ >45 mmHg.

If chronic, the pH can be normal or near normal due to renal compensation. Treat the underlying cause and give proper respiratory support. If severe, intubation and mechanical ventilation may be necessary. If chronic,

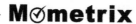

corrections need to be made slowly to avoid overcorrecting. Complications include confusion, seizures, coma, and respiratory failure.

RESPIRATORY ALKALOSIS

Respiratory alkalosis occurs due to an excessive **loss of carbon dioxide** through increased depth or rate of respirations (**hyperventilation**). This can occur with chronic respiratory illnesses or may be acute in nature. It can be caused by hyperventilation from anxiety, pain, fever, pneumonia, sepsis, anemia, hyperthyroidism, hepatic failure, pneumonia, mechanical ventilation, or salicylate toxicity. Initially, the excess bicarbonate is buffered by extracellular H^+, but this is minimal. When chronic, the body will compensate by increasing the excretion of bicarbonate ions (HCO_3^-) through the urine, thus lowering the pH after a few days. **Chronic respiratory alkalosis** usually does not cause patients to experience symptoms. When **acute**, patients may experience light-headedness, dizziness, paresthesias, and syncope due to hyperventilation. On exam, patients may have a fever, may be visibly hyperventilating or short of breath, and may have a positive Chvostek or Trousseau sign.

Diagnose with serum electrolytes and ABGs, which show a pH >7.45 and $PaCO_2 < 35$ mmHg. Treat the underlying cause. With symptomatic respiratory alkalosis, effort should be made to correct the acid-base imbalance by slowing down the respiratory rate and administering oxygen (as needed). If fever is the cause, antipyretics should be given, and the underlying cause of the fever should be treated. Complications include tetany and seizures.

Reproductive System

BREAST DISORDERS

GALACTORRHEA

Galactorrhea refers to an **abnormal milky discharge** from the nipple of one or both breasts that is **not related to lactation** in either a male or a female. This condition is more common in women, but it may occur in men or infants. This condition can be brought on by excessive breast stimulation, side effects of certain medications (oral contraceptives, H2-blockers, antidepressants, blood pressure medications, and some herbal supplements), or pituitary adenomas. It can occur spontaneously or be produced by manual manipulation, and can be continuous or intermittent. Patients presenting with this complaint may also be experiencing dysmenorrhea, headache, or vision changes. If the discharge is other than a milky substance, it may indicate a more significant underlying disease state, such as cancer. Obtain prolactin levels. Discontinue the causative medication or treat the underlying cause.

GYNECOMASTIA

Gynecomastia is the increase of **glandular breast tissue** (not fat) in males; this is not related to normal changes during puberty. It may be idiopathic or caused by medications (e.g., spironolactone, verapamil, cimetidine, finasteride, anabolic steroids), or certain conditions like hypogonadism and hyperthyroidism. This is usually physiological and self-limited; treat cause or discontinue the causative agent.

MASTITIS

Mastitis is a condition in which **bacteria** enter the **breast tissue** through a milk duct or a break in the skin, causing **inflammation, erythema, and pain**. This is usually due to *Staphylococcus aureus* and caused by breastfeeding; but rarely, it occurs in women who are not breastfeeding. Patients present with a painful, erythematous, warm, tender area of the breast and may be accompanied with fever generally >101 °F, fatigue, and an ill appearance. The location of the infection may be indurated and feel hard due to a blocked milk duct. Treat with antibiotics (e.g., dicloxacillin, cephalexin, Augmentin) with attention to the safety of the antibiotic while breastfeeding. Encourage patients to continue breastfeeding and apply warm compresses to the infected area.

192

FIBROCYSTIC DISEASE

Fibrocystic disease (or fibrocystic breast changes) is a common condition in which women develop **bilateral lumps or thickened areas in their breasts**. It is most common in women 20–45 years old but can appear earlier. There is no increased risk of breast cancer in patients who have this condition; it is thought that the fibrocystic masses may be due to **changing hormone levels** during the menstrual cycle. Patients usually complain of breast masses that may change in size and become more painful especially during the menstrual cycle; nipple discharge may also be present, and patients may describe their breasts as feeling full or heavy. These bilateral changes can be described as lumpy, bumpy, ropelike, or having an uneven texture of tissue (e.g., nodular). The lumps are most noticeable in the upper outside area of the breast and maybe into the axillae. Ultrasound exam will show cystic masses within the breasts.

There is no definitive cure for fibrocystic changes. It is thought that caffeine may worsen the condition, so limiting caffeine in the diet may help. These changes are considered a normal deviation and not indicative of any disease. However, it is important to emphasize monthly self-exams (best 1 week after a period, when lumps are smallest) and mammograms because these textures can mask the development of abnormal lumps. Symptoms and palpable changes tend to disappear after menopause.

FIBROADENOMAS AND ABSCESSES

Fibroadenomas are **benign breast masses** that are painless, round, mobile masses that tend to appear during childbearing years (usually <30). They usually appear as solitary lumps. An ultrasound and biopsy may be used for diagnosis; and treatment includes leaving or removing it.

Abscesses are **loculations of infection**. They can be treated with fine-needle aspiration or incision and drainage if necessary, plus antibiotics for 10–14 days (e.g., dicloxacillin, cephalexin, TMP-SMX).

BREAST CANCER

Breast cancer is the **second leading cause of cancer death in women** after lung cancer. Breast cancer is classified as either **carcinoma in situ** or **invasive breast cancer**. Approximately 5–10% of breast cancer is connected to a genetic mutation (BRCA1 or BRCA2) that can be passed on. Other risk factors include a positive family history, increasing age, early menarche, late menopause, or first birth >30 years old, use of HRT, being overweight, smoking, and alcohol use. **Screening mammography** starts at 40–50 years old (depends on the organization) and repeats every 1–2 years until 75 years old.

Monthly breast self-exams are vital to early diagnosis and treatment. Indications of breast cancer include changes in the appearance or texture of the breast and nipple, dimpling of the skin, a retracted nipple, bloody nipple discharge, an obvious lack of symmetry between breasts, and lymphadenopathy. When assessing for signs indicating breast cancer, the practitioner should feel for a painless, hard, fixed (sometimes to the skin), irregular mass in the breast or surrounding tissue. Sometimes clinicians use MRI rather than physical exam to assess those with mutation. The most common locations to find a mass are directly beneath the nipple and the outer-axillary portion of the breast. Workup of a suspicious mass usually begins with an ultrasound to determine if it is solid (possible cancer) or cystic (less likely). If it is solid, a fine-needle aspiration or biopsy and mammogram are performed. Once the cancer is staged, treatment may include surgery (lumpectomy), mastectomy, radiation, hormone therapy (tamoxifen), or chemotherapy. Breast cancer most commonly metastasizes (stage IV) to the bone, liver, brain, and lung. Breast cancer patients face issues associated with body changes, including a perceived loss of femininity, perceived loss of sexual appeal, and loss of sexual function.

CERVICAL DISORDERS

CERVICITIS

Cervicitis is **inflammation or infection of the cervix**. This usually occurs due to **sexually transmitted diseases**, such as chlamydia or gonorrhea. Chemical irritation from lubricants, spermicides, or douching may also cause cervicitis, as well as trauma or malignancy. **Bacterial vaginitis** may also cause a bacterial infection of the cervix. Patients may be asymptomatic or complain of lower pelvic pain that is aggravated during sexual intercourse, as well as bleeding after intercourse or between menses. They may have noticed an increase in vaginal discharge that is yellow or grayish in color with a foul odor. Frequent, burning urination may also be present. Fever may or may not be present depending on the severity of infection. Perform a full pelvic exam (speculum and bimanual); the cervix may appear erythematous, inflamed, or friable. Note type of cervical discharge, which is usually thick and yellowish-green. Perform a Pap smear as needed (e.g., every 3–5 years if ≥21 years old) and HPV testing every 5 years starting at 30 years old.

Obtain gonorrhea and chlamydia cultures for a definitive diagnosis, as well as urine testing. Appropriate empiric antibiotics should be started to prevent spreading the infection (chlamydia: azithromycin and doxycycline; gonorrhea: ceftriaxone and azithromycin), which could lead to pelvic inflammatory disease, a pelvic abscess, or spreading to the patient's sexual partner. Treat sexual partners at the same time as the patient. Adjust antibiotics when culture results are obtained. If the irritation is chemical in nature, patients should stop using the causative agent.

CERVICAL DYSPLASIA AND CERVICAL CANCER

To help screen for **cytology changes on the cervix**, a **Pap smear** is recommended every 3 years if ≥21 years old until about 65–70 years old (not needed if patient has had a non-cancer-related total hysterectomy); starting at 30 years old, another option is a Pap smear plus HPV testing every 5 years. **Cervical dysplasia**, also referred to as cervical intraepithelial neoplasia (CIN), refers to these changes and can be classified as **mild dysplasia** (CIN I; low-grade squamous intraepithelial lesion, LSIL), **moderate dysplasia** (CIN II), or **severe dysplasia** (CIN III; high-grade squamous intraepithelial lesion, HSIL). Severe dysplasia has the highest risk of transforming into invasive cancer (>12 %). Follow-up tests for cervical dysplasia include colposcopy, biopsy, endocervical curettage, or a cone biopsy (loop electrosurgical excision procedure [LEEP], also called large loop excision of the transformation zone [LLETZ]; cold-knife cone biopsy). The LEEP, or LLETZ, is also used for treating dysplastic changes. Treatment depends on the level of dysplasia; 5-fluorouracil (5-FU) may be applied topically for CIN II.

There are several types of **cervical cancer**; the most common is **squamous cell carcinoma** caused by HPV, with adenocarcinoma being the second most common. Cervical cancer is the **third most common cancer in women**. Risk factors for cervical cancer include HPV infection, multiple sex partners, early age at first intercourse, smoking, and being immunocompromised. This is usually caught on Pap smears, but bleeding after sexual intercourse is a common finding by patients. Once the cancer is staged, treatment may involve surgery or radiation and chemotherapy.

OVARIAN DISORDERS
OVARIAN CYSTS

Ovarian cysts are relatively common and occur in or on the surface of the **ovary**. Most do not produce symptoms, but some women have significant symptoms from these cysts. Functional cysts may be either follicular or corpus luteum cysts. **Follicular cysts** occur in the follicle when the egg does not release from the maturing follicle and continues to grow, leading to a cyst; these generally resolve without treatment. A **corpus luteum cyst** occurs after the egg ruptures, and the follicle becomes the corpus luteum. It seals itself off and begins to expand as fluid accumulates in it to form a cyst. The follicular cysts generally do not cause symptoms. The corpus luteum cysts, however, can grow to be >4 cm wide and may cause significant abdominal pain. **Dermoid cysts** (teratoma), which are germ cell tumors that may contain teeth or hair, can grow quite large. Cysts can also rupture, which causes sudden, severe abdominal pain, or even syncope. Diagnose with an ultrasound and rule out cancer. Cysts may be followed by ultrasound for several cycles. Oral contraceptives may prevent cyst formation by regulating hormones. If symptoms are persistent, surgery may be necessary to remove the cyst. If a cyst ruptures, removal of the ovary may be necessary.

OVARIAN TORSION

Ovarian torsion is fairly uncommon but may occur with ovarian cysts/tumors that are usually benign. This occurs more often in cysts >4 cm and on the right side. It typically causes severe, sudden pain and nausea/vomiting. Diagnose with an ultrasound or CT; rule out cancer. Treat with immediate surgical detorsion (try to preserve the ovary) or ovarian removal if the tissue is nonviable.

OVARIAN CANCER

Ovarian cancer has a poor prognosis since it is often not diagnosed until in an advanced stage when it has already spread. The main risk factor is a positive family history of breast or ovarian cancer. CA 125 is increased in ovarian cancer. Surgery is used to stage and treat this, as well as chemotherapy.

POLYCYSTIC OVARIAN SYNDROME

Polycystic ovarian syndrome (**PCOS**) involves dysfunction of the **hypothalamic-pituitary-ovarian axis**. It causes menstrual irregularities, anovulation, infertility, and signs of increased androgens. This is the most common cause of **infertility** within the U.S. and usually starts affecting women in adolescence. Signs and symptoms may include increased weight (in half of patients), hirsutism, acne, acanthosis nigricans, irregular menses, amenorrhea, and insulin resistance/metabolic syndrome. Diagnose clinically and confirm with a transvaginal ultrasound, which shows multiple (>25) cysts or follicles; rule out other causes of the symptoms. Treatment includes lifestyle changes (exercise, weight loss), oral contraceptives (help with menstrual irregularities, acne, hirsutism), metformin for insulin resistance, and infertility treatment for those who desire to have children.

STDS AND INFECTIONS

VAGINITIS

Vaginitis is an **inflammation of the vagina** that is not necessarily due to an infection. Though infection from bacteria (bacterial vaginosis), viruses, or yeast (vaginal candidiasis) can cause this inflammation, it can also be due to decreased estrogen levels following menopause (atrophic vaginitis), causing the vaginal walls to be drier and easily irritated. The symptoms will depend upon the cause of the inflammation, but all types will usually cause vaginal itching or burning and pain with sexual intercourse. **Bacterial vaginosis** causes a foul-smelling, fishy discharge that may be grayish in color; it shows clue cells under the microscope. **Vaginal candidiasis** causes a white curd-like discharge; hyphae are seen under the microscope/KOH preparation.

Trichomoniasis is an STD caused by the parasite *Trichomonas vaginalis*, that can cause a greenish-yellow, frothy vaginal (or penile) discharge. It is often asymptomatic in both men and women. A wet-mount microscopic specimen will show protozoan flagellate motile organisms. **Atrophic vaginitis** causes itching and irritation of the vagina and painful intercourse. There may be pain present during urination, as well. Treatment varies, depending on the cause of the inflammation. Appropriate antibiotics or antifungals are necessary for infections. For bacterial vaginosis: metronidazole 500 mg bid for 7 days OR topical gel. For vaginal candidiasis: clotrimazole 1% cream for 7–14 days OR clotrimazole vaginal tablet for 7 days OR fluconazole 150mg PO × 1. For trichomoniasis (also treat all sex partners): 2 grams of metronidazole OR tinidazole PO × 1 dose. For atrophic vaginitis: estrogen cream or tablets help with the postmenopausal vaginal dryness. Complications of trichomoniasis include urethritis, cystitis, cervical neoplasia, PID, infertility, and preterm birth, and it increases susceptibility to HIV. Screen for other STDs as needed and treat partners accordingly. Counsel patients to avoid douching.

PELVIC INFLAMMATORY DISEASE

Pelvic inflammatory disease (**PID**) is a condition of inflammation and infection in the **upper female reproductive tract** that can lead to infertility. It begins from an infection that moves up from its original source, usually the **cervix or vagina**. The typical causative agents include *Chlamydia trachomatis*, *Neisseria gonorrhoeae*, and *Gardnerella vaginalis* (and other organisms that are found in bacterial vaginosis). PID is often polymicrobial. Risk factors for PID include age <25, engaging in unprotected sex, and having multiple sexual partners.

Signs and symptoms include lower abdominal pain and cramping that is worse after sex/motion, fever, bleeding after sex, vaginal discharge, and possibly nausea/vomiting. Pelvic exam shows cervical motion tenderness and tenderness throughout the reproductive tract, inflammation, and abnormal discharge. This may be diagnosed clinically or may be definitively diagnosed laparoscopically. Test for STDs and order a pregnancy test; rule out an ectopic pregnancy. Treat with empiric antibiotics to cover gonorrhea and chlamydia (ceftriaxone 250 mg IM × 1, PLUS doxycycline 100 mg PO bid for 14 days, and possibly with metronidazole 500 mg PO bid for 14 days); hospitalization may be required to receive IV antibiotics and to monitor the patient. It is important to treat PID to lower the possibility of complications like infertility, future ectopic pregnancies, chronic pain, and tubal or ovarian abscesses.

MENSTRUAL DISORDERS AND MENOPAUSE
PREMENSTRUAL SYNDROME

Premenstrual syndrome (**PMS**) is a condition affecting women during the **luteal phase** of their cycles. This is quite common and usually starts in adolescence, but can be particularly bad when patients are in their 40s. However, PMS completely goes away after menopause. The exact cause is not known, but risk factors include smoking and obesity. The **menstrual cycle** (average 28 days) typically has several phases, including **follicular phase** (FSH stimulates the ovary to prepare a follicle; FSH and LH are low); **ovulatory phase** (about day 13–14 there is a hormonal surge in estrogen, FSH, and LH; LH has the largest surge; ovulation takes place); and **luteal phase** (progesterone surges; estrogen and progesterone remain elevated until they both drop suddenly around day 24, then menses begins, about day 28). Patients present describing symptoms starting in the luteal phase including cravings, anxious feeling, depressive symptoms, sleep issues, bloating/edema, dysmenorrhea, bowel changes, acne, nausea, and mastalgia. Diagnose clinically and treat symptoms with NSAIDs, diuretics, diet and exercise, SSRIs for severe mood issues, and possibly oral contraceptives.

PREMENSTRUAL DYSPHORIC DISORDER

Premenstrual dysphoric disorder (**PMDD**) describes a severe form of premenstrual syndrome that has at least 5 of the following symptoms present (DSM-5) the week before menses (symptoms begin to improve within a few days after menses begins). **Major symptoms:** marked affective lability/mood swings, irritability/anger, depressed mood, anxiety/tension. **Minor symptoms:** reduced interest in typical activities, difficulty concentrating, lethargy/fatigue, appetite changes, sleep disturbances, feelings of being overwhelmed/out of control, breast tenderness/feeling bloated/weight gain/myalgias/arthralgias. At least 1 major symptom must be present for the diagnosis to be made, and symptoms must not be better described by another disorder (e.g., major depressive disorder). Also, this interferes with daily functioning. PMDD is treated with a variety of methods, including diet and exercise, light therapy, relaxation techniques, and cognitive behavior therapy; and medications like NSAIDs, SSRIs, anxiolytics, oral contraceptives, and diuretics.

AMENORRHEA AND DYSMENORRHEA

Amenorrhea refers to the **absence of menses** and may be primary (no menses by age 16 or 2 years after puberty onset) or secondary (menses stops after cycles have started). For **primary amenorrhea**, the workup includes: checking the hypothalamic-pituitary axis for abnormalities, ruling out genetic disorders like Turner syndrome, ruling out ovarian insufficiency like PCOS, and uterine outflow issues like an imperforate hymen. For **secondary amenorrhea**, rule out pregnancy (most common), Asherman syndrome, PCOS, prolactinomas, and possible causes like excessive weight loss or stress, hypothyroidism, and Cushing syndrome. Diagnose with appropriate tests (e.g., β-hCG, FSH, LH, prolactin, TSH; and imaging studies as needed, like ultrasound or MRI); and treat the underlying cause.

Dysmenorrhea refers to **painful menstruation** and may be primary (not due to pelvic abnormalities) or secondary (due to pelvic abnormalities). This can be quite painful and incapacitating and may lead to absence from school or work. **Primary dysmenorrhea** usually starts within 6 months of menarche. Those at increased risk include those with a positive family history, early menarche, or long or heavy menstrual bleeding, and those who smoke. **Secondary dysmenorrhea** usually starts in the 20s or 30s after having cycles without major pain, and has an increased incidence in those with fibroids, endometriosis, PID, and tubo-ovarian abscesses. **Elevated prostaglandins** play a role in both primary and secondary dysmenorrhea. Patients (with primary) present describing cyclical lower abdominal or low back pain (may radiate to the thigh) surrounding their menses.

Diagnose primary dysmenorrhea clinically; use imaging studies (e.g., ultrasound, hysterosalpingography, CT) to determine the underlying cause of secondary dysmenorrhea; rule out infections and pregnancy. Further studies may include hysterosalpingography, laparoscopy, and D&C (dilation and curettage). Treat symptoms with NSAIDs by starting them 24–48 hours before menses and continuing them 1–2 days into menses; sometimes OCs are used. For secondary, treat any underlying causes.

ABNORMAL (DYSFUNCTIONAL) UTERINE BLEEDING

Abnormal uterine bleeding (dysfunctional uterine bleeding) is **irregular uterine bleeding** that is not due to pregnancy or other gynecologic issues. This is common in adolescent and perimenopausal women, and it is usually associated with **anovulation**. Bleeding may be heavy or light and long or short. Patients present describing their irregular bleeding and usually do not have any premenstrual symptoms. Perform a thorough history and physical exam with a Pap smear. This is a diagnosis of exclusion. Rule out pregnancy, bleeding disorders, PCOS, pituitary issues, thyroid issues, and endometrial hyperplasia or cancer. Any bleeding in a postmenopausal woman is a red flag, and diseases like cancer should be ruled out. Treatment involves low-dose oral contraceptives.

MENOPAUSE

Menopause is a natural part of a woman's life in which **menstruation** stops and **ovarian function** decreases. Menopause is reached after menses have stopped for 12 months. Most symptoms occur in the perimenopausal phase, when hormone levels are greatly fluctuating, usually about age 45. Perimenopausal symptoms vary between patients and may last on average 3–8 years. Patients may describe irregular menses, hot flashes/night sweats, weight gain, mastalgia, moodiness, headaches/menstrual migraines, vaginal dryness, urinary symptoms like dysuria and frequency, and sleep issues.

This is a clinical diagnosis; however, it may be confirmed with FSH (>25 mIU/mL indicates perimenopause/menopause). Certain changes take place with menopause, and managing patients after menopause includes protecting against osteoporosis and CVD; screening for breast, cervical, and colorectal cancer; and giving annual influenza vaccines. Hormone replacement therapy (HRT) may be offered to women to help relieve symptoms and to protect from osteoporosis and CAD (may be protective if given early in the course of menopause). HRT should not be started if >60 years old and >10 years since the onset of menopause. Contraindications to HRT include unexplained vaginal bleeding, liver disease, thrombosis, and a history of breast cancer.

PREGNANCY, PRENATAL, DELIVERY, AND POSTNATAL CARE
INITIAL PRENATAL CONSULTATION/VISIT

The first prenatal visit is usually at **8–10 weeks gestation** and includes taking a thorough history and ordering the initial labs. Measure initial height and weight and calculate BMI. **Blood work** should include blood type, Rh factor, antibody screen (Coombs test), CBC, rapid plasma reagin (RPR) for syphilis, hepatitis B antigen (HBsAg), HIV, and rubella antibody. A **pelvic exam** with a Pap smear (may test for HPV), and testing for gonorrhea and chlamydia, may also be necessary. Offer **genetic screening/ testing** (especially if ≥35 years old). To check for **trisomy 18 and trisomy 21**: pregnancy-associated plasma protein-A (PAPP-A) plus β-hCG plus ultrasound for nuchal translucency (11–14 weeks). The **triple screen** (maternal serum α-fetoprotein level, β-hCG, and unconjugated estriol) and **quadruple screen** (same as triple screen but adds inhibin A) in the second trimester screens for trisomy 18, trisomy 21, and neural tube defects. Other tests include **chorionic** villus sampling (CVS), which allows for early testing (11–13 weeks) of multiple chromosome anomalies like CF; **amniocentesis** (usually at 16–18 weeks gestation); and **targeted ultrasounds**.

Feelings and expectations regarding pregnancy are explored at the initial visit, and careful questions regarding **personal safety and abuse** may be proposed. Smoking, alcohol, and recreational drug use should also be addressed. The major components of early prenatal care include identifying patients who are at risk for certain complications; anticipating problems and intervening when able; educating and communicating with the patient; getting early, repeated, and accurate measures of gestational age; and doing ongoing evaluations of the status of the fetus and mother. Visits are scheduled every 4 weeks until 28 weeks gestation, then every 2 weeks until 36 weeks gestation, when weekly visits begin. Routine information to gather during a prenatal visit includes weight and blood pressure; urinalysis for blood, glucose, protein, and bacteria; fundal height; and fetal heart tones, which can begin after 10 weeks gestation.

PRENATAL CARE (RH INCOMPATIBILITY, GESTATIONAL DIABETES, GBS, HYPERTENSION DISORDERS OF PREGNANCY)

Routine prenatal tests include: an ultrasound at 16–20 weeks, a 1-hour glucose tolerance test at 24–28 weeks (screens for gestational diabetes), and a group B streptococcus test of vagina/rectum at 36 weeks.

Rh incompatibility: Mothers with Rh-negative blood can develop **Rho(D) antibodies** against their Rh-positive babies (risk increases after the first Rh-positive baby). RhoGAM is given to the mother at 28 weeks and again within 72 hours of delivery if the baby is Rh-positive.

Gestational diabetes: This can lead to multiple issues, like fetal macrosomia (large babies), shoulder dystocia, and preeclampsia. The 1-hour oral glucose tolerance test (OGTT) is normal if <130 mmol/L; if abnormal results, order a 3-hour OGTT (normal if <140–145). If the 3-hour test is abnormal, start insulin.

Group B streptococcus (GBS): This bacterium is common in the vaginal flora. It may be passed on during delivery and may cause sepsis and meningitis in the newborn baby. If positive, the mother is prophylactically treated: penicillin G or ampicillin. If penicillin allergic, use cefazolin for treatment.

Hypertension disorders in pregnancy: These include preeclampsia, eclampsia, and HELLP syndrome.

Preeclampsia: This is new-onset hypertension and proteinuria occurring after 20 weeks gestation and may even appear up to 6 weeks after delivery. This may be asymptomatic, so screening for proteinuria and blood pressure measurements at prenatal visits are important. Edema may be the only sign. Preeclampsia may become more severe, with headaches, nausea/vomiting, visual issues, and confusion. Close monitoring of patients is vital since this may progress to eclampsia. Delivery of the baby is the only cure.

Eclampsia: Left untreated, this becomes fatal. It involves the same symptoms as preeclampsia but adds seizures. Immediate administration of high-dose magnesium sulfate is needed to treat seizures, and this requires immediate delivery. Close postpartum monitoring is important.

HELLP syndrome: HELLP stands for: H—hemolysis, EL—elevated liver enzymes, LP—low platelets. This is a life-threatening disorder and can be a complication of preeclampsia. Signs and symptoms may include edema, headache, nausea/vomiting, epigastric pain, hematuria, increased bilirubin, increased LFTs, and jaundice. Deliver immediately.

ECTOPIC PREGNANCY

An ectopic pregnancy occurs when a fertilized egg **fails to implant in the uterine lining**. It most often will implant within the **fallopian tube** but can implant within the ovary, abdomen, or uterine cornu, or down low in the neck of the cervix. An ectopic pregnancy often occurs without any known cause, but risk factors include scar tissue, malformation of the tube, previous pelvic inflammatory disease (PID), IUD use, smoking, and history of infertility. Patients may or may not know they are pregnant. They usually present with gradually worsening abdominal pain, usually one-sided, with amenorrhea and vaginal bleeding. **Rupture of the fallopian tube** can occur as the ovum enlarges, which causes severe stabbing pain on the affected side, guarding, and possible syncope and signs of hypovolemic shock (tachycardia, orthostatic hypotension).

Diagnose with ultrasound and check β-hCG levels if the case is not urgent. Treatment includes watchful waiting if the patient is asymptomatic and β-hCG levels are declining; immediate surgical resection if hemodynamically unstable; and a single injection of methotrexate may be used if the ectopic pregnancy is confirmed, unruptured, <4 cm, β-hCG <5,000 mIU/mL, and there is no fetal heartbeat. Follow β-hCG levels until 0. If rupture of the fallopian tube occurs, emergency surgery will be necessary to attempt to repair the tube or remove it.

Cervical Insufficiency (Incompetent Cervix)

The American College of Obstetricians and Gynecologists defines cervical insufficiency or an incompetent cervix as to a cervix that **cannot maintain a pregnancy in the second trimester in the absence of contractions**. The cervix will not remain completely closed during pregnancy, placing the baby at risk for **premature birth**. This insufficiency can be due to past trauma to the cervix, such as from surgery, D&C, induced abortion, cone biopsy, or previous deliveries that were traumatic to the cervix; or genetic anomalies that cause a malformed cervix or reproductive tract (connective tissue disorder, Müllerian defects like a bicornuate uterus). Unfortunately, cervical insufficiency is often asymptomatic and not usually diagnosed until after a second- or third-trimester pregnancy loss. Patients may have some bleeding in the second or third trimester, a feeling of vaginal pressure or fullness, increased discharge, or low back pain.

The cervical dilation may be detected on pelvic exam. Those at risk should receive a **transvaginal ultrasound** at 15–16 weeks. If dilation or a short cervix is found (<2.5 cm), the cervix can be reinforced with a cerclage procedure, which involves placing purse-string sutures in the cervix to draw it closed. This effectively sutures the cervix closed to prevent premature dilation. These sutures are usually removed in the last few weeks of pregnancy (about 37 weeks) when it is safe to deliver the baby. Risk of recurrent cervical insufficiency in future pregnancies is about 30%.

Abruptio Placentae

Abruptio placentae, or placental abruption, occurs when the **placenta** prematurely begins **separating from the uterine wall**. Blood collects between the placenta and the uterus, and it can be a medical emergency that can place the unborn child and mother at risk. It usually occurs after 20 weeks and can be classified as **partial or complete** (emergency), **concealed** (no visible bleeding), or **revealed** (visible bleeding), and as **central or marginal**. Frequently, the cause of the placental abruption is unknown; however, it can occur following some type of trauma, such as a bad fall or car accident in which there is some degree of trauma to the mother. Risk factors include maternal hypertension; previous abruption; cigarette, alcohol, or cocaine use; chorioamnionitis (intra-amniotic infection); and premature rupture of membranes (PROM). Patients may present with vaginal bleeding (80% of cases); decreased fetal movements; abdominal or back pain; uterine tenderness with uterine contractions that are very close together, usually one after another; pain between contractions; and possibly signs of hypovolemic shock.

Diagnose clinically and with an ultrasound; check fibrinogen level and check for a coagulopathy. Treatment depends on the severity of the abruption: admit, manage, and observe; or an emergent C-section may be required. If the mother is preterm and ultrasound determines that the placental abruption is chronic and minor, and the baby is stable, the mother may be closely monitored on bed rest. Monitor signs of maternal or fetal distress. If symptoms should worsen, however, treatment is to deliver the baby as quickly as possible, via emergency C-section. Consult a maternal-fetal medicine specialist, and— if preterm delivery is inevitable—a pediatrician/NICU.

PLACENTA PREVIA

Placenta previa occurs when the **placenta** forms **very close to the cervical os** or may partially or completely **cover the cervix**. Placenta previa is classified as **marginal** (edge of placenta is within 2 cm of the cervical os) or **complete** (covers the cervical os). The cause is not fully understood, but risk factors include scarring of the lining the uterus from previous surgery or trauma, malformation of the uterus or fibroids, multiple gestation, and smoking or cocaine use. Painless bright red bleeding during the third trimester is the most common presenting symptom with placenta previa. The amount and duration of bleeding late in pregnancy will depend upon how much of the cervix is covered by the placenta. There is a risk of massive bleeding and danger to the unborn child if the cervix begins to dilate, causing the placenta to tear prematurely.

Diagnose and follow the progress of a marginal placenta previa with ultrasound(s); rule out abruption. Low-lying placentas usually move to a safe location by 28 weeks as the uterus grows. Treatment depends upon the severity of symptoms. Patients without bleeding can be monitored closely as an outpatient. If bleeding occurs, hospitalize and monitor. The goal is to reach 36–37 weeks before delivering. If bleeding is persistent, the baby should be delivered via C-section as soon as possible, even if premature, to prevent fetal distress, maternal complications, or death. If preterm delivery is inevitable, give corticosteroids if <34 weeks to help promote fetal lung maturity. Placenta previa may be associated with hemorrhage, abruption, and placenta accreta (placenta implanting deeply into uterine wall).

PREMATURE RUPTURE OF THE MEMBRANES (PROM)

Premature rupture of the membranes (**PROM**) is a condition in which the **amniotic sac ruptures** before labor begins. This refers to situations in which the mother is at least at 37 weeks gestation. If this occurs earlier (<37 weeks), it is called **preterm premature rupture of the membranes (PPROM)** and is the leading cause of **preterm birth**. Premature rupture of the membranes can occur because of infection, increased amniotic fluid, a multiple-gestation pregnancy, smoking, history of PROM or amniocentesis, previous surgery or cervical cone biopsy, or abruptio placentae. Patients will experience a trickle or a sudden gush of **amniotic fluid** from the vagina.

Diagnose with a sterile speculum exam (shows vaginal pooling of amniotic fluid) and evaluate fluid (amniotic fluid shows a ferning pattern when dried on a microscope slide, and has an alkaline pH—Nitrazine paper turns blue). Treatment depends on the gestational age and may consist of bed rest and close monitoring, or if term, delivery of the baby. Vaginal delivery can be performed if the baby and mother are stable. Pitocin may be needed to start contractions if they have not started within 24 hours after rupture. Delivery should occur within 24 hours of PROM to decrease the chance of infection.

DYSTOCIA

Dystocia is defined as **difficult, prolonged childbirth or failure to progress**. This is a condition that occurs in approximately 10–15% of pregnancies and is more common in nulliparous/obese women, those with gestational diabetes, and those with a small pelvic diameter. Dystocia can be due to uncoordinated uterine contractions, abnormal fetal presentation or fetal size, or cephalopelvic disproportion (referred to as the 3 P's: power, passenger, or pelvis). A common form of dystocia is **shoulder dystocia**, in which the infant's shoulders are difficult to deliver after the head has already been delivered, due to the size of the infant. This can lead to **brachial plexus injury** or **clavicular fracture** in the newborn. Normal delivery progresses in 3 stages:

- **Stage 1** begins with regular contractions (every 2–3 minutes), until fully dilated to 10 cm (nulliparous women usually progress <1 cm/hour, and multiparous usually dilate <1.5 cm/hour). This has 2 phases:
    - **Latent:** the slow progression of contractions and dilation
    - **Active:** a time of increased dilation and fetal descent
- **Stage 2** begins when fully dilated and lasts until the baby is born.
- **Stage 3** is the delivery of the placenta (usually occurs in about 10 minutes; should occur within 30 minutes post-delivery).

Dystocia is diagnosed clinically when these stages last longer than predicted (e.g., dilated 6 cm with rupture of membranes and no cervical change after 4–6 hours depending on the adequacy of contractions). Treatment may involve Pitocin (oxytocin), assisted vaginal delivery (e.g., forceps, vacuum extraction), or C-section.

POSTNATAL CARE: POSTPARTUM HEMORRHAGE AND ENDOMETRITIS

Postpartum and postnatal care involves **monitoring the mother and baby** in the hours after delivery. Special care for the mother includes monitoring for signs of hemorrhage and for a fever. It is also important to discuss and provide aid for breastfeeding and to discuss the importance of maternal rest, good eating habits, and signs of postpartum depression.

Endometritis is an infection of the uterus following childbirth (most common in the first 24–72 hours; late endometritis may not appear until 6 weeks postpartum), usually due to bacteria ascending from the vagina or from retained placental fragments. It can be life-threatening if not promptly treated and should be considered as a diagnosis in any woman who develops a fever after childbirth. Incidence increases in patients with a C-section, especially if unscheduled, or with PROM, but may also occur after a vaginal delivery. Signs and symptoms include a fever (>38 °C) with chills, lower abdominal or pelvic pain, and nausea/vomiting. The uterus will be tender on palpation, and vaginal discharge present will have a foul odor. The cause is polymicrobial, and IV antibiotics (usually clindamycin and gentamicin) should be started immediately and continued until afebrile for 48 hours. If not improved, consider the possibility of a pelvic abscess.

Postpartum hemorrhage is a leading cause of **maternal mortality** and is usually due to **atony of the uterus**; other causes include lacerations, uterine rupture, and chorioamnionitis. After delivery, the uterus should be massaged to help it contract, which should slow down bleeding; also, any retained placenta should be removed. If massage is not sufficient, oxytocin should be given. Fluid resuscitation is important, and a blood transfusion may be necessary. If blood loss is severe, surgery may be necessary (artery ligation or hysterectomy).

UTERINE AND VAGINAL/VULVAL DISORDERS

ENDOMETRIOSIS

Endometriosis occurs when the **endometrial tissue** that makes up the uterine lining is also present **outside the uterus**. This can occur on areas like the fallopian tubes, ovaries, outside of the uterus, peritoneum, bowel, or bladder. The **ectopic tissue** will thicken with the hormonal changes that occur during the menstrual cycle, and can shed, causing irritation to the surrounding structures. When severe, endometriosis can cause scarring, adhesions, and severe pain. The severity of the endometriosis does not correlate to the amount of pain, and the cause of endometriosis is unknown. Risk factors include a positive family history in a first-degree relative, early menarche, a menstrual cycle <27 days that is heavy and long, and being nulliparous. Patients may be asymptomatic, but the most common presenting symptom is cramping pain (usually starts a few days before menstruation), along with dysmenorrhea, dyspareunia, pain with bowel movements, and low back or inguinal pain. **Infertility** may occur as scar tissue and adhesions form. The physical exam is usually nonspecific and may only reveal pelvic pain.

Diagnosis begins with clinical suspicion and is confirmed with laparoscopic surgery, which can be used to treat it at the same time as the diagnosis; the endometrial tissue is laparoscopically removed, and this may decrease symptoms and increase chances of pregnancy. Medications include NSAIDs for pain, oral contraceptives to help maintain hormone levels and possibly reduce excessive symptoms, and medications to prevent the secretion of hormones by the ovaries (e.g., danazol and GnRH agonists [leuprolide]). As a last resort, hysterectomy may be considered, especially if the patient is finished having children. Endometriosis tends to improve during pregnancy and after menopause.

LEIOMYOMAS

Leiomyomas, or **uterine fibroids**, are very common **benign uterine tumors**. They are formed in the **uterine smooth muscle** and can be **submucosal** (under the inner lining of the uterus), **intramural, subserosal** (under the outer lining of the uterus), or **pedunculated**. They usually form during childbearing years, and incidence increases with age (until menopause); most women are unaware they have them since they are frequently asymptomatic. Risk of leiomyomas is greater for African American women and as well as women with a positive family history, increased weight, and increased estrogen. When leiomyomas do produce symptoms, patients may complain of heavy and prolonged menstrual bleeding, bleeding that may not be associated with menstrual periods, and abdominal or pelvic pain; and, if large enough, those applying pressure to the bowels or bladder may produce constipation and urinary frequency or incontinence.

Diagnosis is made by ultrasound. Treatment may involve medication like GnRH agonists to decrease the size of the fibroids, androgenic agents like danazol to reduce symptoms, NSAIDs for the pain, and surgery such as laser ablation, myomectomy, or fibroid embolization. A hysterectomy can be performed to remove the uterus if the symptoms are severe and the woman is not planning to have any more children.

CYSTOCELE AND RECTOCELE

When the vaginal wall becomes weakened, the bladder or rectum may protrude into the vaginal canal, and a cystocele and/or rectocele result. Muscle weakness can result from straining during childbirth, chronic constipation, coughing, or heavy lifting. In some women, the decrease in estrogen that occurs after menopause may cause laxity of these connective tissues, leading to a cystocele or a rectocele. A **cystocele** or **prolapsed bladder** results when the weakness occurs on the side against the bladder. Patients might present with complaints of pressure within the vagina; a feeling of discomfort when sitting; pain when bearing down, having intercourse, coughing, or lifting; multiple urinary tract infections; or urine leakage. A **rectocele** is a weakness on the **posterior wall of the vagina** against the rectum and results from the same types of injuries. There may be a complaint of vaginal fullness, discomfort when sitting, difficulty passing stool, the sensation that the rectum is not completely emptied following a bowel movement, and possibly chronic constipation. Occasionally, patients may experience episodes of fecal incontinence. However, patients may or may not experience symptoms from a cystocele or rectocele, depending on its severity.

Diagnose these by physical exam while the patient is straining. Treatment involves Kegel (pelvic floor) exercises, and a pessary can be inserted to support the vaginal wall and prevent the bladder or rectum from bulging into the vagina. If symptoms are very bothersome, surgery may be necessary to strengthen the connective tissue and support of these structures.

URETHRAL PROLAPSE, UTERINE PROLAPSE, AND VAGINAL PROLAPSE

Urethral prolapse or a urethrocele is the protrusion of the **distal urethra** into the **urethral meatus** and presents as a urethral mass with vaginal bleeding. This is fairly uncommon, but usually occurs in prepubertal girls or in postmenopausal women. Diagnose clinically per physical exam (the urethral prolapse looks like a donut). Treatment involves topical estrogen cream and, if necessary, surgical repair.

Uterine prolapse occurs when the **uterus** protrudes into the **vaginal canal** and possibly further. This is more common with increasing age and increased weight, and in those who have had multiple births or a hysterectomy. It can be classified as **1st degree** (upper vaginal canal), **2nd degree** (introitus), **3rd degree** (cervix is outside the introitus), and **4th degree** (cervix and uterus are outside the introitus). This also may or may not occur with **vaginal prolapse**. Patients may experience fullness and pressure that increases with straining, and a sensation that their insides are coming out. Other symptoms include constipation and urinary issues like incomplete emptying of the bladder. Smaller prolapses may be asymptomatic. Diagnose per clinical exam, and an ultrasound may be ordered to assess comorbid conditions (e.g., UTIs, bladder outlet obstruction). Treat with estrogen or surgery.

PA Practice Test #1

Want to take this practice test in an online interactive format?
Check out the bonus page, which includes interactive practice questions and much
more: **mometrix.com/bonus948/pance**

1. A 45-year-old male comes to the ER after being involved in a head-on motor vehicle accident earlier in the day. The patient notes that he struck his head, but he did not experience any loss of consciousness. His blood pressure is 190/110, his respirations are irregular, and his electrocardiogram (ECG) shows sinus bradycardia with a heart rate of 42 beats per minute. The patient's symptoms are part of which clinical triad?

    a. Beck triad
    b. Charcot triad
    c. Cushing triad
    d. Bergman triad

2. All of the following are minor manifestations of acute rheumatic fever as described by the modified Jones criteria EXCEPT:

    a. Erythema marginatum
    b. Leukocytosis
    c. Elevated erythrocyte sedimentation rate (ESR)
    d. Arthralgia

3. A 19-year-old woman comes to the office complaining of a painful rash on her elbows and knees. The rash appears as raised erythematous areas topped with silvery, scaling skin. She reports, "The rash is very itchy." She had similar symptoms several weeks before, but they spontaneously resolved without treatment. Which of the following is most likely to be the diagnosis?

    a. Impetigo
    b. Tinea corporis
    c. Rosacea
    d. Psoriasis

4. During a colonoscopy, the gastroenterologist notices that the patient's colon wall has a "cobblestone" appearance. Which of the following is the most likely diagnosis?

    a. Celiac sprue
    b. Crohn disease
    c. Ulcerative colitis
    d. Whipple disease

5. You are evaluating an obese 37-year-old female in the ER. She has been complaining of right-sided abdominal pain and excessive flatulence. She normally has the pain after eating, but it usually resolves on its own. This episode has persisted for several hours. On physical examination, you palpate her right upper quadrant while she takes a deep inspiration. Discomfort during this maneuver is referred to as a positive:

    a. Brudzinski sign
    b. Psoas sign
    c. Murphy sign
    d. Levine sign

6. You are acting as the first assist in the operating room, and the surgeon asks you to close an abdominal incision with an absorbable suture material. Based on the following choices, which suture would be your pick?

    a. Dermabond
    b. Vicryl
    c. Silk
    d. Nylon

7. All of the following are symptoms of esophageal achalasia EXCEPT:

    a. Acid reflux
    b. Dysphagia
    c. Hematochezia
    d. Chest pain

8. Which of the following is NOT part of CREST syndrome?

    a. Calcinosis
    b. Sclerodactyly
    c. Solar urticaria
    d. Esophageal dysmotility

9. A 20-year-old female recently diagnosed with chlamydia comes to your office for swelling and pain in her knees bilaterally. The most likely diagnosis for this woman's complaints is:

    a. Sjögren syndrome
    b. Reiter syndrome
    c. Turner syndrome
    d. Down syndrome

10. A 26-year-old female comes to the ER with complaints of white vaginal discharge and pelvic pain. She admits to having unprotected sex. On physical examination, she has an inflamed cervix and cervical motion tenderness. Which one of the following two-medication pairs should she receive prior to leaving the ER?

    a. Ceftriaxone 250 mg IM and clindamycin 300 mg PO
    b. Clindamycin 300 mg PO and azithromycin 1 g PO
    c. Cefoxitin 2 g IV and azithromycin 1 g PO
    d. Ceftriaxone 250 mg IM and azithromycin 1 g PO

11. A 19-year-old male patient is brought to the ER by his mother for altered mental status. She notes that he "hasn't been acting normally" since the morning. He has a known history of depression and anxiety, for which he does not take medication, and chronic back pain, for which he takes codeine. On physical examination, his pupils are 2 mm bilaterally and he is lethargic, but he is able to be aroused. His heart rate is 44, his blood pressure is 78/44, and his respiratory rate is 8 breaths per minute. Which of the following medications may reverse his symptoms and confirm your suspected diagnosis?

    a.   Oxycodone
    b.   Naloxone
    c.   Prednisolone
    d.   Buspirone

12. You diagnose an adult patient in your clinic with streptococcal pharyngitis. The patient has a known anaphylactic reaction to penicillin. Which of the following medications would be an acceptable substitute?

    a.   Cefepime
    b.   Cephalexin
    c.   Augmentin
    d.   Clarithromycin

13. You are examining a 5-year-old patient for a wellness examination. During the examination, you notice that the child has painful-looking, swollen joints and notching of the maxillary incisors. The child is blind and deaf. Based on his past medical history and examination findings, the patient most likely has a history of:

    a.   Congenital syphilis
    b.   Down syndrome
    c.   Osgood-Schlatter disease
    d.   Turner syndrome

14. A 45-year-old male presents to your clinic with a painful, erythematous bump on his right eyelid of 3 days' duration. The eyeball itself is unaffected. His vision is unaffected. He has no crusting on the eyelids or lashes. The most likely diagnosis is:

    a.   Xanthelasma
    b.   Hordeolum
    c.   Mongolian spots
    d.   Felon

15. A 66-year-old male comes into the office complaining of painless, yellowish, raised patches on his eyelids bilaterally for the past several weeks. He has no other skin lesions and has had no history of these lesions before. He has a known history of hyperlipidemia, for which he is noncompliant with medications. What is the most likely diagnosis?

    a.   Dermoid cyst
    b.   Impetigo
    c.   Mongolian spots
    d.   Xanthelasma

16. Parents of a 5-year-old boy bring him to the ER, noting that he has had worsening ataxia, nausea, vomiting, and headaches. He has no significant medical history. His parents deny recent trauma or recent travel. A magnetic resonance imaging (MRI) scan of the brain shows a tumor in the middle of the cerebellum with mild hydrocephalus. The most likely diagnosis is:

    a. Schistosomiasis
    b. Melanoma
    c. Medulloblastoma
    d. Hygroma

17. A patient in the ER is noted to have right upper quadrant tenderness, a temperature of 102.1 °F, and jaundice. This patient most likely has which one of the following conditions?

    a. Acute cholangitis
    b. Acute appendicitis
    c. Choledocholithiasis
    d. Acute pyelonephritis

18. You have been evaluating a young woman in the office for amenorrhea of 8 weeks' duration. Her urine pregnancy test is positive. During the pelvic examination, you notice a bluish discoloration on the vaginal mucosa. Based on her lab findings and physical examination, this bluish discoloration is called:

    a. Levine sign
    b. Kernig sign
    c. Chadwick sign
    d. Obturator sign

19. A 58-year-old male comes to the ER with a painful, red, swollen big toe. He has a known history of gout. Based on his past medical history and your examination findings, your first-line treatment would be:

    a. Colchicine
    b. Zyloprim
    c. Tetracycline
    d. Amantadine

20. You suspect a patient has benign positional vertigo. Which of the following may help aid in your diagnosis?

    a. Dix-Hallpike test
    b. Electroencephalogram (EEG)
    c. Transcranial Doppler ultrasound (TCD)
    d. Phalen maneuver

21. A 10-year-old child is brought to your office. On physical examination, she is short in stature and has a short, wide neck, broad forehead and tongue, and small ears. She has a medical history of mild cognitive and cardiac defects. Which of the following chromosomal defects is most likely the cause for her condition?

    a. 13
    b. 21
    c. 23
    d. 24

22. A patient comes to the ER complaining of pain with inspiration, fever, and palpitations. He recently underwent a coronary artery bypass graft 2 weeks prior. A cardiology consult is called. The cardiologist tells you he noted "electrical alternans" on your patient's electrocardiogram (ECG). Based on the medical history and ECG findings, you diagnose the patient with:

    a. Pericardial tamponade
    b. Myocardial infarction
    c. Pneumothorax
    d. Heart murmur

23. A patient comes into the ER complaining of dull, constant, left-sided chest pain for the previous 6 hours. He is diagnosed with an inferior-wall myocardial infarction (MI). What do you expect the electrocardiogram (ECG) and troponin levels to show?

    a. ST depression in leads V1 through V6 and normal troponin
    b. ST elevation in leads I, aVL, V5, and V6 and elevated troponin
    c. ST elevation in leads II, III, and aVF and elevated troponin
    d. ST depression in leads V7, V8, and V9 and normal troponin

24. You are evaluating a 72-year-old man in the ER for dizziness and syncope. An electrocardiogram (ECG) shows an increasingly prolonged PR interval on consecutive beats followed by a dropped QRS complex. Based on the ECG findings, you are most likely to suspect what type of heart block?

    a. First-degree heart block
    b. Second-degree heart block
    c. Third-degree heart block
    d. Asystole

25. Management of asymptomatic sinus bradycardia may include:

    a. Continuous telemetry monitoring
    b. Atropine
    c. Epinephrine
    d. Transcutaneous pacing

26. Which of the following is NOT a characteristic of the Beck triad?

    a. Distended jugular veins
    b. Hypotension
    c. Muffled heart sounds
    d. Hypertension

27. All of the following may commonly trigger an asthma attack EXCEPT:

    a. Sinusitis
    b. Allergies
    c. Warm air
    d. Smoke

28. Which of the following cells release insulin?

    a. Alpha cells
    b. Beta cells
    c. Gamma cells (PP cells)
    d. Delta cells

29. Which of the following is NOT a complication of diabetes mellitus?

a.   Atherosclerosis
b.   Renal insufficiency
c.   Neuropathy
d.   Hypotension

30. All of the following combinations of medication are used to treat *Helicobacter pylori* (*H. pylori*) infections EXCEPT:

a.   Clarithromycin, metronidazole, esomeprazole
b.   Amoxicillin, omeprazole, clarithromycin
c.   Omeprazole, metronidazole, tetracycline, bismuth
d.   Pantoprazole, esomeprazole, clarithromycin

31. All of the following are true about peptic ulcers EXCEPT:

a.   Obesity is a major risk factor.
b.   They are commonly caused by *H. pylori.*
c.   They can be diagnosed with a stool antigen test.
d.   Symptoms are exacerbated by the use of nonsteroidal anti-inflammatory drugs (NSAIDs).

32. In Parkinson disease, the deterioration of which neurotransmitter is primarily responsible for its symptoms?

a.   Norepinephrine
b.   Epinephrine
c.   Serotonin
d.   Dopamine

33. A patient presents to the dermatology office for evaluation of a persistent rash. The lesions vary in size. They are vesicular with erythematous bases. A sample is taken and sent to the lab. The Tzanck smear reveals multinucleated giant cells. What is the most likely diagnosis?

a.   Staphylococcus
b.   Herpes simplex
c.   *Trichophyton*
d.   Molluscum contagiosum

34. Which of the following is most likely associated with left bundle branch block?

a.   Pulmonary embolus
b.   Mitral valve prolapse
c.   Severe aortic valve disease
d.   Pericardial tamponade

35. A 26-year-old female is hospitalized for sickle cell crisis. Upon admission, she was also found to have a right-lower extremity deep venous thrombus. While examining the patient, you notice that her oxygen saturation on room air drops to 89%, her heart rate is 122, and her respirations are 35 breaths per minute. She is short of breath and complaining of chest pain. Her arterial blood gas (ABG) is normal, and her electrocardiogram (ECG) shows sinus tachycardia. After administering supplemental oxygen, what is your next course of action?

a.   Order a troponin level and wait for the results
b.   Order a computed tomography (CT) angiogram of the chest
c.   Order a CT of the chest without contrast
d.   Repeat the ABG in 1 hour

36. A 32-year-old male with a known history of tobacco abuse presents to the ER with shortness of breath and chest pain on the right side. The patient's vitals are as follows: temperature 98.6; BP 116/78; HR 102; RR 20; oxygen saturation 99% on room air. His chest x-ray is negative. A CT of his chest shows a right-sided pneumothorax that measures approximately 5%. Which of the following is the most appropriate intervention?

   a. Chest tube
   b. Needle decompression
   c. Bronchoscopy
   d. Serial chest x-rays

37. Which of the following is the most common congenital heart defect?

   a. Ventricular septal defect
   b. Tricuspid atresia
   c. Aortic stenosis
   d. Tetralogy of Fallot

38. What is the most common side effect seen with the use of angiotensin-converting enzyme (ACE) inhibitors?

   a. Liver failure
   b. Hypotension
   c. Erectile dysfunction
   d. Cough

39. Which of the following is a Gram-positive coccus and is frequently the cause of common skin infections and abscesses?

   a. *Haemophilus influenzae*
   b. *Streptococcus pneumoniae*
   c. *Staphylococcus aureus*
   d. *Staphylococcus pseudintermedius*

40. Which of the following is a treatment for Addison disease?

   a. Insulin
   b. Somatropin
   c. Synthroid
   d. Cortisol

41. A patient with a known history of medical noncompliance and chronic obstructive pulmonary disease (COPD) presents with unintentional weight gain over the past week, shortness of breath, and lower-extremity swelling. What laboratory test would be the most useful for this patient's suspected diagnosis?

   a. Alkaline phosphatase
   b. B-type natriuretic peptide
   c. Creatine phosphokinase
   d. Serum sodium

42. A patient is admitted to the hospital with an acute subdural hematoma. The patient has no past medical history. The following day, that patient's serum sodium is 156. The urine specific gravity is <1.005. The patient's Glasgow Coma Scale (GCS) score is 12, so it is difficult to assess his complaints. No change in mental status has been noted. What is the most appropriate treatment for this condition?
   a. Valproic acid
   b. Dexamethasone
   c. Desmopressin
   d. Tolterodine

43. Which of the following is true regarding sickle cell anemia?
   a. It is an autosomal-dominant disease
   b. Heterozygotes are usually asymptomatic
   c. It is due to a defective chromosome 18
   d. It increases the risk of diabetes

44. A 41-year-old female presents to the office with dysuria, frequency, urgency, and lower abdominal discomfort. She denies having fever, chills, back pain, vaginal discharge, nausea, or vomiting. She is in a monogamous relationship and has no history of sexually transmitted diseases. A urine pregnancy test is negative. The urinalysis is positive for leukocytes, bacteria, and nitrites. She has no drug allergies and has not had any antibiotics in the last 3 months. What is the next step in your medical management?
   a. Prescribe ceftriaxone 250 mg IM × 1 dose AND azithromycin 1 g PO × 1 dose
   b. Prescribe ciprofloxacin 500 mg PO BID × 7 days
   c. Prescribe amoxicillin/clavulanic acid 875 mg PO BID × 7 days
   d. Prescribe nitrofurantoin monohydrate/macrocrystals 100 mg PO BID × 5-7 days

45. A 27-year-old patient who is 17 weeks pregnant is symptomatic and diagnosed with a urinary tract infection. She has no drug allergies and has not had antibiotics in the last 3 months. What would be your first-choice antibiotic?
   a. Macrobid
   b. Bactrim
   c. Ciprofloxacin
   d. Moxifloxacin

46. A 26-year-old female is seen in your office and diagnosed with chlamydia. This is her fifth sexually transmitted disease in 2 years. Which of the following interventions is NOT appropriate?
   a. Advise her to avoid telling her partners; they may shun her if they know
   b. Counsel her on the use of condoms and other safe-sex measures
   c. Treat her with ceftriaxone and azithromycin
   d. Order a pregnancy test

47. A 3-year-old male child is brought to the ER for persistent coughing. Prior to the coughing episode, the child had been seen playing with a toy car. The toy car cannot be found. The patient's vitals are as follows: BP 100/55; HR 96; RR 22; oxygen saturation 90% on room air. No object is visible in the child's oropharynx. His breath sounds are diminished on the right. The child is able to speak, but with difficulty. After administering supplemental oxygen, which of the following is the most appropriate next step?
   a. Order a CT of the chest
   b. Perform a finger sweep to attempt to remove the object
   c. Administer nebulizer treatment
   d. Order a pulmonary consult for bronchoscopy

48. A patient recently diagnosed and treated for a urinary tract infection (UTI) by her primary care doctor now presents to the ER with bright-orange urine of 2 days' duration. Her UTI symptoms are improved. She cannot recall the medications she was prescribed, but she notes that her symptoms started after taking the medications. She denies allergies to medications, recent travel, or eating new food. Which of the following is most likely the cause for her symptom?

    a. Pilocarpine
    b. Percodan
    c. Pepcid
    d. Pyridium

49. A woman comes to your clinic for advice on how to help prevent kidney stones. Which of the following is the best advice?

    a. Increase fluid intake, increase carbohydrate intake
    b. Decrease fluid intake, increase calcium intake
    c. Increase fluid intake, limit oxalate intake
    d. Decrease fluid intake, decrease protein intake

50. A 32-year-old woman comes to your office complaining of a several-week history of unexplained sadness and anxiety. She no longer enjoys engaging in her extracurricular activities. She denies traumatic events, phobia, hallucinations, or suicidal ideation. She has no significant past medical history. She's never had these symptoms before. Which of the following medications may be beneficial for your patient?

    a. Levothyroxine
    b. Escitalopram
    c. Amiodarone
    d. Haloperidol

51. Which of the following findings indicates COPD rather than an asthma exacerbation?

    a. Declining forced expiratory volume in 1 second (FEV1)
    b. Partial pressure of arterial oxygen (PaO_2) of 70 mmHg
    c. Focal atelectasis on chest x-ray
    d. Expiratory wheezes

52. A 52-year-old male is brought to the ER after falling 10 feet from a ladder and landing on his buttocks. He notes mild pain but has the feeling of "pins and needles" going down both of his lower extremities. He is also complaining of feeling like he has to urinate but is not able to do so. On physical examination, he has decreased lower extremity reflexes, decreased motor strength, and decreased rectal tone. What is the most likely diagnosis?

    a. Fibromyalgia
    b. Greenstick fracture
    c. Cauda equina syndrome
    d. Kyphosis

53. A 13-year-old child is brought to your office complaining of a several-week history of left hip and knee pain. His parent notices that he has been walking with a progressive limp. The child denies trauma or strenuous activity. He has no significant medical problems. On physical examination, you notice that his left leg is slightly shorter than his right. His joints are not swollen or painful. What is the most likely diagnosis?

    a. Developmental dysplasia of the hip
    b. Paget disease
    c. Slipped capital femoral epiphysis
    d. Osteitis pubis

54. A 66-year-old patient presents to your clinic with progressive bowing of her left femur and tibia as well as pelvis for several months. She notes that she has had two spontaneous leg fractures in the past 4 months. Her only medical issues are diabetes and gout; she is compliant with her medication regimens. On physical examination, she has notable pelvic enlargement on the left side only. She has bowing of the left leg. Her joints are painful, but they are not red or swollen. Her blood work shows that her serum alkaline phosphatase is elevated. Her computed tomography (CT) scan shows multiple bony deformities on her pelvis and left leg. Based on her lab findings and medical history, which of the following medications would NOT be helpful in treating this patient?

    a. Nonsteroidal anti-inflammatory drugs (NSAIDs)
    b. Calcitonin
    c. Fosamax
    d. Colchicine

55. A 55-year-old female presents to the ER with painless vision loss from her right eye of 30 minutes' duration. She denies photophobia, headache, nausea, vomiting, visual disturbances prior to the vision loss, trauma, or periorbital pain. She has a known history of uncontrolled hypertension and transient ischemic attacks. What is the most likely diagnosis?

    a. Acute angle-closure glaucoma
    b. Retinal artery occlusion
    c. Conjunctivitis
    d. Retinal detachment

56. A 72-year-old female with a history of Parkinson disease and congestive heart failure complains of light-headedness, dizziness, and headache for the past several weeks. Her complete blood count, iron studies, complete metabolic panel, thyroid function tests, electrocardiogram, and urinalysis are unremarkable. A CT scan of the brain shows no acute findings. The nurse calls later that day to report that the patient complained of dizziness again today when working with physical therapy to ambulate in her room. Prior to physical therapy, her vital signs were as follows: BP 148/76; HR 70; RR 12; temperature 98.7; and oxygen saturation 100% on room air while supine. Her second set of vitals, taken while sitting up on the side of the bed, are BP 112/50; HR 90; RR 12; temperature 98.7; and oxygen saturation 100% on room air. Which of the following is the most appropriate treatment?

    a. Prescribe diltiazem
    b. Prescribe metoprolol
    c. Prescribe digoxin
    d. Prescribe midodrine

57. A patient is brought to the ER and is diagnosed with cauda equina syndrome. Which of the following is the most likely complication of this condition if treatment is delayed?

    a. Blindness
    b. Hemiparesis
    c. Amputation of the affected extremity
    d. Bladder dysfunction

58. A 12-year-old child comes to the office with right-sided ear pain, purulent otorrhea, and a fever of 100.5 °F. Her father notes that she just returned from a beach vacation, where she spent the majority of her time in the ocean. On physical examination, palpation of her tragus produces pain. Based on her medical history and physical examination, what is your next step?

    a. Stat ear, nose, and throat (ENT) consult
    b. Ofloxacin eardrops
    c. Clindamycin PO
    d. Computed tomography (CT) scan

59. A 64-year-old male is brought to the ER after a motor vehicle accident. He denies head trauma, loss of consciousness, or airbag deployment. His Glasgow Coma Scale (GCS) score is 15. He has a history of atrial fibrillation and takes warfarin. CT scan of his head reveals a 5 mm collection of cerebrospinal fluid (CSF), without blood, located under the dural membrane. Which of the following is the most appropriate treatment for this condition?

    a. Order an MRI of the brain.
    b. No intervention is warranted.
    c. Order an electroencephalogram.
    d. Administer phenytoin.

60. A 33-year-old female presents to the OB-GYN office following her third miscarriage. Her first miscarriage occurred at 13 weeks, her second occurred at 10 weeks, and her last miscarriage occurred at 18 weeks. Other than recurrent spontaneous abortions, she has no medical problems and has no toxic habits. A transabdominal ultrasound is unremarkable. Which of the following is the most likely etiology for her miscarriages?

    a. Leiomyoma
    b. Ectopic pregnancy
    c. Advanced maternal age
    d. Cervical insufficiency

61. A 24-year-old female patient presents to the ER with weakness and paresthesias that started in her legs and progressed to her upper body. Her mother brought her to the ER after she developed dysphagia and dysarthria. The mother notes that her daughter had a viral upper respiratory infection a few weeks prior but is otherwise healthy. The patient's vitals are as follows: temperature 98.6; BP 120/70; HR 82; RR 16; oxygen saturation 92% on room air. A complete metabolic panel, complete blood count, and urinalysis are unremarkable. Blood cultures are drawn and sent to the lab; preliminarily, they are negative. A CT scan of the brain and spine is unremarkable. Which of the following is the least appropriate intervention for this patient's condition?

    a. Plasmapheresis
    b. Intubation
    c. Immunoglobulin therapy
    d. Lumbar puncture

62. A patient comes to your clinic, concerned because his brother has just been diagnosed with type 2 diabetes. His father and paternal grandmother were also diabetics. His fasting blood sugar is 98, and his hemoglobin A1C is 5.2. What is the next step in the management of this patient?

    a. Recheck his hemoglobin A1C in a week
    b. Recommend a low-sugar diet and exercise
    c. Start insulin glargine and metformin
    d. Start metformin only

63. A 35-year-old Caucasian woman comes to your office for her annual wellness visit. Her examination and vital signs are normal. She has no significant past medical history. She states that her father was diagnosed with colon cancer when he was 48 years old. At what time should this patient get her first colonoscopy?

    a. This year
    b. At 38 years old
    c. At 48 years old
    d. At 50 years old

64. A mother brings her unvaccinated child to the ER with a deep whooping cough. The child is diagnosed with pertussis. Which medication can you prescribe to the mother to help prevent the further spread of pertussis?

    a. Augmentin
    b. Clindamycin
    c. Erythromycin
    d. Guaifenesin

65. A father brings in his 3-year-old son to the ER with a cough, runny nose, and a fever of 100.5 °F. The child attends day care. He has no other significant past medical history. On physical examination, he is noted to have a cough, clear rhinorrhea, and mild wheezing bilaterally. He is not in any acute respiratory distress. Based on his physical examination and medical history, what is the most likely diagnosis?

    a. Pneumonia
    b. Cystic fibrosis (CF)
    c. Respiratory syncytial virus (RSV)
    d. Asthma

66. A patient undergoes a mechanical mitral valve replacement and is placed on warfarin 5 mg postoperatively. Today is postoperative day 4, and this morning his INR is 3.0. Which of the following is the most appropriate intervention?

    a. Hold warfarin today, recheck tomorrow
    b. Order a heparin infusion bolus
    c. Order vitamin K
    d. Continue current warfarin dose

67. Parents bring their 3-month-old son to the pediatrician's office for a routine wellness visit. The parents state that the child is developing well, thriving on breast milk, and meeting his milestones. During the physical exam, several 2-4 cm, flat, blue-gray areas of discoloration on his buttocks and lumbar spine are noted. Per the child's medical record, these lesions were present at birth. Which of the following is the most appropriate treatment for this condition?

    a. Refer to a neurologist.
    b. Call child protective services.
    c. Refer to a dermatologist.
    d. No intervention is warranted.

68. A 19-year-old patient comes to your clinic complaining of recurrent nasal congestion. She states that her primary care doctor gave her a nasal spray. It helped her symptoms for the first 3 days. She continued to use it for another 4 days, and the nasal congestion reoccurred. Which of the following medications are most likely to blame for her symptoms?

    a. Oxymetazoline hydrochloride
    b. Benzonatate
    c. Ofloxacin
    d. Guaifenesin

69. A 58-year-old white male patient comes to your office concerned because he has a family history of heart disease and would like to be worked up. His father and older brother died of heart attacks. This patient's fasting total cholesterol is 205, LDL-C is 165, and HDL is 44. His weight, vital signs, fasting glucose, stress test, two-dimensional echocardiogram, and electrocardiogram (ECG) are normal. He has no significant past medical history. What medications would you recommend for this patient?

   a. A baby aspirin and amlodipine
   b. Amlodipine and simvastatin
   c. A baby aspirin and metoprolol
   d. A baby aspirin and simvastatin

70. A mother brings her 1-month-old son into your office for evaluation. He has had poor weight gain, even though he seems to be constantly hungry. She states that the child has an episode of projectile vomiting after almost every feeding. You notice that the child's abdomen is distended, and you palpate an olive-shaped mass in the epigastrium. Based on the medical history and physical examination, what is the most likely diagnosis?

   a. Gastroesophageal reflux disease (GERD)
   b. Gastritis
   c. Pyloric stenosis
   d. Mallory-Weiss tear

71. A 69-year-old male with a history of alcohol abuse comes to the ER after having an episode of hematemesis following binge drinking. Recently he's also been noticing black, tarry stools. He states that he's vomited blood on several occasions, but these episodes have been becoming more frequent. He denies unintentional weight loss or gain, abdominal pain, diarrhea, fever, recent illness, history of bleeding disorders, or lymphadenopathy. His stool guaiac is positive. His physical examination is normal. He currently feels fine. Based on his medical history and physical examination, what is the most likely diagnosis?

   a. Celiac sprue
   b. Whipple disease
   c. Mallory-Weiss tear
   d. Pyloric stenosis

72. A mother brings her toddler to the pediatrician's office for an evaluation. The mother notes that the child's right eye deviates toward her nose. The child has had this condition since she was an infant. Her pupils are equal and reactive. The red reflex test is unremarkable. Which of the following is the most likely complication if treatment is delayed?

   a. Blindness
   b. Depth-perception difficulty
   c. Chronic eye infections
   d. Inability to differentiate colors

73. A 27-year-old female presents to the primary care office for a follow-up visit. She has been complaining of worsening pain and swelling of the knees, elbows, and hips for several months. There is no history of trauma. She has no significant past medical history. Her vital signs are unremarkable. Her laboratory test findings are as follows: Na 136; K 4.9; BUN 35; Cr 1.4; glucose 128. Her urinalysis is positive for trace proteinuria. The enzyme-linked immunosorbent assay (ELISA) test result is positive for antinuclear antibodies. X-rays of the knees, elbows, and hips are normal. She complains of fatigue and has recently lost 10 pounds unintentionally. She has a malar rash, hypertension, and pleural friction rub on assessment. What is the most likely diagnosis?

    a.   Systemic lupus erythematosus
    b.   Scleroderma
    c.   Polymyositis
    d.   Guillain-Barré syndrome

74. A 6-year-old patient comes to the ER and is diagnosed with bacterial conjunctivitis. She has no past medical history and is up-to-date on all of her vaccinations. What is the next step in your medical management?

    a.   Trimethoprim/polymyxin B ophthalmic
    b.   Trifluridine ophthalmic
    c.   Erythromycin ophthalmic ointment
    d.   Famciclovir

75. A 68-year-old female newly diagnosed with hyperlipidemia comes to the ER after she noticed her entire body turning a reddish color and associated mild itching. She was just started on a new medication for her high cholesterol last week, but she cannot remember the name. She denies recent travel, new soaps or detergents, new foods, chest pain, shortness of breath, or palpitations. Other than her generalized flushing and pruritus, her physical examination seems normal. What medication has most likely caused her symptoms?

    a.   Atorvastatin
    b.   Rosuvastatin
    c.   Simvastatin
    d.   Niacin

76. A 58-year-old man presents to the ER with a temperature of 101.5 °F, productive cough with yellow sputum, shaking chills, and mild dyspnea for the past 2 days. His oxygen saturation is 98% on room air. A chest x-ray shows an infiltrate on the lower left lobe. He has no significant past medical history. What is the next step in your medical management?

    a.   Start PO antibiotics and discharge home
    b.   Order a computed tomography (CT) scan of the chest
    c.   Admit to the hospital and start intravenous (IV) antibiotics
    d.   Obtain an arterial blood gas (ABG) test

77. A patient with hyperlipidemia whom you have recently placed on niacin develops mild generalized flushing and pruritus. What would NOT be the next step in your medical management?

    a.   Discontinue the medication immediately.
    b.   Continue the medication and adjust the dosage.
    c.   Give Decadron and Benadryl for symptomatic relief.
    d.   Have the patient take nonsteroidal anti-inflammatory drugs (NSAIDs) prior to niacin dose.

78. A patient arrives in the ER complaining of right-sided abdominal pain. When the PA palpates the patient's right upper quadrant and asks him to inhale, he experiences severe pain. The rest of the physical exam is unremarkable. The patient's vital signs are as follows: temperature 98.9; HR 65; BP 130/76; RR 18; oxygen saturation100% on room air. Which of the following is the most likely diagnosis?

   a. Appendicitis
   b. Cholecystitis
   c. Pyelonephritis
   d. Cholangitis

79. A 14-year-old female patient is brought to the office by her parents complaining of heavy menses, easy bruising, and recurrent nosebleeds. Her mother notes that she had similar but milder symptoms when she was a child. Her hemoglobin level is 9.8. What is the most likely diagnosis?

   a. Von Willebrand disease
   b. Multiple myeloma
   c. Hemophilia
   d. Factor V Leiden

80. A patient presents with a 20-pound unintentional weight loss over the past few months, fatigue, myalgias, nausea, and vomiting. Her complete blood count results are normal. Her remarkable laboratory test values are as follows: Na 128 and K 5.6. While examining the patient, hyperpigmentation of the skin is noted. The patient's vitals are as follows: BP 90/54; HR 86; RR 18; temperature 98.7; oxygen saturation 98% on room air. What laboratory test would be the most useful for this patient's suspected diagnosis?

   a. Lactate
   b. Urine metanephrines
   c. Thyroid-stimulating hormone
   d. Cortisol

81. What is the most effective way to prevent the spread of communicable diseases?

   a. Maintaining a sterile environment
   b. Wearing gloves
   c. Hand washing
   d. Wearing a face mask while working with sick patients

82. A 20-year-old female presents to the ER with worsening left-sided abdominal pain radiating to the back, fever, shaking chills, nausea, and bilious vomiting for the past 3 days. The patient's vitals are as follows: HR 105; RR 20; temperature 100.8; oxygen saturation 99% on room air. On physical exam, she has left epigastric pain with moderate left-sided costovertebral angle tenderness. Her urinalysis is positive for red blood cells only. Her pregnancy test is negative. Her complete blood count is normal except for a white blood cell level of 11.5 without bandemia. The basic metabolic panel, amylase, lipase, and liver function tests are normal. Which of the following is the most appropriate initial diagnostic study?

   a. CT scan of the abdomen and pelvis without contrast
   b. Hepatobiliary iminodiacetic acid scan
   c. Endoscopic retrograde cholangiopancreatography
   d. Obstruction series x-ray

83. **What is the most effective way to prevent rabies infection?**
    a. Immediately obtaining the rabies vaccine
    b. Immediately cleansing the wound
    c. Administering PO Augmentin
    d. Administering IV clindamycin

84. **Which of the following is NOT a way to treat scabies?**
    a. Lotrimin cream
    b. Permethrin cream
    c. Washing linens and clothing in hot water
    d. Avoiding contact with infected people

85. **A woman who is 24 weeks pregnant presents to the office with complaints of nausea, bilious vomiting, non-bloody diarrhea, and fatigue for the past 2 weeks. She has no significant past medical history. She reports going to a picnic about 3 weeks ago and having pasteurized fruit juice, hot dogs, corn, and grilled salmon. Which of the following puts the patient most at risk for listeriosis?**
    a. Fruit juice
    b. Hot dogs
    c. Corn
    d. Salmon

86. **Which of the following is the least likely to cause a cardiac arrest?**
    a. Hyperkalemia
    b. Hypervolemia
    c. Hypokalemia
    d. Hypovolemia

87. **A 19-year-old female presents to the primary care clinic with worsening fatigue, unintentional weight gain, irregular menses, and constipation. The patient's vitals are as follows: BP 102/60; HR 52; RR 12; temperature 98.2; O_2 98% on room air. Her physical exam is generally unremarkable except for a nontender enlarged thyroid gland. Her complete blood count, comprehensive metabolic panel, and urinalysis are unremarkable. A urine pregnancy test is negative. Her thyroid-stimulating hormone (TSH) level is 6.9 mIU/L (the normal range is 0.5-4.0 mIU/L). Her free thyroxine level is 0.12 ng/dL (the normal range is 0.70-1.9 ng/dL). Which of the following is the most appropriate treatment?**
    a. Levothyroxine
    b. Methimazole
    c. Propylthiouracil
    d. Methylprednisolone

88. **A 19-year-old female presents to the ER for a 2-day history of nausea, vomiting, photophobia, and generalized headache. There is no history of trauma. The woman has no significant past medical history. The patient's vitals are as follows: BP 146/88; HR 98; RR 22; temperature 101.8; oxygen saturation 99% on room air. Her complete metabolic panel and complete blood count are unremarkable. Her Glasgow Coma Scale (GCS) score is 13. During physical exam, she flexes her hip and knee with passive flexion of her neck. What is the most appropriate next step?**
    a. Obtain an MRI of the cervical spine.
    b. Initiate hypertonic saline solution.
    c. Send blood cultures.
    d. Perform a lumbar puncture.

89. An 82-year-old male is referred to a gastroenterology office complaining of weight loss, fatigue, abdominal pain, and constipation of several weeks' duration. He has a remote history of tobacco abuse and hypertension that is well controlled with medications. CT scan of the abdomen and pelvis reveals an "apple-core" lesion in the proximal transverse colon. Which of the following is the most appropriate next step?

 a. Sigmoidoscopy
 b. Referral to oncology
 c. Barium enema
 d. Colonoscopy

90. A patient's electrocardiogram (ECG) shows a prolonged PR interval that regularly precedes a QRS complex. The PR interval remains unchanged. What is the most likely diagnosis based on the ECG findings?

 a. First-degree heart block
 b. Second-degree heart block (Mobitz type I)
 c. Second-degree heart block (Mobitz type II)
 d. Third-degree heart block

91. A 28-year-old male came to the office 2 weeks prior. He was diagnosed with an upper respiratory infection, prescribed antibiotics, and advised to follow up in 2 weeks. At the follow-up appointment, the patient reports intermittent dizziness, nausea, tinnitus, and hearing loss. His hearing loss is temporary and then returns to baseline. He notes that although these symptoms are persistent, they are starting to improve. What is the most likely diagnosis?

 a. Labyrinthitis
 b. Ménière disease
 c. Benign positional vertigo
 d. Acoustic neuroma

92. A 28-year-old male patient is brought to your clinic by his brother, who states that the patient's behavior is becoming increasingly erratic. He has intermittent episodes of agitation. The patient has been stating that he has been seeing and talking to his father, even though his father passed away five years ago. The patient has also been having trouble concentrating and often skips through several different topics in a few minutes during a conversation. The patient confides in you that his brother is "part of a conspiracy to lock me away." The patient's labs are all normal, and so are his vital signs. His physical examination is normal as well. A computed tomography (CT) scan of the brain shows no acute abnormalities. Based on his medical history, physical examination, and labs, what is the next step in your management?

 a. Start haloperidol and refer to psychiatry
 b. Start paroxetine and refer to psychiatry
 c. Start escitalopram and refer to psychiatry
 d. Start zolpidem and refer to psychiatry

93. A 58-year-old female is being evaluated by the OB-GYN PA-C in the clinic for mild intermittent vaginal bleeding. She underwent menopause about 10 years prior. The patient's only past medical history is diabetes, which is controlled with metformin and diet. She denies abdominal pain or distension, changes in appetite or weight, dysuria, fever, and back pain. A urinalysis is negative except for blood. Her physical exam and vital signs are unremarkable. A transvaginal ultrasound reveals a right-sided ovarian cyst and thickened endometrial lining. What is the most likely etiology for this patient's symptoms?

    a. Fibroids
    b. Infection
    c. Ovarian cyst
    d. Malignancy

94. One of your pediatric patients has just been diagnosed with thalassemia major. The parents ask you what they can do to limit the severity of symptoms and improve their child's quality of life. What suggestions do you give them?

    a. Blood transfusions and iron supplements
    b. Limiting folate and iron intake
    c. Folate supplements and regular blood transfusions
    d. Avoiding nonsteroidal anti-inflammatory drugs (NSAIDs), legumes, and henna

95. An 18-year-old female presents to the OB-GYN office for a routine visit. She states that she has been noticing scant white vaginal discharge with a fishy odor for the past several days. She states that she has never been sexually active. Her urinalysis and urine pregnancy tests are negative. A swab is taken and sent to the lab. Clue cells are seen on the wet-mount slide. What is the most likely diagnosis?

    a. Bacterial vaginosis
    b. Trichomonas
    c. Vaginal candidiasis
    d. Chlamydia

96. A 35-year-old woman who is 6 weeks pregnant comes to the ER for mild vaginal bleeding and mild low-back pain. Her transvaginal ultrasound is negative for an intrauterine pregnancy. Her serum beta human chorionic gonadotropin (β-HCG) is normal. What is the next step in your medical management?

    a. Stat surgical consult for laparoscopy.
    b. Repeat her β-HCG and ultrasound in 2 days.
    c. Discharge home and recommend bed rest.
    d. Administer methotrexate.

97. A child has been recently diagnosed with impetigo. Which of the following recommendations would NOT prevent the spread of the infection?

    a. You may touch the skin lesions once antibiotics have been started.
    b. Wash hands thoroughly after touching the patient.
    c. Clean all clothes and bed linens in hot water.
    d. Do not share personal-care items with the patient.

98. A 13-year-old male patient is brought to the ER with sudden-onset unilateral testicular pain for the past 2 hours. The patient denies trauma. On physical exam, the right testicle is erythematous and exquisitely tender. There is a loss of the cremasteric reflex on the right. Which of the following is NOT a complication that may occur from delayed treatment?

    a. Malignancy
    b. Infertility
    c. Testicular infarction
    d. Testicular gangrene

99. A father brings his 13-year-old son to the ER. He states that the foreskin of his son's penis is "stuck." The penis is mildly swollen and erythematous. The testes are normal. Upon physical examination, you note that the foreskin cannot be reduced. The most likely diagnosis is:

a. Phimosis
b. Hydrocele
c. Paraphimosis
d. Peyronie disease

100. A 4-year-old boy is brought into the pediatrician's office by his mother, and he is complaining of sores inside his mouth for the past 3 days. He has no past medical history, and his vitals are normal. On physical exam, there are two ulcers inside of his lower lip that have a grayish-yellow base with an erythematous halo. Which of the following is the most appropriate next step?

a. No intervention is needed.
b. Prescribe oral antiviral medication.
c. Prescribe topical antibiotic cream.
d. Recommend an increase in vitamin C intake.

101. A 22-year-old male comes to your clinic with a painless mass on his right testicle of 2 weeks' duration. He denies trauma, lymphadenopathy, or prior infection. His complete blood count (CBC) and chemistry are normal. A physical examination reveals a soft, fluctuant, nontender mass. You shine a flashlight at the mass, which transmits light. Based on his medical history and physical examination, what is the most likely diagnosis?

a. Hydrocele
b. Testicular torsion
c. Varicocele
d. Cryptorchidism

102. A 21-year-old patient in the hospital for sickle cell crisis is newly diagnosed with a pulmonary embolus. She has no past medical history other than sickle cell disease. Which of the following would NOT be part of your medical management once the patient's oxygenation status is stabilized?

a. Consult surgery for an inferior vena cava (IVC) filter
b. Start heparin infusion.
c. Administer analgesics for the chest pain.
d. Repeat D-dimer in 1 week.

103. A 30-year-old patient in your clinic tells you that he seems to get the flu every year. Other than smoking half a pack of cigarettes per day for the past 5 years, he is healthy. He asks you how he can avoid contracting the flu this year. Which of the following is NOT part of your recommendations?

a. Wash hands frequently while at work or at a public venue.
b. Obtain the influenza vaccine in the fall.
c. Avoid the influenza vaccine because he is not in a high-risk group.
d. Decrease tobacco use.

104. All of the following medications will treat atrial fibrillation EXCEPT:

a. Digoxin
b. Furosemide
c. Metoprolol
d. Warfarin

105. A patient visits your office for his annual wellness examination. He tells you he recently became ill after visiting the southwest part of the United States. He had painful red lumps on his lower legs, blood-tinged sputum, loss of appetite, fever, night sweats, and headache. The symptoms spontaneously resolved on their own without treatment. A doctor who saw him in the ER while he was in the southwest said he had valley fever. The patient's vital signs and physical examination are normal. He has no past medical history. Based on his symptoms and medical history, what illness did your patient most likely have?

    a. *Pneumocystis* pneumonia
    b. Tuberculosis
    c. Respiratory syncytial virus (RSV)
    d. Coccidioidomycosis

106. Which of the following can make a definitive diagnosis of ventricular septal defect?

    a. Echocardiogram
    b. Chest x-ray
    c. Electrocardiogram (ECG)
    d. Auscultation with a stethoscope

107. A patient comes to the clinic complaining of persistent right eye irritation for 3 weeks. The conjunctiva is normal. There is no crusting of the lids or lashes. The patient's right lower lid is turned inward. The patient's vision is intact bilaterally. What is the most appropriate treatment for this patient's condition?

    a. Antibiotic drops
    b. Surgical correction
    c. Lubricating ointment
    d. No intervention is warranted

108. A 56-year-old female patient with a history of alcohol abuse presents to the ER with dizziness, chest pain, palpitations, and syncope. A cardiologist viewing her electrocardiogram (ECG) mentions that the QRS complex twists around the isoelectric baseline. What cardiac arrhythmia is the cardiologist most likely describing?

    a. Bundle branch block
    b. Sick sinus syndrome
    c. Torsades de pointes
    d. Atrial fibrillation

109. A 24-year-old woman presents to your clinic with persistent chest pain and shortness of breath, which commonly occur at rest. Exercise does not induce her symptoms. She has been to the ER several times with these symptoms. Her electrocardiogram (ECG), troponin level, chest x-ray, and two-dimensional echocardiogram are all normal. She had a prior cardiac catheterization 1 year ago, which was negative. Her physical examination is normal; palpation of her chest wall does not reproduce symptoms. She has no medical problems. She admits to smoking a pack of cigarettes a day for 5 years. What is the most likely diagnosis?

    a. Prinzmetal angina
    b. Unstable angina
    c. Stable angina
    d. Costochondritis

110. Which of the following can be the cause of syndrome of inappropriate antidiuretic hormone (SIADH)?
    a. Squamous-cell carcinoma
    b. Large-cell carcinoma
    c. Adenocarcinoma
    d. Small-cell carcinoma

111. A patient presents to the ER with suspected infective endocarditis. Which of the following tests would be the least helpful diagnostic aid?
    a. Computed tomography (CT) scan of the chest
    b. Echocardiogram
    c. Chest x-ray
    d. Blood cultures

112. A patient has come to your clinic for multiple visits over the past several weeks with a persistently borderline elevated blood pressure. Today it is 138/88. He has no family history of hypertension. He smokes less than half a pack of cigarettes per day, but otherwise he has no medical problems. Which of the following would be recommendations to help him lower his blood pressure without medications?
    a. Limit tobacco use, increase sodium intake, increase physical activity
    b. Decrease stress, increase tobacco use, increase physical activity
    c. Decrease sodium intake, increase physical activity, limit tobacco use
    d. Limit tobacco use, decrease sodium intake, decrease physical activity

113. A 30-year-old female patient comes to the ER complaining of swelling and pain in her fingers for the past several days. Her past medical history includes obesity, sarcoidosis, and herpes simplex type 2. Grouped vesicular lesions with surrounding erythema are noted at the second, third, and fourth distal phalanges. What is the most appropriate treatment for this condition?
    a. Incision and drainage
    b. Topical acyclovir
    c. Oral clindamycin
    d. MRI of the hand

114. A 61-year-old male walks into the ER with the sudden onset of dull, throbbing, left-sided chest pain radiating to his jaw and back, nausea, vomiting, and diaphoresis. An electrocardiogram (ECG) shows an inferior wall non-ST segment elevation myocardial infarction (NSTEMI). His vital signs are as follows: BP 165/98; HR 92; oxygen saturation 93% on room air; RR 26. The patient is awake and alert, but in moderate pain. After administering oxygen, which of the following would be the next step in your medical management?
    a. Order metoprolol, morphine, and clopidogrel
    b. Order aspirin, morphine, and nitroglycerin
    c. Order an echocardiogram and troponin level
    d. Order metoprolol, aspirin, and clopidogrel

115. A 68-year-old male comes to the ER after having an episode of left-sided chest pain radiating to his left arm for 10 minutes. He was mowing his lawn when the chest pain occurred. It resolved about 5 minutes after he sat down to rest. He states that he often gets similar symptoms during physical activity. The symptoms resolve with rest. He currently has no medical complaints. His past medical history includes hyperlipidemia and obesity. His physical examination is normal. His vital signs are as follows: BP 155/91; HR 88; oxygen saturation 98% on room air; RR 16. Based on his past medical history and physical examination, what is the most likely diagnosis?

- a. Stable angina
- b. Prinzmetal angina
- c. Unstable angina
- d. Aortic aneurysm

116. A 77-year-old female patient comes to your clinic complaining of worsening vision for the past month. She notes that the center of her vision has been deteriorating. It has become incredibly difficult for her to read. Her peripheral vision remains intact. She denies the presence of floaters or flashes of light, photophobia, headache, nausea, vomiting, or trauma. Her past medical history includes osteoarthritis and osteoporosis. She denies recent illness. What is the most likely diagnosis?

- a. Optic neuritis
- b. Macular degeneration
- c. Glaucoma
- d. Retinal artery occlusion

117. A 42-year-old female comes to the ER for right-sided tinnitus, worsening ataxia, right-sided hearing loss, dizziness, and a headache over the last month. She denies trauma or recent illness. She has no significant past medical history. The symptoms are not exacerbated or alleviated by motion. Her physical examination is normal. What is the next step in your medical management?

- a. Order an electromyography.
- b. Order an ear, nose, and throat (ENT) consult.
- c. Perform the Dix-Hallpike maneuver.
- d. Order a magnetic resonance imaging (MRI) scan of the brain.

118. A 56-year-old man with no significant past medical history presents to his primary care physician complaining of worsening toe pain. He denies trauma. He notes that he has had less severe attacks before, but they eventually resolved without treatment. His first toe is red, warm, and swollen with a limited range of motion. What is the most likely etiology for his complaint?

- a. Elevated uric acid levels
- b. Fungal infection
- c. Autoimmune destruction of the joints
- d. Peripheral venous insufficiency

119. A 76-year-old female comes to the ER with nonproductive cough, chest pain with inspiration, and shortness of breath of 2 days' duration. Her vital signs are as follows: BP 144/72; RR 25; HR 101; oxygen saturation 93% on room air. On physical examination, she has diminished breath sounds on the right side. She has dullness to percussion and decreased tactile fremitus on the right side. She has a known history of tobacco abuse and chronic obstructive pulmonary disease (COPD). Based on your physical examination, what is the most likely diagnosis?

- a. Asthma
- b. Pleural effusion
- c. Pneumothorax
- d. Influenza

120. A 27-year-old female with no past medical history other than obesity comes to the primary care clinic with worsening fatigue and frequent urination for the past several weeks. Her urinalysis is positive for glucose and yeast. Her vital signs are unremarkable. Which of the following is the most appropriate next step?

   a. Order ciprofloxacin and phenazopyridine.
   b. Order a urine culture and blood cultures.
   c. Order a repeat urinalysis in 2 weeks.
   d. Order a hemoglobin A1C.

121. A 10-year-old child is brought to the ER by his father for shortness of breath that started about an hour ago. The child has had these symptoms about twice a year, and they are well controlled with medication. The father states that the child uses a "puffer," but he cannot recall the name. The patient's vitals are as follows: HR 85; RR 20; temperature 98.2; O_2 92% on room air. A chest x-ray is unremarkable. Which of the following is the most appropriate treatment?

   a. Ipratropium bromide/albuterol sulfate (DuoNeb)
   b. Budesonide/formoterol (Symbicort)
   c. Fluticasone/salmeterol (Advair)
   d. Formoterol fumarate (Foradil)

122. A 65-year-old male comes to your office with worsening cough and dyspnea of 2 months' duration. He has no other medical problems. He states that he had worked in a coal mine for 30 years, but he has recently retired. On chest x-ray, his lungs show a honeycomb pattern. Based on your findings, what is the most likely diagnosis?

   a. Pneumoconiosis
   b. Schistosomiasis
   c. Coccidioidomycosis
   d. Tuberculosis

123. A 21-year-old male comes to your office after finding a hard, fixed, painless lump on his testicle. He's never had testicular lesions before. He has no past medical history. You shine a penlight at the lesion; it does not transmit light. Based on your physical examination, what is the most likely diagnosis?

   a. Hydrocele
   b. Testicular carcinoma
   c. Varicocele
   d. Testicular torsion

124. A 3-week-old neonate is brought to the pediatrician's office for an evaluation. The baby's parents note that the child has had constipation since birth, and when she does have a bowel movement, her stools are foul smelling and greasy. Chart review reveals that the child has had poor weight gain and growth. A sweat chloride test is positive. Which of the following is NOT a common complication of this condition?

   a. Pancreatitis
   b. Impaired fertility
   c. Diabetes mellitus
   d. Myocardial infarction

125. A mother brings her 6-year-old daughter to the ER for left-sided ear pain of 3 days' duration associated with mild hearing loss, swelling, and fever. She states that her daughter was recently treated for an inner ear infection 1 week prior. The child has no ataxia, vertigo, lymphadenopathy, tinnitus, nausea, or vomiting. Her temperature in the ER is 102.1 °F. On physical examination, you notice mild displacement of the ear caused by swelling of the posterior ear. Her tympanic membrane is erythematous. Based on her medical history and physical examination, what is the most likely diagnosis?

    a. Acoustic neuroma
    b. Cholesteatoma
    c. Mastoiditis
    d. Ménière disease

126. A 50-year-old AIDS patient presents with fever, headache, nausea, and vomiting. The patient's vitals are as follows: BP 163/85; HR 115; RR 24; temperature 102.5; oxygen saturation 97% on room air. His laboratory test values are as follows: white blood cell count 17.5 with 20% bands (the normal level is 0-8%); hemoglobin 16.2; hematocrit 40.1; platelet count 350,000. A basic metabolic panel is unremarkable. A lumbar puncture is performed, and cultures are sent to the laboratory. His India ink stain is positive. Which of the following is the most appropriate treatment?

    a. Vancomycin and piperacillin/tazobactam
    b. Azithromycin and Rocephin
    c. Amphotericin B and flucytosine
    d. Isoniazid and pyrazinamide

127. A 5-year-old child is brought to the ER by his father for an acute asthma exacerbation. Which of the following would NOT be a treatment of choice in an acute asthma exacerbation?

    a. Singulair
    b. Xopenex
    c. Ventolin
    d. Proventil

128. A mother brings her toddler into your office for a multitude of symptoms. Her daughter has been developing nausea, vomiting, fever, and abdominal pain for the past several weeks. During the child's physical examination, you notice that the child has a nontender abdominal mass. The patient also has no right iris (aniridia) and has unilateral swelling on one side of her body. The mother states that she has a family history of cancer, but she can't remember what kind. Based on the child's medical history and physical examination, what kind of tumor is most likely responsible for the child's symptoms?

    a. Hodgkin lymphoma
    b. Lipoma
    c. Wilms tumor
    d. Kaposi sarcoma

129. A mother gives birth to her baby at 28 weeks of gestation. Immediately after labor, the child goes into respiratory distress. No complications have occurred during the pregnancy prior to labor. The mother has no relevant past medical history. What is the most likely diagnosis for the child's respiratory symptoms?

    a. Respiratory syncytial virus (RSV)
    b. Hyaline membrane disease
    c. *Pneumocystis* pneumonia
    d. Pneumoconiosis

130. A 21-year-old male presents to the ER with right-sided eye pain after being involved in a physical altercation. His right conjunctiva has a medial well-circumscribed erythematous area. The extraocular muscles are intact, and the pupils are equal and reactive. He has no vision loss or periorbital swelling. Which of the following is the most appropriate next step?

    a. Administer ofloxacin eye drops.
    b. Obtain a CT scan of the facial bones.
    c. Measure intraocular pressures.
    d. Arrange for follow-up with an ophthalmologist as an outpatient.

131. You are examining a patient in the ER for acute alcohol intoxication. He is well known to the ER for his chronic alcoholism. During your physical examination, you notice that he has white patches on his tongue that cannot be scraped off. This condition is called:

    a. Leukoplakia
    b. Oral thrush
    c. Parotitis
    d. Gingivostomatitis

132. A cardiologist is examining the chest x-ray of a child with a known cyanotic heart defect. He mentions that the child has a "boot-shaped heart." What heart defect does the child most likely have?

    a. Ventricular septal defect
    b. Patent ductus arteriosus
    c. Atrial septal defect
    d. Tetralogy of Fallot

133. A patient presents to your office with various symptoms. Based on the patient's medical history and physical examination, you suspect sarcoidosis. Which of the following tests would you order to confirm the diagnosis?

    a. Computed tomography (CT) scan of the chest
    b. Bronchoscopy with biopsy
    c. Lumbar puncture
    d. Serum phosphorus

134. A 25-year-old female comes to the OB-GYN clinic concerned because she has been developing multiple painful breast lumps over the past several months. They vary in size during the month. On physical exam, there are multiple bilateral soft, tender breast masses. There is no erythema, overlying skin changes, nipple discharge, or lymphadenopathy. Her vital signs are unremarkable. Which of the following is the most appropriate next step?

    a. Schedule a mammogram.
    b. Order an α-fetoprotein level.
    c. Schedule an ultrasound of the breasts.
    d. Refer to an oncologist.

135. A 26-year-old patient has just been diagnosed with a fibroadenoma via biopsy. What is the next step in your medical management?

    a. Monitor for now; no further intervention is needed.
    b. Recommend birth control pills.
    c. Repeat biopsy in 2 months.
    d. Recommend surgical consultation for a mastectomy.

136. Which of the following is NOT a treatment for active tuberculosis?

    a. Clindamycin
    b. Amikacin
    c. Streptomycin
    d. Ethambutol

137. Which of the following remedies would NOT help alleviate the effects of barotrauma?

    a. Chew gum.
    b. Suck on candy.
    c. Yawn.
    d. Ascend quickly.

138. A father brings his 1-year-old daughter in for mild respiratory distress of 1 day's duration. Originally, her symptoms started out like a common cold, but then she developed a noisy, nonproductive cough and low-grade fever. On physical examination, you notice intercostal retractions. Her temperature is 100.5 °F; otherwise, her vitals are normal. Based on her medical history and physical examination, what is the most likely diagnosis?

    a. Hyaline membrane disease
    b. Bronchiolitis
    c. Tuberculosis
    d. Cystic fibrosis

139. Which of the following is a first-line treatment for Hashimoto thyroiditis?

    a. Lantus
    b. Levothyroxine
    c. Lanoxin
    d. Lamisil

140. A 45-year-old man with no history of medical problems has developed worsening, unpredictable mood changes and a decline in cognitive function. He has recently developed an ataxic gait and uncoordinated, jerky body movements. What is the most likely diagnosis?

    a. Tourette syndrome
    b. Guillain-Barré syndrome
    c. Cerebral palsy
    d. Huntington disease

141. A patient presents with myalgia, fatigue, and diffuse bony pain. Further workup reveals the presence of osteoporosis and nephrolithiasis. What is the most likely diagnosis?

    a. Hyperthyroidism
    b. Hypoparathyroidism
    c. Hyperparathyroidism
    d. Hypothyroidism

142. What is the first-line treatment for a scabies infection?

    a. Permethrin
    b. Olanzapine
    c. Phenergan
    d. Ondansetron

143. A patient who presented to the ER after a fall is being evaluated. The x-ray shows a bone fragment separated from the trapezium. What is the most likely diagnosis?

   a. Avulsion fracture
   b. Greenstick fracture
   c. Comminuted fracture
   d. Oblique fracture

144. A 25-year-old female is admitted to the hospital for fever of unknown origin. She is complaining of fever, chills, and diaphoresis. She has a known history of IV drug abuse. The patient's vitals are as follows: BP 102/50; HR 115; RR 22; temperature 103.2; oxygen saturation 98% on room air. The patient has bilateral retinal hemorrhages. She also has nontender, erythematous nodular lesions on the palms and soles that are a few millimeters in diameter. Which of the following is the most appropriate initial diagnostic study?

   a. CT scan of the brain
   b. Blood cultures
   c. Lumbar puncture
   d. Echocardiogram

145. Which of the following medications would you NOT use in a patient with restrictive cardiomyopathy?

   a. Furosemide
   b. Metoprolol
   c. Aspirin
   d. Epinephrine

146. A patient with *Clostridioides difficile* colitis has been experiencing worsening abdominal pain and fever. An abdominal x-ray shows colonic distension. What is the most likely diagnosis based on symptoms and x-ray findings?

   a. Ogilvie syndrome
   b. Toxic megacolon
   c. Intussusception
   d. Hirschsprung disease

147. A patient with a known history of alcoholism comes to the ER with left-sided abdominal pain associated with nausea and vomiting for 1 day after going binge drinking. He states that the pain is worst when lying down. The patient's vitals are as follows: BP 132/66; HR 92; RR 18; temperature 98.2; oxygen saturation 98% on room air. Which of the following is the most diagnostic test for this patient's likely condition?

   a. Lipase
   b. Total bilirubin
   c. Erythrocyte sedimentation rate
   d. Alkaline phosphatase

148. Family members bring a 61-year-old man to your office for the first time for a wellness checkup. As they are filling out paperwork, you notice that he has a resting tremor, slow movements, rigidity, and shuffling gait. What is the most likely diagnosis?

   a. Huntington disease
   b. Alzheimer dementia
   c. Parkinson disease
   d. Guillain-Barré syndrome

149. A 42-year-old female presents to her primary care physician complaining of unintentional weight gain and muscle weakness. She has a known history of asthma and systemic lupus erythematosus. Her medications include fluticasone, prednisone, naproxen, and albuterol. The patient has edematous facies, mild hirsutism, and multiple purple striae on her trunk and legs. Which of the following is the most appropriate test to help diagnose this condition?

a. Adrenocorticotropic hormone (ACTH) stimulation test
b. Ultrasound of the thyroid
c. Dexamethasone suppression test
d. Beta human chorionic gonadotropin

150. A 21-year-old female comes to the ER complaining of a blistering rash and facial swelling that started in the morning. She has never had this rash before. She has no significant past medical history. The only medication she is currently taking is penicillin for streptococcal pharyngitis. On physical examination, you notice a diffuse, dark reddish-purple papular rash on her trunk, face, and extremities with extensive blister formation. Her temperature is 99.9 °F; otherwise, her vitals are normal. Based on her medical history and physical examination, what is the most likely diagnosis?

a. Turner syndrome
b. Stevens-Johnson syndrome
c. Cushing syndrome
d. Guillain-Barré syndrome

151. A mother brings her 6-year-old son in for his annual wellness visit. The child has no past medical history. During the examination, his mother states that about 3 weeks ago, the child had a viral infection. Following the viral infection, she noticed pinpoint reddish-purple dots on his extremities that appeared and spontaneously disappeared. Currently, the child's examination and vital signs are normal. Based on his medical history and physical examination, what is the most likely diagnosis for what caused his dermal symptoms?

a. Immune thrombocytopenic purpura
b. Stevens-Johnson syndrome
c. Von Willebrand disease
d. Glucose-6-phosphate dehydrogenase (G6PD) deficiency

152. A couple brings their 3-year-old daughter to the ER for worsening cough, fever, and sore throat. The child has no past medical history; however, the parents admit that they did not have their daughter vaccinated. On physical examination, you notice that the child is slightly cyanotic. You also see a grayish-black, tough, fiber-like covering of her oropharynx. Based on her medical history and physical examination, what is the most likely diagnosis?

a. Cryptococcosis
b. Shigellosis
c. Cholera
d. Diphtheria

153. A mother brings her 16-year-old daughter to the ER complaining of fever, sore throat, lethargy, and swollen cervical lymph glands. The child's temperature is 100.1 °F; her other vital signs are normal. The child is mildly lethargic but easily aroused and does not appear to be dehydrated. Her physical examination is essentially normal other than her cervical lymphadenopathy. A monospot test is positive. What is the next step in your medical management?

a. Prescribe amantadine.
b. Prescribe Augmentin.
c. Recommend a computed tomography (CT) scan of the abdomen.
d. Recommend rest and fluids.

154. A 71-year-old male comes to your office with a history of multiple nontraumatic fractures over the past 6 months. Blood work reveals hypercalcemia and anemia, and his BUN/creatinine are 36/1.7. Urine studies reveal the presence of the Bence Jones protein. What is the most likely diagnosis?

    a. Acute myelogenous leukemia (AML)
    b. Multiple myeloma
    c. Acute lymphocytic leukemia (ALL)
    d. Paget disease

155. Which of the following would be the least helpful diagnostic test in diagnosing hemolytic anemia?

    a. International normalized ratio (INR)
    b. Coombs test, direct
    c. Complete blood count (CBC)
    d. Lactate dehydrogenase (LDH) test

156. An infant is born with microcephaly, deafness, chorioretinitis, hepatosplenomegaly, and thrombocytopenia. Which of the following diseases would NOT be a likely cause?

    a. Influenza
    b. Rubella
    c. Toxoplasmosis
    d. Cytomegalovirus

157. A 66-year-old female is brought to the ER for headache, anorexia, nausea, and worsening confusion for the past 3-4 days. A CT of the head without contrast is unremarkable. The patient's vital signs are as follows: BP 128/70; HR 66; RR 14; temperature 98.7; oxygen saturation 96% on room air. Her laboratory test values are as follows: Na 122; K 4.9; BUN 24; Cr 0.9; glucose 109. Her past medical history includes hypertension, hyperlipidemia, small-cell lung carcinoma, and tobacco abuse. Which of the following is the most appropriate treatment?

    a. Hydrochlorothiazide
    b. Mannitol IV
    c. Phenobarbital PO
    d. Fluid restriction

158. A 45-year-old patient comes to your clinic with an itchy, purplish rash on her wrists and ankles of 5 days' duration. She's had this rash before, but it usually resolves on its own. Other than the rash, she generally feels well. She has a history of hepatitis C. On physical examination, you notice that her vitals are normal. You note well-defined, pruritic, planar, purple, polygonal papules and plaques on her ankles and wrists. Based on her medical history and physical examination, what is the most likely diagnosis?

    a. Leukoplakia
    b. Impetigo
    c. Psoriasis
    d. Lichen planus

159. Which statement is true regarding Zika virus?

    a. Famciclovir is used to treat Zika virus.
    b. Zika virus can remain in semen longer than in other body fluids.
    c. Zika virus can only be passed during sexual activity if a person is symptomatic.
    d. Due to the small size of the virus, condoms do not decrease the risk of sexual transmission.

160. A 10-year-old patient has just been diagnosed with diabetes mellitus type 1. What is the first-line medication that you would prescribe?

    a. Metformin.
    b. Lantus
    c. Glimepiride
    d. Glyburide

161. A 58-year-old male with a known history of alcohol abuse is brought to the ER for altered mental status. He is oriented to person only, he is vomiting, he is diaphoretic, and you notice a fine tremor. His pupils are dilated, but they are briskly reactive. His vital signs are as follows: BP 166/89; RR 25; HR 119; oxygen saturation 95%. He states that he has not had a drink in 2 days. He denies drug abuse. Based on his medical history and physical examination, what is the most likely diagnosis?

    a. Delusional disorder
    b. Alcohol intoxication
    c. Alcohol withdrawal
    d. Persistent depressive disorder (dysthymia)

162. A mother brings her 12-year-old son to the pediatrician's office for a follow-up visit to evaluate persistent unilateral knee pain of 5 weeks' duration. The child denies any history of trauma. A prior knee x-ray taken in the ER is negative for injury to the bone. There is a painful bony bump just below the affected knee. There is no sign of infection. There is no joint laxity. The child has no other medical problems. Which of the following is the most appropriate next step?

    a. Supply crutches and avoid weight-bearing.
    b. Apply a splint to the knee.
    c. Recommend rest and NSAIDs.
    d. Order an MRI of the knee.

163. A patient is referred to the dermatology office for further evaluation of multiple skin lesions. On physical exam, the PA notes that the fair-skinned, light-eyed patient has multiple similar lesions on the face and upper chest. The lesions are 2-3 mm, symmetrical, pinkish-gray macules with a crusty surface. The patient has no significant past medical history. What is the most appropriate treatment for this condition?

    a. Use antifungal cream.
    b. Stay out of the sun.
    c. Use steroid cream.
    d. Wash all linens in hot water.

164. A patient presents to the ER with a hand laceration that occurred 3 days prior. The wound is clean and dry with no evidence of underlying infection. The date of his last tetanus shot is not known. After administering a tetanus shot, which of the following is the most appropriate next step?

    a. No intervention
    b. Suture repair
    c. Staple repair
    d. Dermabond

165. Patients with a known allergy to penicillin should NOT take which of the following classes of antibiotics?

    a. Sulfonamides
    b. Aminoglycosides
    c. Macrolides
    d. Cephalosporins

166. A 35-year-old woman comes to your office with a myriad of complaints. She has noticed fatigue, progressive ataxia, muscle spasms, dizziness, and difficulty with coordination of fine motor movements. She states that she has recently been diagnosed with optic neuritis. What is the most likely diagnosis?

a. Alzheimer disease
b. Meningitis
c. Multiple sclerosis
d. Huntington disease

167. A 30-year-old male with sickle cell disease comes to the ER with right foot pain, swelling, and fever for the past week. His vital signs are as follows: BP 140/76; HR 102; RR 22; temperature 102.4; oxygen saturation 98% on room air. His white blood cell count is 16.4 with 12% bands. His hemoglobin is 10.2, hematocrit is 35.5, and platelet count is 310,000. His erythrocyte sedimentation rate is 65 mm/hour (the normal range is <15 mm/hour). His C-reactive protein is 22 mg/dL (the normal range is <3.0 mg/dL). An MRI of the foot reveals lytic changes of the first and second metatarsals. What is the most likely etiology for the patient's suspected condition?

a. *Escherichia coli*
b. Salmonella
c. *Enterobacter*
d. *Haemophilus influenzae*

168. A 20-year-old patient presents to the ER with dry cough, runny nose, subjective fever, fatigue, and myalgias for the past 3 days. The patient's vitals are as follows: temperature 99.2; BP 110/76; HR 62; RR 16; oxygen saturation 100% on room air. Several people in his college dorm have similar complaints. His physical exam and complete blood count with differential are unremarkable. A monospot test is negative. His chest x-ray is unremarkable. Which of the following medications may be useful in shortening the course of this patient's suspected infection if it is given early enough?

a. Oseltamivir
b. Gentamicin
c. Famciclovir
d. Augmentin

169. A 13-year-old male patient is brought to the ER with sudden-onset unilateral testicular pain following a trauma that occurred 4 hours previously. What is the next step in your medical management?

a. Recommend warm compresses.
b. Stat surgery consult.
c. Order pain medication to see if it alleviates symptoms.
d. Order intravenous (IV) antibiotics.

170. A patient is admitted to the ICU with a traumatic head injury. Other than the head injury, the patient has no past medical history. The nurse calls you with the morning labs to let you know that the patient's serum sodium is 150 and the serum potassium is 3.2. The serum glucose and urine glucose are normal. The nurse notes that the patient's urine output has increased to over 300 mL per hour. The urine specific gravity is <1.005. The patient has been drinking profusely throughout the night, but she is still complaining of thirst. Based on the lab results and the patient's medical history, what is the most likely diagnosis?

a. Hypothyroidism
b. Diabetes mellitus
c. Hyperthyroidism
d. Diabetes insipidus

171. A 35-year-old female comes to your clinic complaining of a painful sore on her neck of several weeks' duration. It keeps changing in appearance. On physical examination, you notice an asymmetric 9 mm papule on the right side of the patient's neck that has mixed areas of brown, blue, and black. It is moderately tender. No discharge is present. There are no other lesions on her body. Based on the patient's medical history and physical examination, what is the most likely diagnosis?

    a. Impetigo
    b. Basal-cell carcinoma
    c. Melanoma
    d. Squamous-cell carcinoma

172. A 79-year-old nursing home resident is brought to the ER for confusion and agitation for the past 2 days. Her past medical history includes cerebrovascular accident, hypothyroidism, and diabetes. Her vital signs are unremarkable. Her laboratory test values are as follows: white blood cell count 12.2 without bandemia; hemoglobin 12.5; hematocrit 35.2; and platelet count 325,000. Her basic metabolic panel and thyroid function tests are unremarkable. A urinalysis is positive for glucose, trace occult blood, and bacteria, but it is negative for leukocytes and nitrites. A CT scan of the head is positive for atrophy and microvascular ischemic changes. On physical exam, she is oriented to person and place only and displays disorganizing thinking and irrelevant speech. What is the most likely diagnosis?

    a. Normal pressure hydrocephalus
    b. Alzheimer dementia
    c. Delirium
    d. Cerebrovascular accident

173. A 12-year-old male with no known past medical history comes to the pediatric office with his parents, complaining of worsening back pain for several weeks. He denies trauma. During the exam, a C-shaped curvature of his spine is noted. Which of the following is the most likely diagnosis?

    a. Scoliosis
    b. Gibbus deformity
    c. Scheuermann kyphosis
    d. *Amyotrophic lateral sclerosis*

174. A 30-year-old female with a history of obesity and polycystic ovary syndrome comes to the ER complaining of severe headache, pain behind her eyes, and visual changes for the past several days. She denies trauma. Her vital signs, complete blood count, comprehensive metabolic panel, urinalysis, and urine pregnancy tests are unremarkable. An MRI of the brain shows diffuse cerebral edema and papilledema. Which of the following is NOT a treatment for this condition?

    a. Acetazolamide
    b. Ventricular peritoneal shunt
    c. Aneurysm clipping
    d. Frovatriptan

175. A patient is admitted to the hospital for intermittent sharp abdominal pains, excessive belching, and non-bloody emesis. The patient undergoes esophagogastroduodenoscopy (EGD), which reveals gastritis. Which organism is the most likely culprit for the patient's condition?

    a. *Staphylococcus aureus*
    b. *Neisseria gonorrhoeae*
    c. *Helicobacter pylori*
    d. *Shigella*

176. A mother brings her 3-year-old son to the ER for a 3-day history of clear rhinorrhea, fever, and nasal congestion. Today, the child developed a barking cough. The child is not in any respiratory distress, and his appetite, fluid intake, and urinary output have all been normal. The patient's vitals are as follows: HR 85; RR 26; temperature 101.7; oxygen saturation 97% on room air. What is the most appropriate treatment?

    a. Administer oral steroids, discharge home, and humidify the air.
    b. Admit for intravenous steroids and antibiotics.
    c. Discharge home with oral steroids and oral antibiotics.
    d. Consult an ENT specialist immediately.

177. A 45-year-old man comes to the ER with worsening dull non-radiating chest pain, shortness of breath, and dizziness for the past 4 days. The chest pain is not related to activity. The patient's vitals are as follows: BP 96/48; HR 123; RR 24; temperature 98.8; oxygen saturation 95% on room air. A complete blood count is unremarkable. The first two troponins are 0.023 and 0.031, respectively (the normal level is 0.00-0.032). The B-type natriuretic peptide level is 100 pg/mL (the normal level is 50-100 pg/mL). An electrocardiogram shows sinus tachycardia. On physical exam, bulging neck veins are noted. Auscultation of his heart reveals quiet systolic and diastolic sounds. His breath sounds are coarse bilaterally. Based on his symptoms and physical exam, what is the most likely diagnosis?

    a. Cardiac tamponade
    b. Acute congestive heart failure
    c. Aortic dissection
    d. Unstable angina

178. A patient comes to the ER complaining of swelling and pain of the nail bed on her finger for the past several days. The patient states that she had cut her finger several days ago before the symptoms appeared. On physical examination, you notice erythema, tenderness, and swelling of the medial aspect of her nail bed. Scant purulent discharge can be expressed. The patient has no past medical history. What is the most likely diagnosis?

    a. Scabies
    b. Paronychia
    c. Onychomycosis
    d. Condyloma acuminata

179. A 66-year-old patient is brought to the ER by his family for progressing dementia, gait ataxia, and urinary incontinence for the past few months. His only medical issue is hypertension that is well controlled with medication. A CT scan shows rounded ventricles. No other abnormality is noted. A lumbar puncture is performed, but the results are unremarkable. What is the most likely diagnosis?

    a. Alzheimer disease
    b. Huntington disease
    c. Normal pressure hydrocephalus
    d. Hygroma

180. Which of the following medications would NOT be recommended in a patient with a history of fecal impaction?

    a. Colace
    b. Senna
    c. Morphine
    d. Milk of magnesia

181. A 60-year-old female patient developed aphasia, left hemiplegia, and right-sided preferential gaze 4 hours ago. On physical exam she is unable to speak, but she follows most verbal commands on her right side only. She also has a left facial droop. What is the most likely diagnosis?

a. Left middle cerebral artery (MCA) infarction
b. Right posterior cerebral artery (PCA) infarction
c. Right MCA infarction
d. Left PCA infarction

182. A patient presents with shortness of breath, dizziness, and chest pain. An electrocardiogram (ECG) shows sinus bradycardia. The patient's vital signs are as follows: BP 101/55; HR 31; RR 18; oxygen saturation 96% on room air. What is the next step in your medical management?

a. Give atropine
b. Give amiodarone
c. Give vasopressin
d. Give adenosine

183. A 71-year-old female with a history of mild dementia, diabetes, and hypertension comes to the ER complaining of left-sided periorbital pain and diplopia for 1 hour. She also admits to "seeing halos around lights." The visual acuity in her right eye is 20/20, and in the left eye, it is 20/40. Slit-lamp evaluation reveals corneal edema and an irregular, fixed left pupil. A CT scan of the brain is negative for mass, ischemia, or hemorrhage. Which of the following is the most appropriate initial next step?

a. Discharge home and follow up with ophthalmology.
b. Perform fluorescein eye stain.
c. Check a urine drug screen.
d. Administer acetazolamide.

184. A 2-year-old male child is brought to the pediatrician's office for a 4-day history of watery, non-bloody diarrhea and bilious vomiting. The child attends day care, and several children in the class have similar symptoms. The father denies recent travel or a change in diet. The patient's vitals are as follows: temperature, 99.0; HR, 90; RR, 16; oxygen saturation, 99% on room air. The child's exam is unremarkable and his skin has good turgor. What is the most likely etiology for this child's condition?

a. *Escherichia coli*
b. Rotavirus
c. *Campylobacter jejuni*
d. *Shigella*

185. A patient in your office had blood drawn as part of her annual visit. You notice that her thyroid-stimulating hormone (TSH) level is high, her T3 level is normal, and her T4 level is low. Based on her lab values, what is the diagnosis?

a. Addison disease
b. Hypothyroidism
c. Hyperthyroidism
d. Graves disease

186. A primigravida is 28 weeks pregnant and has had no issues thus far in her pregnancy. At a routine OB-GYN visit, she has a type and screen done, which shows that the mother's blood type is O positive. Her husband's blood type is AB negative. Which of the following is the most appropriate intervention?

a. Order a unit of blood to be transfused prior to delivery.
b. Order a transvaginal ultrasound.
c. No intervention is needed.
d. Prescribe RhoGAM.

187. A patient is ambulating with physical therapy in the ICU when one of the therapists tells you that the patient's blood pressure went from 155/88 in the supine position to 131/70 in the sitting position. The other vital signs are as follows: HR 99; RR 18; oxygen saturation 97% on room air. The patient is now complaining of dizziness and headache. The patient's electrocardiogram (ECG) is normal. What is the most likely diagnosis?

a. Sick sinus syndrome
b. Angina
c. Orthostatic hypotension
d. Atrial fibrillation

188. A 68-year-old male presents to the ER with headache and nausea. A computed tomography (CT) scan of his head, electrocardiogram (ECG), and troponin level are normal. The urinalysis shows proteinuria. The patient's vital signs are as follows: HR 98; RR 16; BP 205/121. What is the most likely diagnosis?

a. Stage 2 hypertension
b. Hypertensive crisis
c. Prehypertension
d. Stage 1 hypertension

189. A patient comes to the ER with worsening shortness of breath for 4 days. She is unable to lie down flat and instead has to use several pillows before going to sleep at night. Her B-type natriuretic peptide level is 6,500 pg/mL (the normal level is 50-100 pg/mL). The patient's vitals are as follows: BP 100/60; HR 86; RR 22; oxygen saturation 91% on room air. Troponin and D-dimer test results are unremarkable. After administering diuretics, what is the most appropriate next step?

a. Order a CT angiogram of the chest.
b. Administer antiplatelet therapy.
c. Order an echocardiogram.
d. Apply a nitroglycerin patch.

190. A 21-year-old male comes to the ER with worsening left-sided testicular pain and swelling of 3 days' duration. He denies trauma. He has no past medical history. His vitals are normal. On physical examination, you palpate his scrotum, which feels like there's a mass of worms inside. Based on his medical history and physical, the most likely diagnosis is:

a. Hydrocele
b. Varicocele
c. Testicular torsion
d. Testicular carcinoma

191. A patient comes to your clinic complaining of worsening diaphoresis, palpitations, and generalized tremor for several weeks. On physical examination, you notice that the patient has exophthalmos. What is the most likely diagnosis?

a. Graves disease
b. Addison disease
c. Cushing disease
d. Hashimoto disease

192. A 19-year-old patient is being evaluated in the ER for a wrist laceration. She tearfully admits that the injury was self-induced after she learned she has unintentionally become pregnant. Which of the following is the most appropriate next step?

    a. Call the patient's parents.
    b. Administer a benzodiazepine.
    c. Refer for psychiatric evaluation.
    d. Administer a tetanus shot.

193. A 42-year-old mother with a history of alcoholism gives birth to an infant with low Apgar scores due to central cyanosis. A chest x-ray reveals a boot-shaped heart. An echocardiogram reveals ventricular septal defect, pulmonary artery stenosis, and right ventricular hypertrophy. Which of the following is the most likely diagnosis?

    a. Coarctation of the aorta
    b. Tetralogy of Fallot
    c. Dressler syndrome
    d. Truncus arteriosus

194. You have just examined a patient and suspect that she has Graves disease. What is the next step in your medical management?

    a. Order thyroid function tests.
    b. Order a complete endocrine panel.
    c. Order a cortisol level.
    d. Order a hemoglobin A1C (HbA1c).

195. A 22-year-old female patient presents to the ER with persistent abdominal pain for 3 days. She is admitted to the observation unit for further evaluation. On review of labs the next morning, the following are noted: HBsAg is negative, anti-HBc is negative, and anti-HBs is positive. What can be inferred about the patient's condition based on the laboratory test values?

    a. She is susceptible to being infected with hepatitis B.
    b. She is chronically infected with hepatitis B.
    c. She is immune to hepatitis B due to prior vaccination.
    d. She is acutely infected with hepatitis B.

196. A patient comes to the ER complaining of persistent unilateral shoulder pain that started after his wrestling match at school 2 days prior. The pain is worst at night and when lying on the affected shoulder. The patient states that he has a "crackling" sensation when rotating his shoulder. Which of the following maneuvers helps confirm the diagnosis?

    a. Anterior drawer test
    b. Lachman test
    c. McMurray test
    d. Drop arm test

197. A 30-year-old female presents to the ER with worsening nausea, vomiting, and non-bloody diarrhea. She notes that she's been craving salty foods recently. The patient's vitals are as follows: temperature 98.2; BP 90/50; HR 60; RR 14; O_2 100% on room air. Her laboratory test results are Na 130; K 4.5; BUN 26; Cr 1.2; glucose 114. Patchy areas of hyperpigmentation, which appear as if she had been tanning, are noted. What is the most appropriate treatment?

    a. Levothyroxine
    b. Propranolol
    c. Ketoconazole
    d. Hydrocortisone

198. A patient comes to your office complaining of headache, persistent urinary tract infections, unintentional weight loss, and fatigue. His fasting serum glucose is 161. His hemoglobin A1C (HbA1c) is 6.7. His vitals are normal. His body mass index (BMI) is normal. He has no past medical problems. What is your medical recommendation to this patient?

    a. Lose weight.
    b. Modify diet.
    c. Start metformin.
    d. Start insulin.

199. A patient comes to your office complaining of erectile dysfunction. Which of the following medications would you NOT prescribe for this condition?

    a. Cialis
    b. Levitra
    c. Viagra
    d. Finasteride

200. A patient with no past medical history had a purified protein derivative (PPD) shot 3 days ago and now has an induration of 5 mm. She works as a librarian. What is the next step in your medical management?

    a. Order a chest x-ray.
    b. Order a repeat PPD in 1 month.
    c. No intervention is needed for now.
    d. Start tuberculosis medications.

201. A 24-year-old male comes to your clinic complaining of having epididymitis. He states that he's had several prior epididymitis infections. He notes that he is sexually active and occasionally does not use protection. He denies other medical problems. What would you advise this patient?

    a. Increase fluid intake.
    b. Avoid red meat, seafood, and alcohol.
    c. Use protection when having intercourse.
    d. Recommend urology referral.

202. During a colonoscopy, it is discovered that a patient has multiple areas of outpouching along the colonic wall. What is the most likely diagnosis?

    a. Intussusception
    b. Diverticulosis
    c. Mallory-Weiss tear
    d. Celiac sprue

203. A 70-year-old male with a past medical history of COPD, congestive heart failure (CHF), atrial fibrillation, and rheumatic heart disease, who has had a mitral valve repair, presents to the ER with fatigue and shortness of breath. He is admitted and ultimately diagnosed with a transudative pleural effusion. Which of the following is the most likely etiology for this patient's diagnosis?

    a. CHF
    b. Rheumatic heart disease
    c. COPD
    d. Atrial fibrillation

204. A 60-year-old male with a history of obesity, COPD, and tobacco abuse presents to the ER with increasing fatigue, nonproductive cough, and shortness of breath for 3 weeks. His vital signs are as follows: BP 142/85; HR 104; RR 20; temperature 99.2; oxygen satruation 91% on room air. Physical examination reveals distant heart sounds with S4 gallop, decreased breath sounds at lung bases, and 2+ lower extremity edema. An electrocardiogram and troponin are unremarkable. A B-type natriuretic peptide is 5,025 pg/mL (the normal range is 100-300 pg/mL). Which of the following is the most appropriate initial diagnostic study?

    a. Holter monitor
    b. CT angiogram of the chest
    c. Echocardiogram
    d. Cardiac catheterization

205. A 72-year-old man comes to his primary care office complaining of a burning, painful rash on his side for the past 2 days. He denies fever, chills, sick contacts, or recent travel. The patient has multiple blisters with clear fluid on an erythematous base along his left side. There are no other lesions. The rash is exquisitely painful. Which of the following is the most appropriate next step?

    a. Refer to a dermatologist for punch biopsy.
    b. Prescribe valacyclovir.
    c. Take a skin scraping and send to the lab.
    d. Prescribe ciprofloxacin.

206. A patient comes to her primary care office for follow-up evaluation of progressing unintentional weight loss, fatigue, myalgias, and weakness. She has a history of hepatitis C, for which she does not take medication. Her comprehensive metabolic panel is unremarkable. Her white blood cell count is 14.5 without bandemia; otherwise, the complete blood count is unremarkable. Her erythrocyte sedimentation rate is 78 mm/hr (normal range is <20 mm/hr). She is eventually diagnosed with polyarteritis nodosa. Which of the following is the most appropriate treatment?

    a. Ribavirin
    b. Prednisone
    c. Ampicillin
    d. IV fluids and rest

207. A patient in the intensive care unit (ICU) suddenly becomes unresponsive. There are no carotid or femoral pulses that are able to be palpated. The patient's heart rate on the monitor is 186. There are wide QRS complexes. Which of the following medications would be the most appropriate initial medication while waiting for the defibrillator to arrive?

    a. Magnesium sulfate
    b. Atropine
    c. Epinephrine
    d. Amiodarone

208. A patient has just been diagnosed with benign prostatic hypertrophy. Which of the following medications would you NOT prescribe for this condition?

    a. Proscar
    b. Cardura
    c. Rapaflo
    d. Ramipril

209. A 50-year-old patient comes to a local urgent care center complaining of difficulty speaking and right arm paresthesias for the past hour. His past medical history includes hypertension, obesity, and hyperlipidemia. His home medications include amlodipine and rosuvastatin. The patient's vitals are as follows: temperature 98.2; BP 146/88; HR 86, RR 18; oxygen saturation 99% on room air. He denies alcohol or drug abuse. The PA believes that the patient is having an acute cerebral vascular accident and calls 911. While waiting for emergency medical services (EMS) to arrive, which of the following is the least appropriate action?

  a. Check a fingerstick.
  b. Document the patient's National Institutes of Health (NIH) Stroke Scale score.
  c. Call the patient's emergency contact.
  d. Give aspirin per rectum.

210. A patient is diagnosed with *Clostridioides difficile* colitis. The patient has no allergies to medication. Which of the following medications would you prescribe?

  a. Vancomycin PO
  b. Clindamycin PO
  c. IV azithromycin
  d. IV vancomycin

211. Which of the following medications would help treat a patient in status epilepticus?

  a. Levetiracetam and linezolid
  b. Phenylephrine and Lomotil
  c. Phenytoin and lorazepam
  d. Phenytoin and linezolid

212. Which medical triad comprises three factors thought to contribute to thrombosis?

  a. Beck triad
  b. Virchow triad
  c. Charcot triad
  d. Cushing triad

213. A patient comes to the ER with right-sided foot pain after accidentally striking his foot against a baseboard. He has moderate pain at the first and second metatarsals with mild swelling with palpable deformity. Based on his medical history and physical, what is the most likely diagnosis?

  a. Le Fort fracture
  b. Lisfranc fracture
  c. Monteggia fracture
  d. Colles fracture

214. A patient with cystic fibrosis asks you what medications she can take to help decrease her risk of secondary infection. Which of the following medications would you NOT advise this patient to take?

  a. Motrin
  b. Amiodarone
  c. Mucinex
  d. Albuterol

215. Which of the following is a complication of pulmonary tuberculosis?

  a. Parkinson disease
  b. Hashimoto disease
  c. Cushing disease
  d. Pott disease

216. A patient comes to your clinic complaining of pains all over her body. Multiple lab tests and scans have been negative for acute pathology. She has a history of depression. What is the most likely diagnosis?

   a. Fibromyalgia
   b. Polyarteritis nodosa
   c. Osteoarthritis
   d. Polymyalgia rheumatica

217. Which of the following medications would be used for a person diagnosed with generalized anxiety disorder?

   a. Prednisolone
   b. Promethazine
   c. Permethrin
   d. Paroxetine

218. A 68-year-old woman comes to the primary care clinic complaining of decreasing vision in her left eye for the past several months. She noticed that colors appear to be faded and objects often have halos surrounding them. She is no longer able to drive because her night vision is so poor. She denies headache, trauma, and eye pain, or discharge from the eye. Her past medical history includes diabetes, hyperlipidemia, and tobacco abuse. On physical exam, the patient has a cloudy opacity of her left eye lens. Which of the following is the most appropriate treatment for the patient's likely condition?

   a. Refer for surgical repair.
   b. Prescribe timolol ophthalmic solution.
   c. Refer to a neurologist.
   d. Advise the patient that she needs a stronger eyeglass prescription.

219. You suspect a patient has a deep venous thrombus. Which of the following tests should you initially order?

   a. X-ray
   b. Doppler ultrasound
   c. Computed tomography (CT) scan
   d. Magnetic resonance imaging (MRI)

220. A bleeding defect is seen in the distal esophagus of a patient during an esophagogastroduodenoscopy. The patient has a known history of alcoholism. What is the most likely diagnosis?

   a. Mallory-Weiss tear
   b. Crohn disease
   c. Ulcerative colitis
   d. Whipple disease

221. A 66-year-old female comes to the ER complaining of right calf pain and swelling of 12 hours' duration. She has a past medical history of arthritis and osteoporosis. She states that she had a right hip replacement 4 days ago. On physical examination, you note that she has a positive Homan sign. Based on her medical history and physical examination, what is the most likely diagnosis?

   a. Septic arthritis
   b. Osgood-Schlatter disease
   c. Osteomyelitis
   d. Venous thrombus

222. While reviewing a two-dimensional echocardiography (2D echo) with a cardiologist, you both see that there is backflow of blood from the left ventricle into the left atrium. What is this condition called?

 a. Mitral regurgitation
 b. Pulmonic regurgitation
 c. Tricuspid regurgitation
 d. Aortic regurgitation

223. A patient in the intensive care unit (ICU) suddenly goes into pulseless ventricular tachycardia. What is one of the first medications you would administer?

 a. Magnesium sulfate
 b. Lidocaine
 c. Epinephrine
 d. Amiodarone

224. Parents bring their 12-year-old son to the pediatrician's office for his annual physical evaluation. They have expressed concern because they have noticed that the child has been developing breasts over the past year, which has been a source of anxiety and distress for their son. On physical examination, you notice that the child has enlarged mammary glands bilaterally. The child has no past medical history. The rest of his exam is normal. Which of the following is the most appropriate next step?

 a. Order a urine drug screen.
 b. Obtain a breast ultrasound.
 c. Prescribe testosterone supplementation.
 d. No intervention is warranted.

225. Parents bring in their 2-year-old child to your clinic. They note that he has been tugging on his ears for the past 2 days. He has been getting over a viral upper respiratory infection, but he is otherwise healthy. Upon physical examination, you notice that his left tympanic membrane is erythematous and bulging. His physical examination is otherwise normal. Based on the medical history and physical examination, what is the most likely diagnosis?

 a. Otitis media
 b. Mastoiditis
 c. Otitis externa
 d. Acoustic neuroma

226. A 19-year-old male is referred to the orthopedic clinic for persistent back pain for 4 months. He denies trauma, fever, chills, or toxic habits. The pain started in his low back and has ascended to his cervical spine and descended to his pelvis. X-rays of his thoracic and lumbar spine show mild kyphosis. His complete blood count and basic metabolic panel are unremarkable. His erythrocyte sedimentation rate and alkaline phosphatase are slightly elevated. What is the most likely diagnosis?

 a. Spondylolisthesis
 b. Pott disease
 c. Ankylosing spondylitis
 d. Multiple myeloma

227. A 22-year-old female patient arrives in the ER complaining of left-hand pain and swelling after being involved in a physical altercation several hours earlier. An x-ray shows a transverse and mildly displaced fourth metacarpal fracture. What is the most likely diagnosis?

 a. Boxer's fracture
 b. Monteggia fracture
 c. Buckle fracture
 d. Colles fracture

228. A blood gas test shows the following results: pH, 7.31; PaCO$_2$, 50; HCO$_3$, 25; and PaO$_2$, 94. Which of the following is the most likely diagnosis?

    a. Metabolic alkalosis
    b. Respiratory alkalosis
    c. Metabolic acidosis
    d. Respiratory acidosis

229. A mother brings her 2-year-old son to an urgent care center after he suffered a fall 1 hour before. She states that he fell on the playground earlier and then he stopped using his left arm. On physical exam, the child is holding his left arm flexed and pronated. He is not in any pain or distress as long as his arm is maintained in that position. There is no swelling, deformity, or discoloration of the extremity. His vital signs are unremarkable. An x-ray reveals radial head subluxation. What is the most likely diagnosis?

    a. Tenosynovitis
    b. Colles fracture
    c. Nursemaid's elbow
    d. Tennis elbow

230. A 15-year-old female is brought to your clinic by her mother, who states that her child has not been eating. The girl has no past medical history. Upon further discussion, the child confides in you that she purposely has been skipping meals so she can lose weight. What is the most likely diagnosis?

    a. Anorexia nervosa
    b. Bulimia nervosa
    c. Generalized anxiety disorder
    d. Bipolar disorder

231. A 40-year-old male comes to your clinic and reports that he feels nervous all the time. He has no history of personal loss, disturbing life event, or illness. His physical examination and vital signs are normal. He has no medical problems. What is the most likely diagnosis?

    a. Persistent depressive disorder (dysthymia)
    b. Generalized anxiety disorder
    c. Posttraumatic stress disorder
    d. Phobia

232. A patient in the intensive care unit has the following blood gas results: pH, 7.47; PaCO$_2$, 39; HCO$_3$, 29. What is the most likely diagnosis?

    a. Respiratory acidosis
    b. Respiratory alkalosis
    c. Metabolic alkalosis
    d. Metabolic acidosis

233. A patient with normal pressure hydrocephalus undergoes a lumbar puncture. The patient's symptoms improve. What is the next step in this patient's management?

    a. Obtain a magnetic resonance imaging (MRI) scan of the brain.
    b. Repeat the lumbar puncture in 48 hours.
    c. Prepare for surgical placement of a ventricular peritoneal shunt
    d. Perform an electroencephalogram (EEG).

234. A patient comes to your clinic for an annual physical examination. The patient confesses to you that she has a hard time coming to your clinic, or being outside in general, because of her fear of being outdoors. She reports feelings of extreme anxiety once she leaves her house. She denies any reason for being nervous in crowds of people. What is the most likely diagnosis?

a. Generalized anxiety disorder
b. Posttraumatic stress disorder
c. Persistent depressive disorder (dysthymia)
d. Phobia disorder

235. A patient has hypertrophic cardiomyopathy. What is the most common cause for this condition?

a. Genetic mutation
b. Disease
c. Infection
d. Cancer

236. Parents bring their child into the ER stating that the child has developed rapid, uncontrolled body movements and a fever of 102 °F at home. You notice these body movements during your physical examination as well. You draw blood for lab work, which shows that the patient has a white blood cell count of 17,000 as well as an elevated erythrocyte sedimentation rate (ESR). You suspect the patient has acute rheumatic fever. Which of the following signs/symptoms is NOT among the minor manifestations of rheumatic fever according to the Jones criteria?

a. Fever
b. Chorea
c. Leukocytosis
d. Elevated ESR

237. You are reviewing a two-dimensional echocardiogram when you notice backflow of blood from the right ventricle into the right atrium. The most likely diagnosis is:

a. Aortic regurgitation
b. Mitral regurgitation
c. Pulmonic regurgitation
d. Tricuspid regurgitation

238. Which of the following medications should NOT be given in a patient with pulseless ventricular fibrillation?

a. Amiodarone
b. Lidocaine
c. Vasopressin
d. Atropine

239. A nurse hands you the following arterial blood gas results: pH, 7.49; $PaCO_2$, 20; and HCO_3, 23. Which of the following is the most likely diagnosis?

a. Metabolic alkalosis
b. Respiratory alkalosis
c. Metabolic acidosis
d. Respiratory acidosis

Mometrix

240. A patient is brought to the ER for acute alcohol intoxication. As the patient begins to wake up, you notice persistent, involuntary, horizontal eye movements of both eyes. What is the most likely diagnosis?

    a. Conjunctivitis
    b. Nystagmus
    c. Entropion
    d. Exotropia

241. A patient arrives in the ER complaining of chest pain, dizziness, and shortness of breath. An electrocardiogram (ECG) shows a secondary R wave in lead V1 and a widened QRS complex. What is this conduction disorder called?

    a. Torsades de pointes
    b. Right bundle branch block
    c. Atrial fibrillation
    d. Sinus tachycardia

242. A 65-year-old male patient presents to the ER with dysarthria, ataxia, and left-sided weakness that occurred for about 30 minutes and then spontaneously resolved about 2 hours ago. He has no past medical history. His physical exam is unremarkable. His CBC, chemistry panel, and coagulation studies are normal. His non-contrast head CT and ECG are normal. Which of the following is the most appropriate next step?

    a. Order an electroencephalogram.
    b. No intervention is warranted.
    c. Repeat a CT scan in 24 hours.
    d. Order CT angiography of the brain.

243. A patient with a known history of anxiety and depression is in your clinic for a routine physical examination and confides in you that he wants to commit suicide. He tells you how and when he plans to do it. Which of the following is NOT an appropriate action as a medical professional?

    a. Advise the patient to call a suicide hotline.
    b. Obtain a stat psychiatric referral.
    c. Do not report the patient's actions.
    d. Advise the patient's spouse or parents of his intent.

244. A patient comes to your clinic complaining of persistent right-eye irritation. The conjunctiva is normal. You note that the patient's right lower lid is turned inward. What is this condition called?

    a. Entropion
    b. Exotropia
    c. Ectropion
    d. Esotropia

245. Parents bring in their 5-year-old son for his annual physical examination. The parents state that their son has been having trouble at school and at home with frequent temper tantrums, angry outbursts, short temper, and hostility toward others. He hasn't gone through any life-threatening situations, suffered personal losses, or had any recent changes in his life. His physical examination and vital signs are normal. He has no past medical history. What is the most likely diagnosis?

    a. Adjustment disorder
    b. Persistent depressive disorder (dysthymia)
    c. Attention-deficit/hyperactivity disorder
    d. Oppositional-defiant disorder

Copyright © Mometrix Media. You have been licensed one copy of this document for personal use only. Any other reproduction or redistribution is strictly prohibited. All rights reserved. This content is provided for test preparation purposes only and does not imply an endorsement by Mometrix of any particular political, scientific, or religious point of view.

246. One of your patients has been diagnosed with phlebitis. Which of the following would NOT be a part of your medical management?

    a. Prescribe colchicine.
    b. Recommend compression stockings.
    c. Prescribe analgesics.
    d. Recommend warm compresses.

247. A 21-year-old male comes to the urology office after discovering a lump on his testicle. He has no past medical history. A hard, fixed, 1 cm painless mass on his left testicle is noted. The area is not erythematous. The cremasteric reflex is intact. The lesion does not transilluminate. The right testicle is unremarkable. Which of the following lab studies would be the least helpful in confirming the diagnosis?

    a. Lactate dehydrogenase (LDH)
    b. Human chorionic gonadotropin (HCG)
    c. Alpha-fetoprotein (AFP)
    d. Complete blood count (CBC)

248. A 16-year-old female patient arrives in the ER complaining of headache, nausea, and photophobia. She is diagnosed with a migraine headache. Which of the following medications would you prescribe for this patient to help prevent and treat future episodes?

    a. Fluvastatin
    b. Frovatriptan
    c. Fluoxetine
    d. Fexofenadine

249. A female patient was diagnosed with gestational diabetes 2 weeks previously, and the OB-GYN PA recommended light exercise and dietary modifications. Today, her 1-hour postprandial glucose is 223 mg/dL (the normal level is 127-140 mg/dL). Earlier in the week, her 1-hour postprandial glucose levels were 259 mg/dL and 211 mg/dL when measured on separate occasions. Her laboratory test values are as follows: Na 137; K 4.2; BUN 21; Cr 0.8; glucose 299. Her urinalysis is positive for glucose, but it is otherwise unremarkable. What is the most appropriate initial step in her medical management?

    a. No intervention is necessary.
    b. Initiate pioglitazone.
    c. Refer to an endocrinologist.
    d. Initiate regular insulin.

250. A 21-year-old male patient arrives in your office for the first time for a routine physical examination. While talking to him, you note that he has involuntary facial tics. His cognitive function is normal. What is the most likely diagnosis for his behavior?

    a. Huntington disease
    b. Tourette disorder
    c. Alzheimer disease
    d. Multiple sclerosis

251. You are examining a patient with suspected chronic obstructive pulmonary disease (COPD). Which of the following is the best test to help aid your diagnosis?

    a. Spirometry
    b. Chest x-ray
    c. Auscultation with a stethoscope
    d. Electrocardiogram (ECG)

252. A 45-year-old male patient who was diagnosed with a stroke, and received tissue plasminogen activator (tPA) 5 hours previously, has urinary incontinence. The patient has moderate left-sided weakness and blurred vision, but he remains cognizant. Which of the following is the most appropriate intervention?

    a.   Order a bladder ultrasound.
    b.   Have the nurse apply a Texas catheter.
    c.   Order the nurse to insert a Foley catheter.
    d.   Have the patient ambulate to the commode.

253. A patient arrives in the ER complaining of worsening hemoptysis, fever, chills, and weakness for the past week. This patient has a history of HIV. A chest x-ray is ordered, which shows a fungal ball in the right lung. What is the most likely diagnosis?

    a.   Cystic fibrosis
    b.   Pneumoconiosis
    c.   Sarcoidosis
    d.   Aspergillosis

254. A mother brings her 18-month-old son to your clinic, noting that he has been displaying progressively deteriorating social and communication skills and repetitive behaviors. This triad of symptoms best defines which of the following disorders?

    a.   Oppositional-defiant disorder
    b.   Attention-deficit/hyperactivity disorder
    c.   Autism spectrum disorder
    d.   Adjustment disorder

255. A mother, pregnant with her first child, is Rh positive. The child is Rh positive. What is the next step in medical management?

    a.   Prescribe antibiotics.
    b.   Order an ultrasound.
    c.   No intervention is needed.
    d.   Prescribe RhoGAM.

256. A woman who is 36 weeks pregnant develops eclampsia. Her liver function tests and complete blood count are normal. What would be the next step in medical management?

    a.   Observe on telemetry monitor.
    b.   Discharge home and monitor as an outpatient.
    c.   Induce labor.
    d.   Order a stat blood transfusion.

257. A 56-year-old man with a history of chronic obstructive pulmonary disease (COPD) comes to the ER complaining of worsening shortness of breath and chest pain. A chest x-ray shows blunting of the right costophrenic angle. What is the most likely diagnosis?

    a.   Pleural effusion
    b.   Aspergillosis
    c.   Pneumoconiosis
    d.   Pneumothorax

258. Which of the following chest x-ray findings is most consistent with the diagnosis of a pneumothorax whose size is approximately 5%?

   a. Honeycomb appearance of the lungs
   b. Granulomas
   c. Area on chest x-ray with no lung markings
   d. Normal chest x-ray

259. Which of the following conditions would NOT be a contributing factor to the development of obesity?

   a. Graves disease
   b. Hypothyroidism
   c. Cushing syndrome
   d. Menopause

260. Which of the following is NOT a treatment for allergic rhinitis?

   a. Decongestants
   b. Antihistamines
   c. Antibiotics
   d. Corticosteroids

261. Which of the following would NOT be used in the treatment of a patient with a phobia disorder?

   a. Xanax
   b. Metoprolol
   c. Lexapro
   d. Ritalin

262. Which of the following treatments is NOT an intervention for a patient going through withdrawal from alcohol?

   a. Zofran
   b. Narcan
   c. Thiamine
   d. Ativan

263. A 37-year-old female patient comes to the ER complaining of worsening fever, dysphonia, and dysphagia of 3 days' duration. She notes recently having a tooth infection, but she did not seek medical attention for it. While you are talking to the patient, a family member says, "She sounds like she has a hot potato in her mouth." Her tongue is swollen and out of place, and she has swelling and erythema of her proximal neck. What is the most likely diagnosis?

   a. Oral leukoplakia
   b. Acute pharyngitis
   c. Ludwig angina
   d. Aphthous ulcers

264. A patient being seen in the ER is diagnosed with a blowout fracture. Which of the following would NOT be an intervention for this patient?

   a. Irrigation
   b. Antibiotics
   c. Steroids
   d. Surgery

265. A patient comes to the ER complaining of facial pain and swelling after being physically assaulted. A computed tomography (CT) scan reveals a fractured maxilla. What is the most likely diagnosis?

    a. Boxer's fracture
    b. Lisfranc fracture
    c. Colles fracture
    d. Le Fort fracture

266. What is the most common preventable cause of pelvic inflammatory disease?

    a. Appendicitis
    b. Ectopic pregnancy
    c. Childbirth
    d. Venereal disease

267. A patient is diagnosed with gastroesophageal reflux disease. Which of the following medications is the most appropriate treatment for this condition?

    a. Ketoconazole
    b. Metronidazole
    c. Fluconazole
    d. Esomeprazole

268. Which of the following statements is NOT true regarding Meckel diverticulum?

    a. It is more common in females than males.
    b. It is usually found about 2 feet from the ileocecal valve.
    c. Initial presentation is more common in toddlers than adults.
    d. It affects approximately 2% of the population.

269. A patient comes to your clinic complaining of worsening gastroesophageal reflux symptoms, as well as abdominal pain and hematemesis. A serum gastrin level is high. A computed tomography (CT) scan of the abdomen shows multiple small tumors in the head of the pancreas and the duodenum. What is the most likely diagnosis?

    a. Celiac disease
    b. Zollinger-Ellison syndrome
    c. Whipple disease
    d. Crohn disease

270. A patient comes to the ER with increasing left shoulder pain and decreased range of motion after a heavy box fell on his shoulder. On physical examination, he has limited abduction. A shoulder x-ray is negative for fracture or dislocation. What is the next step in your medical management?

    a. Order a repeat x-ray in 2 weeks.
    b. Order a magnetic resonance imaging (MRI) scan of the shoulder.
    c. No intervention is necessary.
    d. Administer electromyography (EMG).

271. A patient is admitted to the hospital for multiple right leg fractures following a motor vehicle accident. His leg is splinted, and the patient is sent to the medical floor for monitoring. A nurse from the hospital unit calls later that day to report that the patient's right foot has become pale and cool. An arterial ultrasound shows limited flow. His creatine phosphokinase (CPK) test result is 14,000 U/L (the normal range is 22 to 198 U/L). Which of the following is the most appropriate initial intervention?

    a. Order a repeat CPK in 24 hours.
    b. Administer a bolus of IV fluids.
    c. Remove the splint.
    d. Consult a vascular surgeon.

272. An 18-year-old female is in the primary care office for her annual wellness exam. She has no significant past medical history. She mentions that she develops abdominal cramping, non-bloody diarrhea, and flatulence when eating foods such as yogurt and cheese. Which of the following tests is the least helpful in evaluating the patient's suspected condition?

 a. Lactose tolerance test
 b. Serum calcium
 c. Lactose-hydrogen breath test
 d. Lactose-restricted diet

273. A patient comes to your clinic stating that she has noticed skin changes over her right breast. During the physical examination, you note that her skin has an erythematous, swollen, pitted surface. What is the most likely diagnosis?

 a. Carcinoma
 b. Abscess
 c. Gynecomastia
 d. Fibroadenoma

274. A 43-year-old female with a history of COPD and atrial fibrillation presents to the ER complaining of shortness of breath and palpitations for the past 2 days. Her medications include theophylline and digoxin. Her vital signs are as follows: BP 140/80; HR 122; RR 18; temperature 98.2; O_2 98% on room air. Her basic metabolic panel, thyroid function tests, troponin, and complete blood count are unremarkable. Her theophylline level is 13 mcg/mL (the normal range is 5-15 mcg/mL), and her digoxin level is 3.2 ng/mL (the normal range is 1.5-2.5 ng/mL). Her electrocardiogram reveals a regular narrow complex tachycardia. The PA instructs the patient to make a forceful exhalation while closing her mouth and pinching her nose shut. The patient converts to normal sinus rhythm. Which of the following is the most appropriate diagnostic study to establish a definitive diagnosis in this patient?

 a. Transesophageal echocardiogram
 b. 2D echocardiogram
 c. CT angiogram of the chest
 d. Electrophysiology study

275. A patient is scheduled for a coronary artery bypass graft the following morning. He is a type 2 diabetic who is currently receiving metformin, Lantus, and regular insulin on a sliding scale regimen. He is ordered to be NPO past midnight. When reviewing preoperative orders for this patient, the PA would expect to find which of the following treatment plans?

 a. Give metformin the morning of surgery with a sip of water.
 b. Use long-acting insulin the morning of surgery.
 c. Use insulin infusion starting early the morning of surgery.
 d. Hold all antihyperglycemic medications.

276. Which of the following is the best way to prevent beriberi?

 a. Increase calcium intake.
 b. Increase thiamine intake.
 c. Increase folate intake.
 d. Increase iron intake.

277. Which of the following is the best way to prevent osteoporosis?

 a. Increase calcium intake.
 b. Increase thiamine intake.
 c. Increase folate intake.
 d. Increase iron intake.

278. A 20-year-old female patient comes to the ER with nausea, vomiting, and constipation for a duration of 2 days. The patient was discharged from the hospital a week before after having a laparoscopic appendectomy. She has no other pertinent past medical history. The patient's vitals are as follows: temperature 98.8; BP 116/70; HR 55; RR 16; oxygen saturation 100% on room air. A complete blood count and basic metabolic panel are unremarkable. On physical exam, the patient's abdomen is softly distended with hypoactive bowel sounds and mild epigastric tenderness. An abdominal x-ray shows distended bowel without evidence of obstruction. Which of the following is the least appropriate intervention?

    a. IV fluids
    b. Resuming regular diet
    c. Bowel regimen
    d. Antiemetics

279. A woman who is 35 weeks pregnant presents to the ER with continuous contractions, abdominal pain, back pain, and bright-red vaginal bleeding. What is the most likely diagnosis?

    a. Endometriosis
    b. Premature rupture of the membranes
    c. Placental abruption (abruptio placentae)
    d. Placenta previa

280. A 2-month-old baby girl born 6 weeks premature is referred to the cardiology office for further evaluation of a heart murmur. The parents admit that the child seems frequently tired and her growth has been poor. A 2D echocardiogram shows flow between the aorta and pulmonary artery. Which of the following is the most appropriate next step?

    a. Recommend surgical closure.
    b. No intervention is necessary for now.
    c. Prescribe aspirin 81 mg.
    d. Prescribe warfarin.

281. A patient comes to the ER complaining of left wrist pain after falling on an outstretched hand. An x-ray shows a fracture of the distal radius and a dislocation at the radioulnar joint. What is the most likely diagnosis?

    a. Le Fort fracture
    b. Colles fracture
    c. Galeazzi fracture
    d. Monteggia fracture

282. A 36-year-old primigravida is 30 weeks pregnant. She has a past medical history of stage II endometriosis and obesity. During her routine office visit, she was diagnosed with preeclampsia. Which of her medical issues puts the patient at greatest risk for preterm labor?

    a. Advanced maternal age
    b. Endometriosis
    c. Obesity
    d. Preeclampsia

283. A 24-year-old female who is 12 weeks pregnant comes to the ER complaining of sudden-onset abdominal pain and vaginal bleeding. She has had a prior transvaginal ultrasound, which showed an intrauterine pregnancy (IUP). An ultrasound cannot visualize the IUP. A urine pregnancy test is negative. What is the most likely diagnosis?

   a. Threatened abortion
   b. Missed abortion
   c. Completed abortion
   d. Dysmenorrhea

284. An 80-year-old female comes to her primary care clinic complaining of worsening pelvic, leg, and neck pain for the past several weeks. X-rays of her femurs show bowing, and x-rays of the neck and pelvis show multiple bony deformities. Her vital signs are unremarkable. Her laboratory test findings are as follows: Na 135; K 4.5; BUN 26; Cr 1.0; glucose 136; Ca 13.1. Her liver function tests are unremarkable except for her alkaline phosphatase, which is 450 IU/L (the normal range is 44 to 147 IU/L). Which of the following is the most appropriate treatment?

   a. Calcium gluconate
   b. Zoledronic acid
   c. Percolone
   d. Calcium carbonate

285. Which of the following would NOT be an appropriate treatment for giardiasis?

   a. Furosemide
   b. Ondansetron
   c. Loperamide
   d. Metronidazole

286. A 26-year-old female patient comes to her primary care office complaining of alternating episodes of diarrhea and constipation that get worse after eating. The symptoms are not caused by one particular type of food. Her medications include sertraline. Her vital signs and physical exam are unremarkable. She is negative for stool occult blood, and her stool culture, fecal lactoferrin, complete blood count, basic metabolic panel, and thyroid function test results are unremarkable. She had a CT scan of the abdomen and pelvis that was unremarkable. What is the most likely diagnosis?

   a. Whipple disease
   b. *Hirschsprung* disease
   c. Celiac sprue
   d. Irritable bowel syndrome

287. Which of the following tests is the most diagnostic for monitoring the course of choriocarcinoma and its response to therapy?

   a. Complete blood cell count
   b. Bence Jones protein
   c. Computed tomography (CT) scan of the abdomen and pelvis
   d. Beta human chorionic gonadotropin (β-HCG)

288. All of the following are therapies used to treat leiomyomas EXCEPT:

   a. Nonsteroidal anti-inflammatory drugs (NSAIDs)
   b. Birth control pills
   c. Antibiotics
   d. Iron supplements

289. A 21-year-old obese African American female presents to her OB-GYN clinic complaining of menorrhagia and pelvic pain associated with her menses for the past several months. Other than obesity, she has no past medical history. She does not take any medications. A transvaginal ultrasound shows a well-defined, hypoechoic intramural lesion. Which of the following would be the least helpful in treating this patient's condition?

    a. NSAIDs
    b. Birth control pills
    c. Chemotherapy
    d. Iron supplements

290. A 40-year-old male patient comes to the ER for shortness of breath and palpitations for 2 days. He's never had these symptoms before. His past medical history includes tobacco abuse and hypertension. His vital signs are as follows: BP 142/85; HR 136; RR 14; temperature 98.6; oxygen saturation 99% on room air. An electrocardiogram shows atrial fibrillation (AF). The patient is given Cardizem for rate control, and he notes a bit later that he is feeling much better. A repeat electrocardiogram shows conversion to sinus rhythm. Which of the following is the most appropriate intervention?

    a. Evaluate for the underlying cause.
    b. Prepare for cardiac catheterization
    c. Consult for cardioversion.
    d. Admit to ICU.

291. A 71-year-old female with a history of well-controlled diabetes and hypertension is admitted for a first-time embolic stroke. Her home medications include amlodipine, aspirin 81 mg, metoprolol succinate 100 mg, and metformin 500 mg. Further investigation reveals that the patient has paroxysmal atrial fibrillation. It has been 12 hours since administration of tissue plasminogen activator (tPA). Which of the following is the most appropriate next step?

    a. Prescribe aspirin 325 mg.
    b. Start IV heparin and PO warfarin.
    c. Prescribe clopidogrel 75 mg.
    d. Plan to start dabigatran 24 hours after tPA.

292. Which of the following is NOT an appropriate intervention for a partial small-bowel obstruction?

    a. Antibiotics
    b. Intravenous (IV) fluids
    c. Nasogastric tube
    d. Antiemetic medications

293. A 36-year-old nulliparous female comes to the OB-GYN clinic for post-coital bleeding for the past several weeks. She admits to having unprotected sex with multiple partners. She has a known history of tobacco abuse, hypothyroidism, obesity, and diabetes, but is noncompliant with medical follow-up. She has been on oral contraceptives since her teens. She is ultimately diagnosed with cervical cancer. Which of the following is a risk factor for her diagnosis?

    a. Diabetes
    b. Oral contraceptives
    c. Nulliparity
    d. Age

294. A 20-year-old female with no significant past medical history complains of intermittent dizziness associated with certain body positions. The symptoms usually resolve with rest or changing position. She denies change in vision, focal motor deficit, ataxia, facial asymmetry, or change in hearing. What is the etiology for her diagnosis?

    a. Cerumen impaction
    b. Inner ear disturbance
    c. Parkinson disease
    d. Acoustic neuroma

295. A 16-year-old male is referred to a gastroenterology office for intermittent grayish, oily, foul-smelling diarrhea, flatulence, abdominal cramping, and anorexia for the past several months. There has been no recent travel, and there have been no sick contacts. His vital signs, stool culture, complete blood count, and comprehensive metabolic panel are unremarkable. The patient has the presence of serum immunoglobulin A (IgA)-class endomysial antibodies (EMA). An esophagogastroduodenoscopy (EGD) confirms the diagnosis. Which of the following is the most appropriate next step?

    a. Prescribe antibiotics.
    b. Order blood cultures.
    c. Refer for surgery.
    d. Refer to a dietician.

296. What is the primary underlying cause of spondylolisthesis?

    a. Incorrect alignment of the disk
    b. Insufficient calcium
    c. Unknown cause
    d. Infectious etiology

297. Which of the following is the least effective method of preventing unwanted pregnancy?

    a. Intrauterine device
    b. Birth control pills
    c. Withdrawal method
    d. Condoms

298. Which of the following medications is the most appropriate in treating rheumatoid arthritis?

    a. Metronidazole
    b. Meropenem
    c. Metformin
    d. Methotrexate

299. Which of the following is a major contributing factor to the development of osteoarthritis?

    a. Immune disorder
    b. Degenerative disease
    c. Congenital disorder
    d. Infectious etiology

300. An 82-year-old male with a known history of osteoarthritis comes to your clinic complaining of worsening back pain. During the examination, you notice he has a C-shaped curvature of his spine, causing him to look like a hunchback. What is the most likely diagnosis for this condition?

    a. Kyphosis
    b. Cauda equina syndrome
    c. Avascular necrosis
    d. Sciatica

Answer Key and Explanations for Test #1

1. C: The Cushing triad is a clinical triad defined as hypertension, bradycardia, and irregular respirations. It suggests rising intracranial pressure due to intracranial pathology such as hemorrhage. The Beck triad is the combination of distended jugular veins, hypotension, and muffled heart sounds. It occurs as a result of pericardial effusion. The Charcot triad is the combination of jaundice, fever, and right upper quadrant abdominal pain. It occurs as a result of ascending cholangitis. The Bergman triad is the combination of dyspnea, petechiae, and mental status changes. It occurs when a patient has a fat embolism.

2. A: Major manifestations of acute rheumatic fever include the following:

- Erythema marginatum: raised, nonpruritic, pink rings on the trunk and inner surfaces of the limbs
- Carditis: inflammation of the heart muscle
- Chorea: rapid, uncontrolled body movements
- Subcutaneous nodules: painless, firm collections of collagen fibers over bones or tendons
- Polyarthritis: temporary migrating inflammation of the large joints

Minor manifestations of acute rheumatic fever include the following:

- Fever (101 °F to 102 °F)
- Arthralgia: joint pain without swelling
- Elevated ESR or C-reactive protein (CRP)
- Leukocytosis
- Prior episode of rheumatic heart disease or rheumatic fever
- Heart block seen on an electrocardiogram (ECG)

3. D: Psoriasis causes cells to build up rapidly on the surface of the skin, forming itchy, dry, red, raised patches covered with grayish silvery lesions that are easily friable. Psoriasis is sometimes painful. Plaques frequently occur on the skin of the elbows and knees, but they can affect any area. This is a chronic condition. Impetigo is a bacterial infection that is most commonly caused by *Staphylococcus aureus* or *Streptococcus pyogenes*. It causes lesions that can occur anywhere on the body. They are small, red, and pus-filled and can crack open and form a thick yellow or honey-colored crust. They occur most commonly in young children. Tinea corporis, also known as "ringworm," is a fungal infection that develops on the superficial layer of the skin, occurring anywhere on the body. It is characterized by an itchy, red, circular rash with a central clearing. Rosacea is a chronic inflammatory skin condition characterized by redness of the face, most commonly on the cheeks, nose, forehead, and chin.

4. B: In Crohn disease, the colon wall may have a "cobblestone" appearance due to the intermittent pattern of affected and nonaffected colonic tissue. Celiac sprue is an immune reaction that damages the lining of the small intestine and prevents it from absorbing important nutrients. A diagnosis can be made by an upper endoscopy with biopsy. Ulcerative colitis usually affects continuous stretches of the colon and rectum. Whipple disease is rare chronic disease caused by a bacterial infection (*Tropheryma whipplei*). The affected bowel is usually swollen with raised, yellowish patches.

5. C: A positive Murphy sign aids in the diagnosis of acute cholecystitis. The Brudzinski sign is positive when flexion of the neck usually causes flexion of the hip and knee. This maneuver is used to help diagnose meningitis. The psoas sign is positive when a patient experiences abdominal pain when he or she actively flexes the leg at the hip and knee. This maneuver is used to help diagnose appendicitis. The Levine sign is positive when a patient is holding a clenched fist over his or her chest to describe dull, pressing chest pain consistent with the discomfort of angina pectoris.

6. B: Vicryl sutures are absorbable. They take anywhere from 42 to 70 days to completely absorb. Other examples of absorbable sutures include Monocryl, PDS, and chromic gut. Prolene, silk, and nylon sutures are all nonabsorbable sutures. Other examples of nonabsorbable suture materials include polyester sutures and stainless-steel sutures. Dermabond is a type of skin adhesive meant for superficial skin lacerations; it should never be used on any other surface besides the skin.

7. C: Esophageal achalasia is a dysmotility issue involving the lower esophageal sphincter not relaxing properly. This impairs the smooth passage of food and liquids from the lower esophagus into the stomach. Acid reflux, dysphagia, and chest pain are symptoms of esophageal achalasia. Hematochezia is when a person has bright-red blood coming from the rectum. This occurrence is commonly associated with gastrointestinal (GI) bleeding.

8. C: CREST syndrome includes five main features: **C**alcinosis, **R**aynaud phenomenon, **E**sophageal dysmotility, **S**clerodactyly, and **T**elangiectasia. The CREST syndrome is part of the autoimmune disorder systemic sclerosis (scleroderma). This immune disorder causes skin and body tissues to improperly tighten. Solar urticaria is the development of hives when the skin is exposed to sunlight; it is not related to CREST syndrome.

9. B: Reiter syndrome causes inflammation of the urinary tract, eyes, skin, mucous membranes, and joints. Chlamydia is the most common cause of Reiter syndrome. Sjögren syndrome is a disorder of the immune system that causes a decrease in the production of mucus and moisture. Turner syndrome is a genetic condition in which females are missing all or part of an X chromosome. Some of the symptoms may include infertility, amenorrhea, short stature, and webbed neck. Down syndrome is a genetic condition in which there is a chromosomal abnormality on chromosome 21 (trisomy 21). Some signs of Down syndrome may include broad forehead and tongue, slanted eyes, small ears, and cognitive and cardiac defects.

10. D: Ceftriaxone 250 mg IM injection in a single dose plus azithromycin 1 g PO in a single dose (or in place of azithromycin, doxycycline 100 mg PO BID for 7 days) is the recommended regimen for treating gonorrhea (GC)/chlamydia infections. Clindamycin is not given as treatment for either gonorrhea or chlamydia. The patient should be treated in the ER for suspected GC/chlamydia infection to prevent the patient from potentially spreading the disease.

11. B: Naloxone (Narcan) is an opiate antidote to treat potential or confirmed narcotic overdoses. Oxycodone is an opiate. Prednisolone is a corticosteroid drug. It is useful for the treatment of a wide range of inflammatory and autoimmune conditions. Buspirone is an anxiolytic used for short-term relief of anxiety symptoms. Although this may be useful as an occasional maintenance drug for the patient's history of anxiety, he is not anxious during the examination.

12. D: Augmentin is a penicillin, and cefepime and cephalexin are cephalosporins. Approximately 10% of patients with a penicillin reaction may also have an allergy to the cephalosporins. In patients with a documented allergy to penicillins, the use of cephalosporins is contraindicated. Clarithromycin is a macrolide and may be safely administered to a patient with a penicillin allergy.

13. A: Pegged teeth, swollen joints, gummatous ulcers, deafness, and blindness are characteristic of congenital syphilis. Down syndrome patients have a myriad of physical signs, such as broad forehead and tongue, eyelid creases, small ears, short stature, and a flat head. They do not have pegged teeth and generally have unusually flexible joints. Osgood-Schlatter disease is characterized by chronic knee pain in young children and adolescents. Turner syndrome is a genetic condition in which females are missing all or part of an X chromosome. Some of the symptoms may include infertility, amenorrhea, short stature, and a webbed neck.

14. B: A hordeolum, or stye, appears as a red, swollen, tender pimple on the edge of the eyelid. It is caused by an infected eyelash follicle. Xanthelasmas are raised, yellow patches on the eyelids. The incidence of occurrence increases with age; they are common in patients with hyperlipidemia and are not painful. Mongolian spots are a non-raised, grayish-blue skin lesion most commonly seen on the sacrum or buttocks. A felon is an infection/abscess inside the fingertip that can expand and affect adjacent tissues if left untreated.

15. D: Xanthelasmas are raised yellow patches on the eyelids. The incidence of occurrence increases with age. They are common in patients with hyperlipidemia. Dermoid cysts are growths or outpouchings that may contain miscellaneous structures such as skin, hair, or teeth. They are not lesions that begin later in life; they are slow-growing/present at birth. Impetigo is a bacterial infection that is most commonly caused by *Staphylococcus aureus* or *Streptococcus pyogenes*. It causes lesions that can occur anywhere on the body. They are small, red, and pus-filled and can crack open and form a thick yellow or honey-colored crust. They occur most commonly in young children. Mongolian spots are flat, blue or blue-gray skin markings near the buttocks that commonly appear at birth or shortly thereafter.

16. C: Medulloblastomas are the most common malignant brain tumor and are significantly more common in children than in adults. They usually occur in the cerebellum. A hygroma is a collection of cerebrospinal fluid in the subdural space. Acute hygromas are usually caused by head trauma or a recent neurosurgical procedure. Schistosomiasis is a chronic parasitic infection due to eating improperly cooked pork. On an MRI scan of the brain, it can appear as multiple enhancing nodules occurring on bilateral cerebral hemispheres. Melanoma is a malignant skin cancer.

17. A: The Charcot triad is the combination of jaundice, fever, and right upper quadrant abdominal pain. It occurs as a result of acute cholangitis (ascending cholangitis), which involves bile duct obstruction and infection (usually due to bacteria ascending the GI tract). Acute appendicitis usually presents as periumbilical, epigastric, or right lower quadrant abdominal pain, fever, nausea, vomiting, and extreme sensitivity to movement. Choledocholithiasis is the presence of stones within the common bile duct but without infection. The pain is colicky, but patients do not always display symptoms. Acute pyelonephritis usually presents as fever, shaking chills, costovertebral angle pain, nausea, vomiting, and urinary tract infection (UTI) symptoms.

18. C: In early pregnancy, high levels of estrogen cause increased venous pressure, causing the mucosal surfaces of the genitals to turn a purplish or bluish color (Chadwick sign). The obturator sign is positive when abdominal pain is elicited with the internal rotation of the flexed right leg. This maneuver helps diagnose appendicitis. The Levine sign is positive when a patient is holding a clenched fist over his or her chest to describe pressing or squeezing chest pain consistent with the discomfort of angina/ischemia chest pain. The Kernig sign is positive when a patient is unable to extend his or her leg when the hip is flexed. This maneuver helps diagnose meningitis.

19. A: Colchicine is used only in acute gout attacks. Allopurinol (Zyloprim) is used for the treatment of chronic gout, and is used to prevent rather than treat gout attacks. Other treatments for gout include nonsteroidal anti-inflammatory drugs (NSAIDs) and steroids. Tetracycline is an antibiotic and is not used to treat gout. Amantadine has been used in the treatment of the influenza virus and for Parkinson disease.

20. A: The Dix-Hallpike test or maneuver checks for positional vertigo (BPPV) and involves a patient sitting upright with his or her head laterally rotated to one side. The patient is helped to lie down quickly with his or her head slightly extended beyond the end of the table. The test is considered positive if this maneuver reproduces symptoms of vertigo or nystagmus. An electroencephalogram (EEG) helps diagnose seizures or abnormal brain activity. The transcranial Doppler (TCD) ultrasound measures the presence of vasospasm in the brain's blood vessels. The Phalen maneuver is a diagnostic tool used to help diagnose carpal tunnel syndrome by flexing the wrist for 30 seconds, which reproduces symptoms.

21. B: This child has Down syndrome, which is caused by an extra chromosome 21 (trisomy 21). Chromosome 23 is the sex chromosome. Patients with abnormalities on chromosome 13 (also known as Patau syndrome) usually have serious brain, pulmonary, and circulatory defects that are often fatal. Few patients survive infancy. Those that survive have severe intellectual and physical disabilities. Turner syndrome is a genetic condition in which females are missing all or part of an X chromosome. Some symptoms may include infertility, amenorrhea, short stature, and webbed neck. Klinefelter syndrome patients have an extra Y chromosome, leading to poor muscle strength, decreased fertility or infertility, gynecomastia, and low testosterone levels. There is no chromosome 24. All humans have 23 chromosomal pairs, totaling 46 chromosomes.

22. A: Electrical alternans is the alternation of the amplitude or axis of the QRS complex between beats, most commonly seen with pericardial tamponade or severe pericardial effusion. Given the patient's history of recent surgery and his diagnosis of pericardial tamponade, this patient most likely has Dressler syndrome. This can occur days to months after a cardiac injury when the body mistakenly attacks healthy heart tissue.

23. C: Severe ischemia can result in ECG changes within minutes of the occurrence. Other helpful diagnostic aids would include troponin level, creatine phosphokinase-MB (CPK-MB) level, and a two-dimensional echocardiogram (2D echo). These aids can be more diagnostic than an ECG, but an ECG result is obtained much quicker than blood work or a 2D echo. It takes a minimum of 3 hours for a cardiac insult to be reflected in blood tests. Choice A would show an anterior MI. Choice B would show a lateral-wall MI. Choice D would show a posterior-wall MI.

24. B: There are two types of second-degree heart block. Mobitz type I (Wenckebach block) is characterized by progressive prolongation of the PR interval on beats followed by a blocked P wave/dropped QRS complex. The PR interval resets, and the cycle repeats. Mobitz type II heart block is characterized by intermittently nonconducting P waves. The PR interval remains unchanged. In first-degree heart block, there is a prolonged PR interval that regularly precedes a QRS complex. In third-degree heart block (complete heart block), there is no apparent relationship between P waves and QRS complexes. Asystole is a state of no cardiac electrical activity.

25. A: The other modalities would be used if the patient had symptomatic bradycardia. Choice A may be a part of the workup, although an ECG is usually all that is necessary. Symptoms of bradycardia may include pallor, weakness, dizziness, altered mental status, fatigue, and shortness of breath. If the patient had been symptomatic, atropine would have been the first-line agent used. In the event that atropine is ineffective, epinephrine and dopamine may be used. If the patient continues to display signs of poor perfusion, he or she may be a candidate for transcutaneous pacing.

26. D: Hypertension is not a factor in the Beck triad. The Beck triad is the combination of distended jugular veins due to increased venous pressure, hypotension due to low arterial pressure, and muffled heart sounds due to excessive fluid around the heart. It occurs as a result of pericardial effusion. Aside from physical examination findings, an electrocardiogram (ECG) and/or a two-dimensional echocardiogram may help diagnose this condition.

27. C: Warm air does not commonly cause an asthma exacerbation, although extreme heat or humidity may cause an asthma attack. Cold air usually triggers an asthma attack because it can irritate the airways. Sinusitis, or any upper respiratory infection that affects breathing, can cause irritation and induce an asthma attack. Allergens such as dust and pollen can aggravate the airways, which can induce an asthma attack. Cigarette smoke is a common trigger that can cause irritation and inflammation in the airways, which can aggravate asthma. Patients who live around tobacco smokers are predisposed to developing asthma.

28. B: All the choices are a part of the islets of Langerhans, which are responsible for the endocrine function of the pancreas. Beta cells secrete insulin, which stimulates the cells to use and store glucose, lowering the blood sugar levels. Alpha cells produce glucagon, which stimulates cells to break down their glucose reserves to raise the serum glucose level. Gamma cells (or PP cells) of the pancreas secrete a specialized type of peptide, which is thought to reduce one's appetite. Delta cells of the pancreas secrete somatostatin, which plays a role in food absorption by the small intestine.

29. D: Diabetics are at risk for hypertension, not hypotension. Diabetics have higher levels of blood sugar because the pancreas produces insufficient or no insulin. High levels of blood glucose stimulate systemic inflammation and atherosclerosis formation, causing a multitude of other pathologies. Atherosclerotic plaques decrease the lumen of blood vessels, causing hypertension. Excessive deposits in the renal tubules can cause chronic renal insufficiency and potentially renal failure. The systemic inflammation caused by diabetes can also lead to neuropathy.

30. D: The most effective treatment of *Helicobacter pylori* is the combination of two antibiotics (amoxicillin and clarithromycin, or metronidazole) plus a proton pump inhibitor. Two antibiotics are recommended due to potential antibiotic resistance. In areas with increased resistance (>15%) to clarithromycin, quadruple therapy is used (PPI plus bismuth, metronidazole, and tetracycline). It is recommended that the patient be treated for 10 to 14 days to increase the chances of complete recovery.

31. A: Obesity is not a major risk factor. More than half of the diagnosed cases of peptic ulcers are caused by *Helicobacter pylori. H. pylori* may be diagnosed with a stool antigen test, a blood antibody test, and a carbon urea breath test, as well as other modalities. Major risk factors include smoking, alcohol consumption, and nonsteroidal anti-inflammatory drug (NSAID) use.

32. D: Parkinson disease destroys dopamine-producing neurons in the substantia nigra and causes motor symptoms (dyskinesia, tremor, rigidity) as well as cognitive symptoms. Approximately 80% of the substantia nigra is destroyed prior to the onset of symptoms. Norepinephrine and epinephrine are major components in the body's fight-or-flight response. Serotonin is involved with a multitude of functions, including mood, cell growth, and hemostasis.

33. B: The Tzanck smear is a quick, inexpensive test that helps diagnose diseases caused by herpes simplex viruses. A viral culture is much more sensitive, but the result takes longer.

34. C: Left bundle branch block acts as a red flag for four conditions: severe aortic valve disease, ischemic heart disease, chronic hypertension, and cardiomyopathy. Pericardial tamponade generally has abnormalities with QRS complexes on the ECG. Pulmonary emboli are generally diagnosed by ventilation-perfusion (VQ) scan or computed tomography (CT) angiogram of the chest. In some patients with a pulmonary embolus, the ECG may be normal. The most common ECG findings are T-wave abnormalities. Mitral valve prolapse is generally not diagnosed on an ECG. It is usually diagnosed by the patient's history, auscultation with a stethoscope, and two-dimensional echocardiogram.

35. B: This patient may have a pulmonary embolus, which is best diagnosed with a CT angiogram of the chest. Sickle cell disease increases the risk of pulmonary embolus, stroke, heart attack, pulmonary hypertension, skin ulcers, priapism, and other health problems. A CT scan of the chest without contrast would most likely be nondiagnostic. Waiting for a troponin level or an ABG would increase the risk of mortality in this patient.

36. D: Small pneumothoraxes (approximately 5% to 10% in size) can be monitored on a telemetry floor with daily chest x-rays. No intervention may be warranted, and they may resolve without invasive measures.

37. A: According to the American Heart Association, the most common congenital heart defect is ventricular septal defect. The hole may be small and may spontaneously close on its own. If the hole is small but remains patent, the patient may be asymptomatic. If the hole is large enough to cause symptoms, it may warrant surgical intervention. The occurrence of aortic stenosis increases with age, but it is not the most common heart defect. Tricuspid atresia is one of the most uncommon cyanotic congenital heart defects. Tetralogy of Fallot is the most common type of cyanotic congenital heart defect.

38. D: A persistent, dry cough is the most common side effect of taking ACE inhibitors. The development of a cough is not serious and does not have any long-term health complications. In the event that the cough persists, the patient should be placed on a different medication regimen. Switching to another ACE inhibitor would not be helpful because if one ACE inhibitor causes a cough, all medications of this class would likely cause the same symptom.

39. C: *Staphylococcus aureus* is a gram-positive coccus that is responsible for common skin infections as well as other illnesses. *Staphylococcus pseudintermedius* is a gram-positive coccus. It is very common in animals, especially dogs, but it is rare in humans. *Haemophilus influenzae* is a gram-negative coccobacillus. It is a main cause of pneumonia, meningitis, and other pathologies. It does not commonly cause skin infections.

Streptococcus pneumoniae is one of the main causative organisms in pneumonia, meningitis, and other pathologies. It is much less common in skin infections.

40. D: Addison disease is caused by a lack of cortisol. Giving cortisol exogenously helps alleviate the disease's symptoms, which include hyperpigmentation and hypotension. Diabetes is caused by insufficient (or complete lack of) insulin production. Many diabetic patients depend on insulin injections in order to help control their disease. Patients with insufficient growth hormone depend on somatropin injections to help correct their symptoms. Synthroid (levothyroxine) is a medication taken by patients with hypothyroidism.

41. B: The patient's noncompliance with COPD management has caused the patient to develop cor pulmonale (right-sided heart failure; "blue-bloater"). B-type natriuretic peptide is produced by the cardiac ventricles and helps monitor fluid balance; it becomes elevated in cases of heart failure. COPD increases the right ventricle's afterload, which causes the ventricle to swell and become dilated. Perfusion becomes more strenuous, and the body's blood pressure increases to keep pace. This patient's workup should also include a CBC and chemistry panel, chest x-ray, ECG, pulse oximetry, arterial blood gases, and an echo.

42. C: Desmopressin is another name for antidiuretic hormone (ADH), used in treating those who have diabetes insipidus. This patient most likely has diabetes insipidus caused by their traumatic head injury. Diabetes insipidus is caused by insufficient ADH, which causes the body to conserve little if any water. This condition may be caused by trauma, surgery, or infection.

43. B: Sickle cell disease is an autosomal-recessive genetic blood disorder caused by a defect on chromosome 11. Patients who have only one recessive allele have sickle cell trait; they are usually asymptomatic and do not suffer the same medical complications as those with the disease. Sickle cell disease increases the risk of stroke, heart attack, pulmonary hypertension, skin ulcers, priapism, and other health problems. Sickle cell disease does not increase the risk for diabetes.

44. D: The patient has a urinary tract infection (UTI) and needs an antibiotic to cover gram-negative organisms. The most common cause of UTIs is *Escherichia coli*. Appropriate first-line treatment for uncomplicated UTIs in females includes nitrofurantoin, TMP-SMX, fosfomycin, and pivmecillinam. Choice A would be used to treat potential gonorrhea (GC)/chlamydia infections. Ciprofloxacin 250 mg PO BID × 3 days is second-line and reserved for complicated cases due to increased resistance. Augmentin is a second-line treatment. Patients with an uncomplicated UTI should be treated for a minimum of 3 days and up to 7 days, depending on the antibiotic.

45. A: Macrobid is a category B medication; these are generally considered safe for use in pregnant women. The other choices are category C medications. Category C medications have shown potential adverse effects in prior research studies, but they may sometimes be used depending on the importance of the indication. Because the patient has a urinary tract infection—which is important, but not life-threatening—and she has no drug allergies, there are safer alternatives to category C medications. Other safe antibiotic choices in pregnancy include cephalexin, amoxicillin, and Augmentin.

46. A: You should advise all patients with presumed or confirmed venereal disease to inform their partner(s) as soon as possible so they can also get tested. This helps to prevent others from spreading the disease and potentially infecting more people. As a medical provider, you cannot tell the patient's family or loved ones without permission; doing so would break Health Insurance Portability and Accountability Act (HIPAA) privacy laws.

47. D: The child has likely aspirated his toy. Because the patient is hypoxic, a stat bronchoscopy should be performed to confirm the diagnosis and remove the object. While waiting for a pulmonologist to evaluate the patient, the patient should be maintained on a non-rebreather mask.

48. D: Pyridium is often given in conjunction with an antibiotic to help alleviate dysuria. The most common side effect of Pyridium is bright-orange urine. Other common side effects may include headache and rash.

Although the decision to discontinue the medication must be based on the severity of the side effects, a change in urine color should not be the reason to discontinue the medication. The urine will go back to its normal color once the medication course has been completed.

49. C: Increasing one's fluid intake is the most important way to help prevent kidney stones. Kidney stones are usually made up of calcium oxalate, which can be found in dairy, fruits such as apples and grapes, vegetables such as broccoli and turnips, beer, and several other foods. Those who suffer from kidney stones may find it advisable to limit foods high in calcium oxalate.

50. B: Escitalopram (Lexapro) is a selective serotonin reuptake inhibitor (SSRI) commonly used to treat anxiety and depression. Levothyroxine is a synthetic thyroid hormone medication used for those with hypothyroid disease. Amiodarone is used to treat cardiac arrhythmias such as atrial fibrillation and ventricular fibrillation. Haloperidol is an antipsychotic medication. Because this woman has no history of psychotic episodes, this medication would not be appropriate.

51. A: The hallmarks of COPD are airflow obstruction with a persistent and productive cough, and progressively declining pulmonary function tests (progressive decline in FEV1 over time). Hypoxia on an arterial blood gas test (PaO_2 <75 mmHg) can be seen in both COPD and acute asthma exacerbations. Expiratory wheezes and atelectasis are nonspecific findings that can be seen in both.

52. C: Cauda equina syndrome can be caused by disease, trauma, or infection. It is caused by severe compression of the nerve roots below the termination of the spinal cord (below L1), which can cause motor dysfunction, urinary retention, and saddle anesthesia, among other neurologic issues. It can be diagnosed clinically and by exam and is confirmed with a computed tomography (CT) scan or magnetic resonance image (MRI). A spinal surgeon or neurosurgeon will decide whether or not the patient needs surgical decompression based on the presentation and radiological findings. Kyphosis is a curvature of the thoracic spine, causing a "hunchback" appearance. Fibromyalgia is a disease that causes chronic pain, which is potentially due to oversensitive nerves. A greenstick fracture is most commonly seen in children due to the flexibility of their bones. It occurs when the bony cortex bends abnormally, causing a partial break.

53. C: Slipped capital femoral epiphysis is when the femoral head is displaced from the acetabulum, causing hip and knee pain as well as gait disturbances. Once diagnosed, it is usually surgically corrected to prevent avascular necrosis of the femoral head. It is usually seen in prepubescent and pubescent children who are going through a growth spurt. Osteitis pubis is a noninfectious inflammation of the pubic symphysis, causing lower abdominal or groin pain. This condition is normally seen in athletes. Developmental dysplasia of the hip is when a child is born with instability of one or both femoral heads, which can become displaced from the acetabulum. This is typically diagnosed when the child is a newborn by checking for a hip "clunk" using the Ortolani and Barlow maneuvers. However, this may occur at any time during the growth process. Paget disease is the abnormal degeneration of bone tissue and replacement with new, but weaker bone tissue usually in a localized area in the body. It is extremely uncommon in children.

54. D: Bisphosphonates (such as Fosamax), NSAIDs, and calcitonin are the mainstays of treatment for Paget disease. Paget disease is the abnormal degeneration and formation of bone, usually in a localized area of the axial skeleton. Alkaline phosphatase is found in bone; after bony destruction or injury, it is released into the blood, increasing serum levels. It is one way to diagnose this disease. The diagnosis can also be made on CT scan, magnetic resonance imaging (MRI), or bone scan. Colchicine would provide little value because it is used to treat acute gout exacerbations.

55. B: Retinal artery occlusion causes sudden, painless loss of vision and is commonly caused by a clot that blocks the blood flow to the eye. It is common in patients with coagulopathy disorders, hypertension, diabetes, or advanced atherosclerosis. Conjunctivitis is the bacterial, viral, or allergy-induced inflammation of the conjunctiva, which may cause a foreign-body sensation, redness, visual disturbances, itching, tearing, and discharge. It does not cause sudden, painless blindness. Acute angle-closure glaucoma occurs when the intraocular pressure is so high that it damages the optic nerve, which can impair vision and cause severe eye pain. Prior to actually losing their vision, patients usually note visual disturbances, such as seeing halos around objects. They may also present with headache on the same side as the vision loss, orbital or periorbital pain, nausea, and vomiting. Retinal detachment is painless and commonly caused by trauma, but it can also be caused by advanced age or disease processes such as diabetes. Immediately prior to losing vision (which is described as being like a curtain closing), patients usually have partial vision loss or visual disturbances such as the appearance of flashes and floaters, which is different from this patient's presentation.

56. D: Midodrine is an inotrope that can be used to treat orthostatic hypotension. It works by limiting the ability of the blood vessels to expand, which in turn raises blood pressure. Orthostatic hypotension is a condition in which the systolic blood pressure drops by >20 mmHg and/or the diastolic blood pressure drops by >10 mmHg when the patient goes from the sitting/supine position to an upright position.

57. D: The collection of nerve roots that exit the base of the spinal cord below L1 is known as the cauda equina. Cauda equina syndrome occurs when these nerve roots are compressed and disrupt motor and sensory function to the lower extremities and bladder. It is a medical emergency that requires surgical intervention within 24-48 hours. Delay in treatment can result in permanent sensory deficits, paralysis, erectile dysfunction, and bladder or bowel dysfunction.

58. B: Antibiotic eardrops and pain medications are the mainstays of medical management of otitis externa. Oral antibiotics are generally not prescribed. Imaging of the brain or the ears is generally not indicated unless abscess or osteomyelitis is suspected; these complications are very rare. An ENT consult is not necessary for otitis externa. It is a very common condition that usually resolves with antibiotics.

59. A: If there has not been any acute trauma or severe neurologic symptoms, a small subdural hygroma on a CT scan of the head will be an incidental finding. However, because this patient has a history of trauma and is on anticoagulation, an MRI of the brain should be ordered to differentiate a subdural hematoma from a subdural hygroma.

60. D: Approximately 80% of miscarriages occur during the first trimester and are caused by chromosomal abnormalities. Miscarriages that occur in the second or third trimester are usually caused by drug or alcohol abuse, trauma, severe infection, or uterine or cervical abnormalities. Cervical insufficiency (previously incompetent cervix) may cause the cervix to dilate prematurely, causing a spontaneous abortion. Treatment for cervical insufficiency is a cerclage.

61. D: Guillain-Barré syndrome is an autoimmune disorder in which the body attacks its own nervous system; this is a medical emergency. The cause is generally unknown, but having certain viral or bacterial infections increases the risk of developing this disorder. Symmetric weakness and paresthesias usually begin distally and move upwards. A lumbar puncture may help diagnosis this, but it is not used as a therapeutic aid, a preventative aid, or a way to speed up recovery. Interventions include supportive care, intubation, plasmapheresis, and treatment with IVIG.

62. B: Although the patient is at risk for developing diabetes, his fasting blood sugar and hemoglobin A1C are normal. Medications at this point are unnecessary. Rechecking the hemoglobin A1C in 1 week would be useless because it is a calculation of an average blood sugar level over a 3-month period. This patient's hemoglobin A1C doesn't need to be checked for at least another 3 months.

63. B: This woman should be checked when she is 38 years old. The current recommendation in the US (ACP, ACG, USPSTF) is to get screened 10 years prior to the age of a first-degree relative who was diagnosed with colon cancer. If no risk factors are present, then it is recommended to obtain a colonoscopy by 50 years of age. Because her father was 48 years old when he was diagnosed, she should get screened at age 38. If she had no significant family history, then her first colonoscopy should be when she is 50 years old, or 45 years old if she were African American. The latest recommendation of the American Cancer Society (ACS) now states that screening should begin at 45 years old.

64. C: Erythromycin should be given to prophylactically treat close contacts (e.g., household) of those with pertussis (given within 21 days of the start of the cough in the patient). Prophylaxis should also be given within 21 days to high-risk people who are exposed (e.g., <12 months old, in third trimester of pregnancy, immunodeficient, asthmatic). Prophylaxis is the same as the treatment for pertussis (adults: erythromycin 500 mg QID × 14 days). Alternative antibiotics: clarithromycin, azithromycin, TMP-SMX. Augmentin, clindamycin, and guaifenesin play no role in the treatment or prevention of pertussis. The most important way to prevent pertussis is to get vaccinated.

65. C: The patient has RSV. It is an acute, self-limiting, usually non-life-threatening virus that most commonly presents with a cough and wheezing. It is more prevalent in children who attend day care and in children <2 years old. The patient's fever and other presenting symptoms make asthma a less likely diagnosis. Pneumonia usually presents with a high fever (above 101.5 °F), productive cough, myalgia, shortness of breath, as well as a myriad of other symptoms. A barking cough is usually not present. Patients with cystic fibrosis display signs and symptoms very early in life, such as abdominal discomfort from chronic constipation, poor weight gain, steatorrhea, salty-tasting skin, poor appetite, fatigue, fever, and pancreatitis. It would not develop suddenly in a 3-year-old child with no prior symptoms.

66. D: The goal INR for a mechanical mitral valve is 2.5-3.5. This patient is subtherapeutic and should be given warfarin.

67. D: Mongolian spots are flat, blue or blue-gray skin markings near the buttocks and lower spine that commonly appear at birth or shortly thereafter in babies with darker skin. No intervention is needed; they commonly fade by the time the child reaches elementary school. If neurologic symptoms or spots are extensive, further workup is needed.

68. A: Oxymetazoline hydrochloride is a nasal decongestant that may cause rhinitis medicamentosa or rebound nasal congestion. Patients should be advised to discontinue the medication after 3 to 5 days to prevent this from happening. Benzonatate is an antitussive that does not cause rhinitis medicamentosa. Ofloxacin is an antibiotic eardrop used to treat infections of the ear canal (otitis externa). Guaifenesin is an expectorant used to treat cough and chest congestion.

69. D: This patient is at an intermediate risk for atherosclerotic cardiovascular disease (ASCVD). He should be given a baby aspirin for prophylaxis against potential future heart attacks, as well as simvastatin for his hyperlipidemia (since his LDL is >160 and he has a positive family history), and he should initiate lifestyle modifications. It is recommended that one's total cholesterol should be <150 and LDL level should be ≤100. His blood pressure, heart rate, fasting glucose, two-dimensional echocardiogram, and stress test are normal; prescribing antihypertensive medications such as metoprolol and amlodipine is unnecessary.

70. C: Pyloric stenosis commonly presents in neonates, but presentation of symptoms may start when the child is several months old. The chief symptoms are abdominal pain, dehydration, swollen abdomen, and, most notably, projectile vomiting. The narrowed pylorus may feel like a small "olive" mass in the epigastrium. A Mallory-Weiss tear in the esophageal junction is often seen in alcoholic patients. It is caused by persistent episodes of vomiting; however, any pathologic process that causes forceful coughing or vomiting may cause a Mallory-Weiss tear. GERD and gastritis may cause abdominal discomfort and occasionally vomiting, but they would not cause projectile vomiting or failure to thrive, or be associated with an abdominal mass.

71. C: A Mallory-Weiss tear in the esophageal junction is usually seen in alcoholic patients, and is caused by persistent episodes of vomiting; however, any pathologic process that causes forceful coughing or vomiting may cause a Mallory-Weiss tear. Pyloric stenosis commonly presents in neonates, but presentation of symptoms may start when the child is several months old. It does not suddenly present in the seventh decade of life. Celiac sprue is an immune reaction that damages the lining of the small intestine and prevents it from absorbing important nutrients. It presents with nausea, vomiting, diarrhea, and abdominal pain, which occur after ingesting gluten products. Whipple disease is a bacterial infection of the bowel. It is a rare infection that presents with fever, abdominal pain, non-bloody vomiting, diarrhea, and arthralgia.

72. B: Esotropia is a condition in which the eye deviates medially (usually one eye is affected). The result is that one eye fails to properly communicate visual images to the brain. Improper vision development, especially with depth perception, may occur. Patching the stronger eye, wearing glasses, and surgical correction for severe cases are treatments for this condition.

73. A: Systemic lupus erythematosus (SLE) is an autoimmune disorder that causes inflammation in joints and organs. There are multiple signs and symptoms, such as polyarthralgia, hair loss, and oral ulcerations; but a unique sign is a malar rash that is butterfly-shaped and covers the nose and cheeks. Patients are positive for antinuclear antibodies. Other antibodies, like antiphospholipid and anti-Sm, may be present. Evaluating renal function in SLE patients is important since early detection and treatment of renal involvement can significantly improve renal outcome.

74. A: Trimethoprim/polymyxin B ophthalmic drops have good coverage, especially against *Streptococcus pneumoniae* and *H. influenzae*, so it is an excellent choice for treating children. Erythromycin ophthalmic ointment may be used in a child with bacterial conjunctivitis, but resistance is increasing, and compliance is low due to the difficulty parents have using ophthalmic ointment. Erythromycin ophthalmic is most often used for prophylactic treatment of neonatal gonococcal infections. Trifluridine ophthalmic is used to treat keratitis caused by herpes simplex. Famciclovir is an oral antiviral used to treat keratitis caused by herpes zoster.

75. D: Niacin's most common side effect is flushing, which may be associated with pruritus. If these symptoms develop, the dosage may need to be adjusted, but the drug does not have to be discontinued. Simvastatin, atorvastatin, and rosuvastatin may possibly cause pruritus; but generally, they may cause jaundice, not flushing. Other side effects of statin medications may include fever, abdominal pain, myositis, and arthralgia.

76. A: The patient is not in any respiratory distress, and he is not hypoxic. He most likely has a bacterial pneumonia, which requires PO antibiotics. The chest x-ray shows the infiltrate: a CT scan of the chest exposes the patient to more radiation that he does not need. If he had a significant past medical history or appeared toxic, then hospitalization and IV antibiotics might be needed. The diagnosis of pneumonia can be made based on physical examination, medical history, and a chest x-ray. The patient does not need an ABG test because he is saturating 98% on room air.

77. A: Niacin may cause flushing or pruritus, but it does not have to be discontinued unless symptoms are severe. Niacin should originally be prescribed at the lowest dose possible to help prevent these symptoms; if the patient tolerates the dosage, it can always be titrated up. If flushing and pruritus do occur, patients can take medications such as Decadron and/or Benadryl. Nonsteroidal anti-inflammatory drugs (NSAIDs) taken 30-60 minutes prior to the niacin dose can help minimize flushing. It is important to monitor LFTs.

78. B: Based on the information provided and the choices given, the patient most likely has acute cholecystitis. In cases of suspected cholecystitis, an examiner may ask a patient to take a deep breath while the examiner palpates the right upper quadrant. If this maneuver elicits pain, then the patient has a positive Murphy sign. Altered mental status, jaundice, and fever are generally present in patients with ascending cholangitis. Appendicitis is located in the right lower quadrant at the McBurney point. Pyelonephritis is a kidney infection with pain at the costovertebral angle.

79. A: Von Willebrand disease (VWD) is a hereditary bleeding disorder caused by factor VIII clotting deficiency. It is a much milder form of hemophilia. Desmopressin, recombinant Von Willebrand factor (VWF), and VWF/factor VIII concentrates are treatments. Factor V Leiden leads to a hypercoagulable state with an increased risk of thrombosis. Multiple myeloma is a cancer of the plasma cells that leads to bone pain and pathologic fractures.

80. D: Addison disease (primary adrenal insufficiency) occurs when the adrenal glands produce insufficient amounts of cortisol and aldosterone. This may be due to trauma, infections like tuberculosis, or malignancy. Administration of exogenous cortisol is the mainstay of treatment. Lactate tests for the presence of lactic acidosis. Testing urine for the presence of metanephrines evaluates for the possibility of a pheochromocytoma or other tumors that produce excess catecholamines (epinephrine and norepinephrine). Thyroid-stimulating hormone tests for thyroid issues.

81. C: Hand washing is the most important measure in preventing communicable diseases. Maintaining a sterile environment at all times is not plausible. Wearing gloves is important, but the gloves may rip. If the gloves touch a contaminated surface and then touch someone's mouth or face, the gloves will not prevent illness. Wearing a face mask may help, but it does not fully prevent spreading diseases. If someone's hands are contaminated and he or she touches the mouth or eyes, wearing a face mask will not prevent the person from getting ill.

82. A: The patient most likely has a kidney stone (nephrolithiasis). Calcium stones are the most common, followed by struvite, then uric acid stones. An abdominopelvic CT scan should be ordered to confirm the diagnosis (gold standard); an ultrasound or kidney, ureter, and bladder (KUB) radiographs can also be helpful in assessing patients. Costovertebral angle tenderness is usually a sign of a kidney infection. A urine culture should be ordered, and IV fluids should be initiated.

83. B: Immediately cleansing the wound is the number one way to help prevent rabies. The rabies vaccine will prevent rabies, but it usually takes longer to obtain the vaccine than it does to wash the wound. If the animal is caught, it would have to be tested for rabies prior to subjecting the bite victim to a series of vaccinations. Administration of antibiotics may be necessary if a secondary infection develops, but this would not be useful in preventing rabies from occurring.

84. A: Lotrimin cream helps treat fungal infections, not scabies. Mites burrowing underneath the skin cause scabies infections. Topical creams such as permethrin can be used to treat infections. Pills are available for persistent infections refractory to topical treatment. Washing clothing and linens in hot water and avoiding infected people are ways to help prevent the spread of infection.

85. B: Listeriosis is spread through contaminated food. It is recommended to thoroughly wash produce, cook meat and fish prior to eating it, avoid unpasteurized milk or juice, and limit processed foods such as hot dogs and deli meats during pregnancy (should heat these to 165 °F). Hot dogs and deli meats may be contaminated after they are cooked and prior to being packaged. Pregnant women infected with listeriosis may only exhibit mild symptoms, but the infection may result in death of the fetus.

86. B: Hypervolemia is the least likely to cause cardiac arrest. There are 12 main causes of cardiac arrest (six H's and six T's): hypovolemia, hypoxia, hydrogen ions (acidosis), hyperkalemia, hypokalemia, hypothermia, toxins, tamponade, tension pneumothorax, thrombosis, thromboembolism, and trauma. Hypervolemia may increase the heart's preload, which may eventually lead to heart failure, but it is much less likely to cause a myocardial infarction.

87. A: Levothyroxine is a synthetic thyroid hormone used to treat hypothyroidism. An abnormally high TSH indicates hypothyroidism: The thyroid gland is trying to make more thyroxine (T4) because there isn't enough T4 in the blood. The free T4 index measures how much unattached T4 is in the blood and available to get into cells.

88. D: The patient likely has acute meningitis. The triad of meningitis is fever, nuchal rigidity, and headache. Photophobia, lethargy, nausea, vomiting, anorexia, and flu-like symptoms are also common. The patient has a positive Brudzinski sign. Brudzinski sign is positive when flexion of the neck causes flexion of the hip and knee due to inflammation of the meninges. A CT scan or MRI of the brain may show diffuse inflammation and cerebral edema. A lumbar puncture will help detect the specific organism. Blood cultures should be sent, but a lumbar puncture is the priority.

89. D: A colonoscopy will directly visualize the lesion. A biopsy of the lesion can show practitioners what type of malignancy is present and can direct their care. Sigmoidoscopy cannot visualize a lesion in the proximal transverse colon.

90. A: In first-degree heart block, there is a prolonged PR interval that regularly precedes a QRS complex. There are two types of second-degree heart block. Mobitz type I, or Wenckebach block, is characterized by progressive prolongation of the PR interval on beats followed by a blocked P wave/dropped QRS complex. The PR interval resets, and the cycle repeats. Mobitz type II heart block is characterized by intermittently nonconducting P waves. The PR interval remains unchanged. In third-degree (complete) heart block, there is no apparent relationship between P waves and QRS complexes.

91. A: Labyrinthitis is the most likely diagnosis. It usually follows a viral infection such as the flu or the common cold. It differs from Ménière disease because hearing and balance does not deteriorate after each episode. In cases of labyrinthitis, inner ear functions return to baseline after every episode. In Ménière disease, there is a chronic deterioration of inner ear function. Benign paroxysmal positional vertigo (BPPV) is vertigo that can be elicited with head movement and confirmed with an abnormal Dix-Hallpike maneuver. An acoustic neuroma is a slow-growing tumor that causes unilateral tinnitus.

92. A: Haloperidol is an antipsychotic medication. This patient most likely has schizophrenia. Schizophrenia is a mental disorder that makes it hard for a person to differentiate between what is real and not real. It also affects one's concentration, mood balance, sleep, and ability to maintain appropriate behavior. Choices B and C are selective serotonin reuptake inhibitors (SSRIs), which are used to treat anxiety, depression, panic disorder, and posttraumatic stress disorder. They may provide some relief of symptoms, but they should be used in conjunction with other antipsychotic medications. Choice D is a sedative. This may provide some relief of symptoms, but it should not be the only medication used in a schizophrenic patient.

93. D: Postmenopausal bleeding in conjunction with thickened endometrial lining suggest that the patient may have endometrial cancer. A biopsy should be done to confirm the diagnosis.

94. C: The mainstays of treatment for thalassemia major are folate supplements and regular blood transfusions. In cases of severe disease, chelation therapy (removal of excess iron from the blood) and a bone marrow transplant are necessary. Thalassemia major is a rare genetic blood disorder in which the hemoglobin is defective and causes severe hemolytic anemia. Patients with thalassemia should avoid iron because they are already at risk for iron overload in their blood due to regular blood transfusions, which can cause tissue damage due to iron deposits (versus hemochromatosis—a genetic cause of iron overload). Avoiding legumes, NSAIDs, and henna would be suggestions for those with G6PD deficiency, not those who have thalassemia major.

95. A: Bacterial vaginosis (BV) is a vaginal infection due to an imbalance of bacterial flora. It is not considered to be a sexually transmitted infection. A positive whiff (amine) test and clue cells point to BV. Metronidazole or clindamycin is the treatment for this condition.

96. B: This woman may have an ectopic pregnancy versus a threatened abortion. Because she is only 6 weeks pregnant, the intrauterine pregnancy (IUP) may be too small to see. If the repeat β-HCG increases normally and an IUP is seen after 2 days, then the diagnosis is most likely threatened abortion. If the β-HCG levels become higher than normal and an IUP still cannot be seen, then methotrexate or a surgical consult may be needed to treat the ectopic pregnancy.

97. A: Impetigo is a bacterial infection that is most commonly caused by *Staphylococcus aureus* or *Streptococcus pyogenes*. It causes lesions that can occur anywhere on the body; they are small, red pustules that can crack open and form a thick yellow or honey-colored crust. They most commonly occur in young children. These lesions are contagious, and family members and friends should avoid touching them until they are completely healed. Family members should wash bed linens in hot water and avoid sharing personal-care products (such as razors and towels) with the patient to prevent the spread of the disease. Hand washing is strongly recommended as well.

98. A: Testicular torsion is a surgical emergency that should be corrected within 6 hours of onset. Although it is usually caused by a traumatic event, in some cases, the cause is unknown. Failure to receive prompt treatment can result in infarction, gangrene, and infertility. Malignancy is not a complication of torsion.

99. C: Paraphimosis is when the foreskin gets trapped behind the glans penis and cannot be brought back to its original position. If it cannot be resolved at the bedside with conservative methods, then surgical intervention may be necessary. This can lead to a medical emergency due to constriction. Phimosis is when the foreskin cannot be retracted. A hydrocele is the collection of fluid around the testicle, which is usually due to a patent processus vaginalis but may be due to trauma or infection. Peyronie disease occurs in adults due to fibrosis around the corpus cavernosum, which causes painful bending of the penis when erect. This may be due to trauma, but the exact cause is unknown.

100. A: The patient has aphthous ulcers, which are non-life-threatening and do not require antibiotics or antiviral medication. Topical corticosteroids and vitamin B12 are the mainstays of treatment. The cause is unknown, but stress, trauma, and dietary deficiencies in iron and folate are believed to be linked to this condition.

101. A: A hydrocele is the collection of fluid around the testicle, which is usually due to a patent processus vaginalis but may be due to trauma or infection. It is not harmful and has no serious long-term complications. Testicular torsion is a *medical emergency*. It occurs when the spermatic cord becomes twisted and blood flow to the testicle is severely diminished or absent. It presents with acute onset of pain and swelling of the affected testicle. A varicocele is an enlargement of the veins in the scrotum, causing testicular aching and/or swelling to occur. The venous enlargement is usually due to faulty valves in the veins or compression of a neighboring vein disrupting blood flow in nearby veins. Cryptorchidism is a condition in which one or both testicles have not descended into the scrotum.

102. D: A D-dimer test is a highly sensitive but nonspecific blood test for detecting the presence of clots. If the person is already diagnosed with a pulmonary embolus (PE), then the D-dimer will be positive. It will take weeks to months to get the clot to dissolve. Because the patient has sickle cell disease and is at high risk for developing future clots, placing her on a heparin infusion, sending her home on warfarin, and placing an IVC filter are viable treatment options. Because the patient has a PE that is causing chest pain, administering analgesics would be appropriate management.

103. C: He should be getting the influenza vaccine every year. Though he is not in a high-risk group (e.g., very young, very old, healthcare worker, or immunocompromised), the vaccine still provides modest protection against contracting the influenza virus. Conservative measures such as frequent hand washing are also recommended. His tobacco abuse increases the risk of contracting pulmonary diseases such as influenza, and it raises the complication rates in the event that he does contract the disease. Therefore, severely limiting tobacco use or quitting altogether is recommended.

104. B: Furosemide is a loop diuretic used to treat congestive heart failure and edema, but it is not a treatment used in atrial fibrillation. Metoprolol is a β-blocker that helps slow the heart rate down. Warfarin is a blood thinner that helps prevent the heart from sending clots to the lungs or brain. Digoxin is an inotropic agent that increases the force of the heart's contraction and reduces strain on the heart. It is used to treat hypertension, cardiomyopathy, and atrial fibrillation.

105. D: Coccidioidomycosis, also known as "valley fever," is a self-limiting respiratory infection caused by a fungus endemic to southwestern soil in the United States. It may present with cough with or without hemoptysis and flu-like symptoms. It may also present with erythema nodosum (painful erythematous lumps). *Pneumocystis jirovecii* pneumonia usually occurs in immunocompromised patients (e.g., those with HIV). Symptoms are similar to the influenza virus, and patients most commonly have a nonproductive cough. PO and sometimes IV antibiotics are needed to treat this opportunistic infection. Symptoms of tuberculosis may include fever, night sweats, hemoptysis, nausea, vomiting, anorexia, and fatigue. This disease does not go away on its own. RSV is an acute, self-limiting, usually non-life-threatening virus that most commonly presents with a cough and wheezing. It is more prevalent in children who attend day care and in children <2 years old.

106. A: A two-dimensional echocardiogram can make a definitive diagnosis of ventricular septal defect (VSD). VSD is the most common congenital heart defect after bicuspid aortic valves. Smaller defects may need no further treatment. Larger defects can cause heart failure and pulmonary hypertension, as well as other complications, and require surgical repair. A chest x-ray may show cardiomegaly, but it is not a definitive test for VSD. An ECG may show left ventricular hypertrophy, but it is not used as a definitive test for VSD. Auscultation with a stethoscope may reveal a heart murmur (harsh, holosystolic murmur at lower left sternal border), but it is not a dependable diagnostic aid for VSD.

107. B: Entropion is a condition in which the eyelid turns inward so that the eyelashes rub against the eye surface, causing chronic irritation. Artificial tears and lubricating ointments can help relieve symptoms of entropion. However, surgery is needed to fully correct the condition. Left untreated, entropion can cause chronic eye infections, scarring, and vision loss.

108. C: Torsades de pointes literally means "twisting of the points." It is a polymorphic ventricular tachycardia that can be caused by congenital disease, electrolyte abnormalities caused by malnourishment or alcoholism, or adverse drug interactions. Administering antiarrhythmic medications and reversing the electrolyte abnormalities, if applicable, are the mainstays of therapy. Bundle branch block shows a wide QRS. Sick sinus syndrome shows sinus bradycardia. Atrial fibrillation has a "sawtooth" pattern.

109. A: Prinzmetal variant angina is a condition that is thought to be more common in women. It is much more common in people who smoke cigarettes. It is due to vasospasm of coronary arteries; it spontaneously resolves without treatment. Typically, it will occur at rest, and no ECG changes may be seen unless the test is performed during an acute episode. Unstable angina is a condition in which chest pain occurs at rest and during activity due to severe atherosclerosis. Stable angina is chest pain—alleviated with rest—that is due to mild to moderate atherosclerotic disease. Costochondritis occurs when the chest wall is strained due to strenuous physical activity, trauma, or idiopathic cause. Palpation reproduces symptoms.

110. D: Small-cell carcinoma is responsible for causing a number of paraneoplastic syndromes, such as SIADH, Cushing syndrome, and limbic encephalitis. Paraneoplastic syndromes are a localized or systemic response to the presence of tumor cells in the body. The other three choices are subtypes of non-small-cell carcinoma, which is not commonly a cause of paraneoplastic syndromes.

111. C: A chest x-ray may be ordered in a case of infective endocarditis, but it is one of the least helpful tests compared to the other choices. A chest x-ray may show cardiomegaly or a pyogenic abscess, but it can also be normal in some cases. Blood cultures would be positive, which shows that the patient has bacteremia. An infection needs to be present in order to make the diagnosis of infective endocarditis. A CT scan of the chest would show a fluid collection, abscess, or inflammation around the endocardium. An echocardiogram would show one or more vegetations on the heart; this is the preferred diagnostic aid.

112. C: Limiting one's tobacco use (or preferably quitting smoking altogether), limiting sodium intake, and increasing physical activity are all recommendations a healthcare professional should make to a patient with prehypertension. Prehypertension is defined as systolic blood pressure of 120 to 139 mmHg and diastolic blood pressure 81 to 89 mmHg on 3 visits, 4-6 weeks apart. Medication regimens may be avoided if patients take conservative measures to lower their blood pressure.

113. D: Herpetic whitlow is an intensely painful infection of the hand involving one or more fingers. It typically affects the terminal phalanx and is caused by herpes type 1 or 2. The primary infection is typically the most severe. Topical antiviral medications such as acyclovir may shorten the clinical course. Deep surgical incision is contraindicated because this may lead to complications.

114. B: The *immediate* treatment in the presence of an MI (whether NSTEMI or STEMI) is morphine, oxygen, nitrates, and aspirin. Remember the mnemonic: MONA. Also start β-blockers and heparin (or other anticoagulant). β-blockers such as metoprolol decrease the workload of the heart and should be given within 24 hours for an NSTEMI. Antiplatelet medications, such as aspirin, are used to help prevent clot formation. Clopidogrel is used if aspirin is not tolerated, but in most situations, aspirin is the first-line antiplatelet regimen. Nitroglycerin helps as a vasodilator to decrease the workload of the heart and so decrease pain. A troponin level should be immediately ordered, but an echocardiogram may wait.

115. A: This patient has stable angina. Stable angina is present when a patient experiences chest pain that is alleviated with rest. This condition occurs with mild to moderate atherosclerotic disease. A patient may develop chest pain during periods of physical activity caused by cardiac ischemia. During rest, the body's demands on the heart lessen and the blood flow becomes adequate to perfuse the heart. Prinzmetal variant angina is a condition that is thought to be more common in women with or without atherosclerosis. It is much more common in people who smoke. It is due to vasospasm of coronary arteries, typically occurs at rest, and spontaneously resolves without treatment. Unstable angina is a condition in which chest pain occurs at rest and during activity due to severe atherosclerosis. An aortic aneurysm is an outpouching of part of the vessel wall, or it may be a circumferential outpouching of the vessel wall caused by disease or trauma. Patients may be asymptomatic, but as the aneurysm becomes significantly large or ruptures, the patient will display severe abdominal or back pain. Symptoms do not resolve with rest.

116. B: Macular degeneration is an age-related eye disease that irreversibly affects central vision, while peripheral vision is preserved. About one-third of patients age >75 suffer from this. The macula, which is located in the center of the retina, is responsible for central vision. There are some dietary modifications that can slow the progression, but once macular degeneration occurs, there is no cure. The dry form has a gradual loss of vision, while the wet form has rapid vision loss. Optic neuritis is the inflammation of the optic nerve due to infectious or immunologic disorders. It presents with sudden-onset eye pain and loss of vision. Open-angle glaucoma presents with worsening unilateral or bilateral painless visual field loss. Acute-angle closure glaucoma occurs when the intraocular pressure is so high that it damages the optic nerve, which can impair vision and cause severe eye pain, redness, and halos. Retinal artery occlusion occurs when a clot blocks blood flow to the eye, causing sudden, painless, unilateral vision loss. It is common in patients with coagulopathy disorders, hypertension, diabetes mellitus, or atherosclerosis.

117. D: The patient may have an acoustic neuroma; an MRI scan of the brain is an essential diagnostic tool. Acoustic neuromas are tumors of the acoustic nerve that may cause facial droop or unilateral facial paresthesias/pain, ataxia, tinnitus, hearing loss, dizziness, and receptive aphasia. An electromyography (EMG) test might be considered if muscle weakness or facial droop were present, to test the activity of muscles and the nerves. This patient's physical examination is normal, so an EMG is of little use. An ENT consult would be appropriate once a workup has been done and tests have been completed. The Dix-Hallpike maneuver helps to confirm the diagnosis of benign positional vertigo. Movement does not exacerbate the patient's symptoms, so this condition can be ruled out.

118. A: Gouty arthritis is caused by high levels of uric acid (serum uric acid >6.8 mg/dL). The elevated uric acid levels cause crystal deposits to form in the joint spaces, causing pain, erythema, and swelling. These deposits can cause tophi, which are red, swollen areas found on a joint or on the skin. Treatments may include steroids, NSAIDs, or medications that reduce the production of uric acid, such as allopurinol.

119. B: The patient has a right-sided pleural effusion, most likely due to her COPD. It is a pathologic fluid collection in the pleural space. It may develop postoperatively, but more commonly it is caused by infection or disease. Pleural effusions may present with dyspnea, pleuritic chest pain, fever, and cough. In instances of a large pleural effusion, breath sounds will be diminished due to the fluid collection in the pleural space. Tactile fremitus is decreased, and there is dullness to percussion due to the fluid. In cases of a pneumothorax, the symptoms may present similarly to those with pleural effusion. On physical examination, breath sounds and tactile fremitus are decreased due to the decreased lung space/size, but percussion is hyperresonant due to the extra air in the thoracic cavity. Thus, hyperresonance helps distinguish a pneumothorax from a pleural effusion. Acute asthma exacerbation and influenza may present with similar symptoms, but there would be no decreased tactile fremitus or dullness to percussion.

120. D: The patient may have diabetes mellitus and needs further workup to confirm the diagnosis. A hemoglobin A1C is a monitor of the average serum glucose for the past 3 months. A complete blood count, basic metabolic panel, and urine culture should also be checked. The patient should be given a topical or oral antifungal such as fluconazole to treat her vaginal candidiasis.

121. A: Short-acting β-2 bronchodilators are some of the first-line agents in treating an acute asthma exacerbation. The anticholinergic, ipratropium bromide, may also be useful in an acute exacerbation. The other three choices are long-acting medications that are to be used for maintenance therapy, and are not efficacious in an acute episode. Also, formoterol (long-acting β-2 agonist) should not be used as monotherapy due to an increased risk of asthma-related death.

122. A: This patient most likely has pneumoconiosis, also known as "miner's lung" due to a miner's prolonged coal-dust exposure. It presents as an upper respiratory infection that does not resolve. The honeycomb appearance on chest x-ray is a common finding. There is no medical treatment other than to remove the causative agent. Schistosomiasis is a chronic parasitic infection caused by eating improperly cooked pork. On a brain MRI, it appears as multiple enhancing nodules occurring in bilateral cerebral hemispheres. Coccidioidomycosis, also known as "valley fever," is a self-limiting respiratory infection caused by a fungus endemic to soil of the southwestern United States. It may present with cough, with or without hemoptysis and flu-like symptoms. It may also present with erythema nodosum, which is characterized by painful erythematous lumps. Tuberculosis is a bacterial infection of the lungs, causing symptoms such as night sweats, lymphadenopathy, fever, chills, hemoptysis, nausea, vomiting, anorexia, and fatigue.

123. B: Testicular carcinomas present as a hard, painless, fixed, solid testicular lesion that does not transilluminate; it is the most common cancer in males ages 15-35. Your next step should be to order imaging studies and blood work to confirm the diagnosis. Prognosis is good with early treatment. A hydrocele is a soft, painless, fixed testicular mass. It is due to a collection of fluid around the testicle, and is usually due to a patent processus vaginalis but may be due to trauma or infection. Hydroceles are not harmful and have no serious long-term complications. A varicocele is an enlargement of the veins in the scrotum, causing testicular aching and/or swelling to occur. The venous enlargement is usually due to faulty valves in the veins or compression of a neighboring vein disrupting blood flow in nearby veins. Testicular torsion is a *medical emergency*. It occurs when the spermatic cord becomes twisted, and blood flow to the testicle is severely diminished or absent. It presents with acute onset of pain and swelling of the affected testicle.

124. D: Cystic fibrosis (CF) is a disease that causes thick, sticky mucus to build up in the lungs, the digestive tract, and other areas of the body. It is an autosomal recessive inherited condition. The sweat chloride test is the standard diagnostic test for CF. Common complications include recurrent respiratory infections, respiratory failure, impaired fertility, liver disease, and heart failure.

125. C: Mastoiditis is an infection of the mastoid bone of the skull. It is generally a complication of inner ear infections. Symptoms may include fever, ear pain, ear discharge, swelling behind the ear (where the mastoid bone is located), hearing loss, headache, and erythema. Imaging studies such as MRI and CT scans can make the definitive diagnosis. Acoustic neuromas are tumors of the acoustic nerve. They are much more common in adults than in children. Symptoms include gradual hearing loss, dizziness, headache, tinnitus, facial droop, and ataxia. They do not cause fever or swelling behind the ear. A cholesteatoma is a cyst-like collection of squamous epithelia in the middle ear, which is usually due to chronic otitis media infections but may be congenital. Symptoms usually include painless ear drainage and hearing loss. It does not cause swelling behind the ear. Ménière disease is a usually chronic disorder of the inner ear, causing a mild to severe sensation of fullness in the affected ear, vertigo, dizziness, and hearing loss. The exact cause is unknown, but it is most likely multifactorial. Ménière disease is much more common in adults than in children. It does not cause fever or swelling behind the ear.

126. C: A *Cryptococcus* species is the pathogen causing this patient's meningitis. It is one of the defining opportunistic infections of patients with AIDS; their CD4 count is usually less than 200. It can be a common fungal pathogen in immunocompromised patients such as those with cancer or AIDS. Diagnosis is made by a CSF culture, and an India ink stain may be used to quickly identify the pathogen under the microscope. Treatment includes PO and IV antifungal medications.

127. A: Singulair is a leukotriene inhibitor. It is used to help prevent asthma exacerbations and seasonal allergies. Since it is a preventative, it will not help during an acute episode. Xopenex and Ventolin are short-acting β-2 bronchodilators. These medications are some of the first-line agents in treating an acute asthma exacerbation.

128. C: Wilms tumor is the most common renal tumor in pediatric patients. The exact cause is unknown, but incidence does increase with family history, suggesting there is a genetic component. Symptoms may include abdominal pain, abdominal mass, nausea, vomiting, constipation, and changes in urine color. Signs such as hemihypertrophy and aniridia (complete or partial absence of the iris) may be associated with this disease. Hodgkin lymphoma is a malignancy of the white blood cells. A lipoma is a benign tumor created by the overgrowth of fatty tissue. Kaposi sarcoma is related to HIV/AIDS and generally appears as multiple cutaneous lesions, but it may affect the internal organs as well.

129. B: Hyaline membrane disease, also known as infant respiratory distress syndrome, is a common cause of respiratory distress in premature infants. It is due to insufficient surfactant. Treatments include supplemental oxygen and the administration of synthetic surfactant. RSV is an acute, self-limiting, usually non-life-threatening virus that most commonly presents with a cough and wheezing. It is prevalent in children <2 years old and is usually more serious in the neonatal period (and in those <6 months); it may require hospitalization. *Pneumocystis* pneumonia usually occurs in immunocompromised patients. Symptoms are similar to the influenza virus. Patients most commonly have a nonproductive cough. Pneumoconiosis, also known as "miner's lung," is a disease caused by prolonged dust exposure.

130. C: This patient has a hyphema, considering his symptoms and history of recent trauma. A hyphema is a localized hemorrhage in the eye due to rupture of blood vessel(s). If the visual field is unaffected and the exam is primarily benign (and no sign of globe rupture), then the patient should have intraocular pressures measured and should have an immediate ophthalmology consult. Close follow-up with an ophthalmologist is recommended to ensure resolution of symptoms.

131. A: Leukoplakia is a condition in which white patches may develop on the tongue or inside the mouth. It is similar in appearance to oral thrush, except that in cases of thrush, the white lesions may be scraped off. The causes of leukoplakia are unknown, but it is commonly seen in alcoholics and those who smoke or chew tobacco. Thrush is a yeast infection seen in patients who are poorly controlled diabetics, those who have been on long-term steroids or antibiotics, and immunocompromised patients. Parotitis is an infection of the parotid gland, which produces facial swelling and pain. Gingivostomatitis is a herpesvirus infection of the mouth and gums, appearing as painful ulcers and sores.

132. D: Out of the choices given, tetralogy of Fallot is the only cyanotic congenital cardiac defect. It is the most common congenital cyanotic heart defect, usually associated with chromosomal abnormalities. Tetralogy of Fallot is most commonly caused by infections during pregnancy or by excessive alcohol intake during pregnancy. The radiological sign "boot-shaped heart" or "coeur en sabot" is most commonly associated with tetralogy of Fallot. The heart looks like a boot due to right-ventricular hypertrophy and pulmonary stenosis.

133. B: Bronchoscopy with biopsy would provide definitive confirmation of the diagnosis. Patients with sarcoidosis have multiple granulomas in their lungs, as well as in other organs. Sarcoidosis is a systemic inflammatory disease that can attack any organ, but it most commonly attacks the lymph nodes and lungs. A CT scan and serum phosphorus may aid in the diagnosis, but they are not definitive tests. A lumbar puncture would provide no diagnostic value.

134. C: This patient most likely has fibrocystic breast disease. It is a benign condition in which single or multiple breast cysts develop. They may change in size and become more painful with each menstrual cycle. People placed on hormone replacement therapy or birth control pills generally have less severe symptoms. A breast ultrasound should be ordered to further evaluate the patient. If the patient were 40 years of age or older, a mammogram would be the preferred diagnostic test.

135. A: A fibroadenoma is a benign breast mass that usually does not cause pain. It can be monitored; no intervention is necessary unless it becomes large and the patient requests removal. Birth control pills are not useful in treating fibroadenomas. Repeating a biopsy would not be helpful unless changes occur with the mass. Fibroadenomas are benign lesions that do not become malignant. There is no reason for a mastectomy because fibroadenomas are benign lesions.

136. A: Clindamycin is not a medication that would be used in the treatment of tuberculosis. There are a multitude of medications used to treat tuberculosis; they are used in a variety of combination therapies. The first-line medications are isoniazid, rifampin, pyrazinamide, and ethambutol. Less common drug remedies include amikacin, ethionamide, moxifloxacin, para-aminosalicylic acid, and streptomycin. Affected patients are usually on multiple medications for 6 months or longer.

137. D: Ascending or descending quickly will exacerbate the effects caused by barotrauma. Barotrauma is when the pressure in the middle ear is higher than that of the outer ear. Symptoms can include ear pain, hearing loss, and dizziness. The goal of treatment or prevention is to keep the eustachian tubes open so the pressure between the outer ear and the inner ear remains normalized. Actions such as chewing gum, yawning, or sucking on candy can help keep the pressures normalized.

138. B: Bronchiolitis is a common viral upper respiratory infection in children. It usually starts with mild symptoms similar to those of the common cold and then progresses to wheezing and breathing difficulties causing intercostal retractions, and in extreme cases, cyanosis due to respiratory insufficiency. It is commonly caused by RSV. Hyaline membrane disease, also known as infant respiratory distress syndrome, is a common cause of respiratory distress in premature infants. It is due to insufficient surfactant. Treatments include supplemental oxygen and the administration of synthetic surfactant. Tuberculosis symptoms may include fever, night sweats, hemoptysis, nausea/vomiting, anorexia, and fatigue. Cystic fibrosis is a chromosomal disorder that causes the lungs to become chronically plugged with mucus. Symptoms may include abdominal discomfort from chronic constipation, salty-tasting skin, poor appetite, fatigue, fever, delayed growth, poor weight gain, clay-colored stools, and frequent episodes of pneumonia. The diagnosis is usually made shortly after birth (newborn screen).

139. B: Levothyroxine is a synthetic thyroid hormone used to treat Hashimoto thyroiditis, which causes hypothyroidism. Lantus is a type of exogenous insulin used to treat patients with diabetes. Lanoxin (digoxin) is an antiarrhythmic agent used to treat conditions such as atrial fibrillation. Lamisil is medication used to treat fungal infections.

140. D: Huntington disease is a progressive neurologic disorder caused by an autosomal-dominant chromosomal abnormality. It most commonly occurs in people 30-40 years old. Tourette syndrome is first noticed in childhood and is characterized by involuntary verbal sounds or motor movements. It does not cause cognitive impairment, although it may be seen in the presence of cognitive disorders. Guillain-Barré syndrome is an autoimmune disease that causes ascending muscle weakness or paralysis; it does not cause cognitive impairment. Cerebral palsy is a neurologic disorder that causes motor and cognitive impairment. It is diagnosed in infancy or childhood. It may be caused by infection or trauma, but the most common cause is prenatal hypoxia.

141. C: This patient is suffering from hyperparathyroidism. Elevated serum calcium can cause a multitude of nonspecific symptoms, such as weakness and fatigue, depression, bone pain, myalgia, constipation, polyuria, polydipsia, cognitive impairment, nephrolithiasis (kidney stones), and osteoporosis. Hyperthyroidism causes an increase in metabolism, producing symptoms such as unintentional weight loss, high blood pressure, tremor, palpitations, and weakness. Hypoparathyroidism will also cause many nonspecific symptoms; the most common is perioral and extremity paresthesias. Hypothyroidism causes a slowing in metabolism and potentially impaired cognitive function, producing symptoms such as unintentional weight gain, low blood pressure, bradycardia, weakness, myxedema, and slow speech.

142. A: Permethrin cream is an insecticide used to treat skin infections caused by scabies and lice. Olanzapine is an antipsychotic medication used to treat psychiatric disorders. Phenergan is an antihistamine used to treat allergic reactions and to alleviate pruritus and nausea. Ondansetron is an anti-nausea medication used to help prevent and/or treat nausea and vomiting that is due to illness or induced by certain medications such as chemotherapy agents.

143. A: An avulsion fracture is when one piece of bone is separated from the whole. Many avulsion fractures are small and heal well without surgical intervention. Conservative management includes placing an Ace wrap or splint, offering pain medications, and applying ice for swelling.

144. D: This patient has infective endocarditis caused by her drug use. Endocarditis causes a number of symptoms, including fever, chills, dyspnea, nonproductive cough, and diaphoresis. Common causes are indwelling triple-lumen catheters or peripherally inserted central catheter (PICC) lines, dental procedures, and IV drug abuse with contaminated needles. The signs indicating the diagnosis are the presence of Roth spots and Janeway lesions. Roth spots are retinal hemorrhages with pale centers. Janeway lesions are non-painful erythematous nodules on the palms and soles.

145. D: Restrictive cardiomyopathy is the inability of the heart to relax between beats. Epinephrine is a vasoconstrictor, which would increase the workload of a heart that is already impaired. Furosemide and metoprolol help lower the heart rate and also lower the preload and afterload on the heart. The blood is being squeezed through restricted vasculature, which raises the risk of developing clots. Aspirin helps prevent the formation of clots and is commonly used in the treatment of restrictive cardiomyopathy.

146. B: Toxic megacolon is a complication of *Clostridioides difficile* colitis. It is the pathologic distension of the colon caused by *C. difficile*, Crohn disease, and ulcerative colitis. Signs and symptoms may include tachycardia, abdominal pain, abdominal distension, leukocytosis, and fever. The treatment is to decompress the colon either by rectal tube or by surgical intervention. Ogilvie syndrome is a condition in which a patient presents with signs and symptoms of intestinal obstruction without actually having an obstruction. The bowel loses its ability to contract and to pass food and waste products along the gastrointestinal (GI) tract; this commonly occurs after surgery or in severely chronically ill patients. Intussusception is when one part of the bowel folds in on itself, causing an obstruction. This is common in children. Symptoms include nausea, vomiting, lethargy, and "red currant jelly" stools. Hirschsprung disease is a congenital condition in which the bowel cannot contract and move food and waste products along the GI tract due to lack of nerve innervation of portions of the bowel.

147. A: This patient has alcohol-induced pancreatitis. Alcohol is the leading cause of acute pancreatitis; stones are the second most common cause. Therapies include cessation of alcohol, rest, IV fluids, thiamine and folic acid, pain medications, and keeping the patient NPO until symptoms improve. An abdominal ultrasound, CT scan, or magnetic resonance cholangiopancreatography (MRCP), as well as an elevated lipase level, are diagnostic tools for confirming the condition.

148. C: This patient most likely has Parkinson disease. The classic four signs of Parkinson disease are resting tremor, rigidity, slow movements, and shuffling gait. These are due to the deterioration of the substantia nigra, which decreases levels of dopamine. Huntington disease is a progressive neurologic disorder caused by an autosomal-dominant chromosomal abnormality. Signs include progressive decline in cognitive function; ataxic gait; and uncoordinated, jerky body movements. Alzheimer disease is the development of progressive cognitive decline; the underlying cause is not fully understood, but it is known to exhibit amyloid deposits and neurofibrillary tangles in the brain. Motor skills are much less affected until late stages of the disease. Guillain-Barré syndrome is an autoimmune disease that causes peripheral neuropathy with ascending muscle weakness or paralysis. It does not cause resting tremor or rigidity.

149. C: This patient has an excess of cortisol due to her exogenous steroid use, causing Cushing syndrome. Signs and symptoms of Cushing syndrome include buffalo hump (posterior cervical fat pad), swelling of the face, myalgias, unintentional weight gain, irregular menses, striae, hirsutism, and bone loss. Diagnostic tests include blood cortisol levels, a low-dose dexamethasone suppression test, and a 24-hour urine free cortisol test.

150. B: This patient is most likely suffering from Stevens-Johnson syndrome caused by a reaction to penicillin. It is a reaction of the skin and mucous membranes to medication. It begins with vague, flu-type symptoms for a few days followed by progressive dermal manifestations (epidermal detachment). It can be life-threatening if not treated immediately; patients need hospitalization. Cushing syndrome is caused by too much cortisol, causing symptoms such as buffalo hump (posterior cervical fat pad), swelling of the face, myalgia, unintentional weight gain, irregular menses, striae, hirsutism, hyperglycemia, and bone loss. Guillain-Barré syndrome is an autoimmune disease that causes muscle weakness or paralysis. Turner syndrome is a genetic condition in which females are missing all or part of an X chromosome. Some of the symptoms may include infertility, amenorrhea, short stature, and webbed neck.

151. A: The child most likely had immune thrombocytopenia, a.k.a. immune (or idiopathic) thrombocytopenic purpura (ITP), caused by his viral syndrome. It is characterized by petechiae (a pinpoint rash) seen on the extremities. In children, ITP usually resolves on its own without treatment. Stevens-Johnson syndrome begins with flu-like symptoms for a few days and then progresses to dermal manifestations. The rash is a diffuse, dark red macular and papular rash with extensive blistering (epidermal detachment in <10% of the body), usually requiring hospitalization. It can be life-threatening if not treated immediately and adequately. Von Willebrand disease is a milder form of hemophilia. It is caused by factor VIII deficiency. Symptoms include prolonged bleeding after dental or surgical procedures, minor injuries, and menorrhagia. G6PD deficiency is an X-linked recessive hereditary disease in which the defect of this enzyme causes red blood cells to break down prematurely. It causes pallor, dark urine, jaundice, and failure to thrive. It is generally diagnosed in infancy. Symptoms do not spontaneously resolve.

152. D: The child has diphtheria. It is a respiratory infection, very rare in developed countries due to the diphtheria, tetanus, and pertussis (DTaP) vaccine, but children can still get diphtheria if they are not vaccinated. Signs and symptoms include a grayish-black, tough, fiber-like covering of the oropharynx, fever, chills, sore throat, cyanosis, and in severe cases, drooling and stridor. Cryptococcus infections are generally seen in patients who are immunocompromised. Cryptococcus is a fungus that people with normal immune systems can handle. There is no vaccine to prevent against cryptococcus infections. Shigella causes bacterial gastroenteritis. Cholera is a rare bacterial gastroenteritis that may cause severe dehydration and lead to death.

153. D: The child has mononucleosis caused by the Epstein-Barr virus. Conservative treatment such as rest, fluids, and refraining from physical activity to prevent splenic rupture are recommended. Amantadine is an antiviral medication used within 1-2 days after the onset of flu symptoms to help shorten the duration of the illness. Augmentin would be used if the child had a bacterial upper respiratory infection. A CT scan of the abdomen is not recommended if splenic rupture is not suspected.

154. B: This patient has multiple myeloma, which is a type of cancer of the plasma cells. The most common signs and symptoms are bone pain and pathologic fractures. Multiple myeloma can also cause damage to the kidneys, causing anemia. The presence of the Bence Jones protein in the urine distinguishes this from Paget disease, which can also cause bone pain and pathologic fractures. Acute myelogenous leukemia (AML) is a cancer of the blood and bone marrow, usually presenting with bleeding, bruising, fatigue, and weight loss. AML is more common in adults. Acute lymphocytic leukemia (ALL) is a cancer of the white blood cells, usually presenting with weight loss, fatigue, petechiae, and fever. ALL is more common in children.

155. A: The INR is used to monitor or measure the effectiveness of the anticoagulant medication Coumadin. The INR is calculated from the prothrombin time (PT). An INR is not used in the workup of hemolytic anemia. The Coombs test looks for antibodies that may attach themselves to red blood cells and cause premature apoptosis. It is used in diagnosing hemolytic anemia from an immune-mediated cause. A CBC may be able to indicate what type of anemia is present, whether the patient is pancytopenic, or whether an underlying infection is present. LDH is present in blood cells; increased levels of LDH indicate hemolytic anemia.

156. A: Influenza is not responsible for causing the abnormalities seen in this infant. Microcephaly, deafness, chorioretinitis, hepatosplenomegaly, and thrombocytopenia are common signs and symptoms of TORCH infections that are contracted in utero. TORCH infections can be caused by **T**oxoplasmosis (avoid contact with cat feces), **O**ther (syphilis, varicella-zoster, parvovirus B19 [erythema infectiosum], HIV, Zika virus), **R**ubella, **C**ytomegalovirus, and **H**erpes simplex virus type 2 (HSV-2). The infant's prognosis depends on which type of infection she has. Some TORCH infections can be prevented with vaccines, and others can be treated with antibiotics, but because most infections are viral, there is no cure.

157. D: Small-cell carcinoma is responsible for causing a number of paraneoplastic syndromes, such as syndrome of inappropriate antidiuretic hormone (SIADH). The treatment of SIADH is slow correction of hyponatremia. For more severe cases with seizures or the presence of cerebral edema, 3% hypertonic fluids may be carefully used. In milder cases, restriction of fluids is the mainstay of treatment. Loop diuretics may be used, but thiazide diuretics should be avoided since they exacerbate the hyponatremia.

158. D: This patient has lichen planus, which is commonly described as well-defined, pruritic, planar, purple, polygonal papules and plaques. It may occur on mucous membranes or on the skin. It is a benign condition and the exact cause is unknown. It is linked to some chronic diseases, such as hepatitis C. Leukoplakia is a condition in which white patches may develop on the tongue or inside the mouth. Impetigo is a bacterial infection that is most commonly caused by *Staphylococcus aureus* or *Streptococcus pyogenes*. It causes lesions that can occur anywhere on the body. The lesions are small, red pustules and can crack open and form a thick yellow or honey-colored crust. They occur most commonly in young children. Psoriasis causes cells to build up rapidly on the surface of the skin, forming itchy, dry, red, raised patches covered with grayish silvery lesions that are easily friable. Psoriasis is sometimes painful. Plaques frequently occur on the skin of the elbows and knees, but they can affect any area. This is a chronic condition.

159. B: Zika virus is transmitted through the *Aedes* mosquito. Symptoms include fever, headache, conjunctivitis, rash, myalgias, and arthralgias. People may only have mild symptoms and may not be aware they have the virus. It may be transmitted sexually and can cause severe birth defects, including microcephaly. Zika can remain in semen longer than in other body fluids. Therefore, it is recommended that pregnant women abstain from sex or use condoms throughout their pregnancy to prevent transmission by a partner who has contracted the virus or traveled to an area with a risk of Zika. There is currently no vaccine or treatment for Zika virus.

160. B: Lantus (insulin glargine, long-acting) would be a first-line treatment in a patient with newly diagnosed type 1 diabetes mellitus. The patient would also need a second preprandial insulin (rapid-acting, before meals). Type 1 diabetes is an autoimmune disease in which the body attacks the islets of Langerhans of the pancreas. The islets of Langerhans have beta cells, which produce insulin. Patients who are type 1 diabetics are insulin dependent their whole lives. Biguanides and sulfonylureas are not effective in type 1 diabetes mellitus. Insulin is the gold-standard treatment for type 1 diabetes mellitus.

161. C: The patient is suffering from acute alcohol withdrawal. He states that he has not had an alcoholic beverage in 2 days. Some symptoms may start as soon as a few hours (6 hours) after the last drink or may take

2-3 days to appear. Signs and symptoms may include tachycardia, nausea, vomiting, diarrhea, diaphoresis, confusion, headaches, seizures, fine motor tremor, and dilated pupils. The patient is confused, but he is not delusional. Persistent depressive disorder (dysthymia) is a milder form of major depressive disorder.

162. C: The patient has Osgood-Schlatter disease, which is an inflammation of the anterior tibial tubercle due to overuse while the bone is still growing. It is most commonly seen in prepubescent boys. Pain medications may be used, and rest is recommended, but no intervention is warranted. Symptoms will resolve eventually.

163. B: Actinic keratoses can appear as flesh-toned, pink, gray, or reddish macules or papules with a scaly surface caused by overexposure to the sun. They increase with age. These lesions have a propensity for becoming squamous cell carcinomas, so it should be recommended to patients to avoid prolonged sun exposure and to use sunscreen. The lesions may be removed with various techniques, such as curettage, freezing with liquid nitrogen, and keratolytics.

164. A: This wound should heal by secondary intention because it is 3 days old. Small superficial wounds more than 24 hours old should not be closed due to the increased risk of infection. Large wounds should be referred to a plastic surgeon.

165. D: Approximately 10% of patients with a penicillin reaction will also have an allergy to cephalosporins, especially the older first-generation cephalosporins (e.g., cephalexin, cefadroxil). In patients with a documented allergy to penicillin, cephalosporins should be avoided.

166. C: This patient most likely has multiple sclerosis (MS). One of the most common presenting symptoms is persistent fatigue. One of the most common signs is optic neuritis. Approximately 40-50% of MS patients will experience optic neuritis during the course of their disease. Patients may also present with progressive ataxia, muscle spasms, dizziness, incoordination of fine motor movements, urinary frequency, incontinence, nystagmus, and depression. Alzheimer disease is a progressive cognitive decline. The underlying cause is not fully understood, but it is known to exhibit amyloid deposits and neurofibrillary tangles in the brain. Motor skills are much less affected until late stages of the disease. Meningitis is an infection that classically presents with nuchal rigidity, photophobia, and headache. Huntington disease is a progressive neurologic disorder caused by an autosomal-dominant chromosomal abnormality. Signs include progressive decline in cognitive function; ataxic gait; and uncoordinated, jerky body movements.

167. B: Osteomyelitis is an infection of the bone that can be caused by blood-borne pathogens from open wounds, cellulitis, trauma, artificial joints or heart valves, diabetes, and sickle cell disease. Salmonella is the most likely pathogen in sickle cell patients.

168. A: Oseltamivir, or Tamiflu, is an antiviral medication used to shorten the course and lessen the severity of flu symptoms (type A or B) if given early enough during the course of infection (within 48 hours of symptom onset). Antibiotics play no role in the treatment of influenza.

169. B: If testicular torsion is suspected, a stat surgical consult is warranted because the only correction of torsion is surgery. Surgery should be performed within 6 hours of the trauma in order to save the testicle. If blood flow is compromised for too long, the testicle may need to be removed. Warm compresses would help if the patient had an abscess or testicular swelling without torsion, but they would provide very little benefit in this scenario. Pain medications should be given, but a surgical consult should be called first. The patient may need preoperative antibiotics for prophylaxis, depending on the surgeon's preferences, but it should not be the next step in management because testicular torsion is not due to an infection.

170. D: This patient most likely has diabetes insipidus caused by her traumatic head injury. Diabetes insipidus is caused by insufficient antidiuretic hormone (ADH), which causes the body to conserve little, if any, water. This condition may be caused by trauma, surgery, or infection. In this case, it is most likely caused by the patient's traumatic brain injury. Diabetes mellitus occurs when the body's insulin production is insufficient to meet a patient's glucose intake. Patients with diabetes mellitus will have high glucose levels in their blood and urine; those with diabetes insipidus do not. Hypothyroidism causes a slowing in metabolism and potentially impaired cognitive function, producing symptoms such as unintentional weight gain, low blood pressure, bradycardia, weakness, myxedema, and slow speech. Hyperthyroidism causes an increase in metabolism, producing symptoms such as unintentional weight loss, high blood pressure, tremor, palpitations, and weakness.

171. C: This patient most likely has melanoma. The definitive way to make the diagnosis is via biopsy. The way to help diagnose melanoma on physical examination is to think of the mnemonic ABCDE: **a**symmetry, **b**orders, **c**olor, **d**iameter, and **e**volving over time. Melanoma frequently occurs as asymmetric lesions with irregular borders, with multiple colors within one lesion, with a diameter greater than 6 mm, and whose appearance changes or evolves over time. Impetigo is a bacterial infection that is most commonly caused by *Staphylococcus aureus* or *Streptococcus pyogenes*. It causes lesions that can occur anywhere on the body. They are small, red pustules that can crack open and form a thick yellow or honey-colored crust. They occur most commonly in young children. Basal-cell carcinoma is the most common type of skin cancer. It is usually described as a pearly pink or flesh-colored lesion that is easily friable and does not heal. Squamous-cell carcinoma is usually described as a light-colored, scaly crust on an erythematous base. It is usually found on sun-exposed areas.

172. C: This patient is experiencing delirium due to her urinary tract infection. A urine culture should be sent, and the patient should be started on intravenous antibiotics.

173. C: Scheuermann kyphosis refers to the abnormally excessive convex curvature of the thoracic spine (>40-45°) that usually appears in adolescents around 10-15 years old. Normal kyphosis is <40°. The mainstay of treatment includes braces and then surgical correction if severe (>75°).

174. C: This patient has idiopathic intercranial hypertension (pseudotumor cerebri), which is an idiopathic increase in intracranial pressure. Risk factors include obesity, polycystic ovary syndrome, systemic lupus erythematosus, and hypoparathyroidism; but the cause is unknown. Treatments include glaucoma medications such as acetazolamide, triptans, diuretics, and pain medications. If symptoms persist, a ventricular peritoneal shunt may be warranted.

175. C: *Helicobacter pylori* is a type of bacteria that lives in the gastrointestinal tract and may cause gastritis and duodenal ulcers. Various treatment regimens (triple or quadruple therapy) include combinations of 2-3 antibiotics (clarithromycin, amoxicillin, metronidazole, tetracycline), a proton pump inhibitor, and bismuth.

176. A: The child has croup, which is most commonly caused by the parainfluenza virus. Antibiotics would be of no value because it is a viral illness. IV steroids would be prescribed if the patient was in respiratory distress or unable to take orally. The mainstays of therapy in uncomplicated cases of croup are humidified air (cool-mist vaporizer), oral steroids, rest, and maintaining adequate hydration.

177. A: The patient most likely has a cardiac tamponade—the abnormal collection of fluid in the pericardial sac, which compresses the heart. This can be due to injury or prior disease like pericarditis, cancer, or previous surgery. The patient's symptoms are consistent with the Beck triad (signs of cardiac tamponade), which is the combination of hypotension, muffled heart sounds, and distended jugular veins.

178. B: Paronychia is an abscess adjacent to the nail bed. This can occur on the fingers or the toes. The cause may be idiopathic, but there is usually a history of trauma or a break in the skin prior to the onset of symptoms. Treatment includes warm compresses, antibiotics, and sometimes incision and drainage of the wound. Onychomycosis is a fungal infection of the nail, which causes the nail to thicken, become yellow or gray, and occasionally fall off. Condyloma acuminata is the appearance of genital or anal warts due to a viral sexually transmitted disease (human papillomavirus [HPV]).

179. C: This patient has normal pressure hydrocephalus (NPH), which is more common in the elderly. The common triad seen with NPH patients is abnormal gait, urinary incontinence, and dementia. The opening pressure of a lumbar puncture is normal (hence, "normal pressure" hydrocephalus). The ventricles, however, are enlarged on CT scan or MRI. The treatment is a lumbar puncture to see if the symptoms resolve or improve. If they do not, then the patient will need a CSF shunt (e.g., ventricular peritoneal shunt). NPH may be idiopathic or may be due to trauma, infection, meningitis, tumor, or postsurgical complication.

180. C: Morphine is a narcotic medication that can cause constipation. This medication would not be recommended in a patient with a history of fecal impaction because it may precipitate bowel motility issues. Senna and Colace are stool softeners that may help make it easier to pass a bowel movement in a patient with a history of constipation. Milk of magnesia helps prevent water from being reabsorbed in the intestines. Because it increases the amount of water that remains in the bowels, it helps promote bowel movements.

181. C: This patient had a right MCA stroke. The brain has contralateral control over the body. If the patient has a right-sided cerebral abnormality, then he or she will have left-sided symptoms. The language centers are primarily located in the temporal regions of the brain, which are perfused by the MCA.

182. A: Atropine, dopamine, and epinephrine are medications that can be given for a patient experiencing symptomatic bradycardia. The other choices given are antiarrhythmic agents, which are used to slow down a patient's heart rate. Amiodarone may be given to patients having pulseless ventricular tachycardia/ventricular fibrillation or atrial fibrillation. Vasopressin, like amiodarone, slows down the heart rate and is given in the presence of ventricular tachycardia or ventricular fibrillation. Adenosine is given to a patient experiencing supraventricular tachycardia.

183. D: Acute angle-closure glaucoma is a medical emergency that can cause permanent loss of vison if it is not addressed immediately. Once diagnosed, the initial intervention includes oral acetazolamide to lower intraocular pressure, as well as administration of pressure-lowering eyedrops (e.g., pilocarpine, timolol) to prepare for surgery. Then treat with laser iridotomy.

184. B: Rotavirus is one of the most common viral diarrheal illnesses that affect infants and toddlers. It usually presents with non-bloody diarrhea, vomiting, low-grade fever, and anorexia. The mainstay of treatment is hydration. It usually resolves within a week.

185. B: This patient has hypothyroidism. Her TSH is attempting to stimulate the thyroid gland to make more thyroid hormone, but the thyroid is unable to produce sufficient thyroid hormone for the body. The pituitary recognizes that there is insufficient thyroid hormone circulating, so it produces more TSH in hopes of stimulating the thyroid more. The T3 levels may be normal or at the lower end of normal range in hypothyroidism because T4 is the active form of thyroid hormone made available to the body.

186. C: No intervention is needed for an Rh-positive mother with an Rh-negative baby or an Rh-positive mother with an Rh-positive baby. If a pregnant mother is Rh negative, RhoGAM needs to be administered at 28 weeks and within 72 hours of birth or miscarriage.

187. C: This patient most likely has orthostatic hypotension, which is defined as a drop in systolic blood pressure of ≥20 mmHg and a drop in diastolic blood pressure of ≥10 mmHg within 3 minutes of a patient moving from a supine to sitting position. Symptoms may include weakness, dizziness, headache, and syncope. Orthostatic hypotension may be caused by medications, or it may be due to prolonged bed rest, especially if it occurs in a hospital setting.

188. B: The patient is in hypertensive crisis. Hypertensive crisis is defined as a systolic BP >180 and a diastolic BP >120; with evidence of organ damage, it is a hypertensive emergency. The patient has proteinuria, which means the kidneys are showing signs of damage; he requires emergency treatment.

Standard classifications of hypertension in adults (from JNC 7; based on 2 or more readings):

- Normal blood pressure is defined as <120/80.
- Prehypertension is defined as a systolic BP from 120 to 139 and a diastolic BP from 80 to 89.

- Stage 1 hypertension is defined as a systolic BP from 140 to 159 and a diastolic BP from 90 to 99.
- Stage 2 hypertension is defined as a systolic BP ≥160 and a diastolic BP of ≥100.

Guidelines from American College of Cardiology and American Heart Association in 2017 lower these:
Normal = <120/80; **Elevated** = 120-129 and <80; **Stage 1** = 130-139 or 80-89; **Stage 2** = ≥140 or ≥90.

189. C: The patient is in congestive heart failure (dyspnea, orthopnea, increased B-type natriuretic peptide) and would benefit from supplemental oxygen, diuresis, an echocardiogram, and a cardiology consult. A basic metabolic panel should be ordered regularly to monitor the patient's kidney function once diuresis is initiated. The patient's weight should be measured daily to help monitor the efficacy of treatment.

190. B: A varicocele is an enlargement of the veins in the scrotum, causing testicular aching and/or swelling to occur. The venous enlargement is usually due to faulty valves in the veins or compression of a neighboring vein disrupting blood flow. Palpation of the affected testicle is often described as feeling like "a bag of worms." Testicular torsion is a *medical emergency*. It occurs when the spermatic cord becomes twisted and blood flow to the testicle is severely diminished or absent. It presents with acute onset of pain and swelling of the affected testicle. Testicular carcinomas present as hard, painless, fixed testicular solid lesions. A hydrocele is the collection of fluid around the testicle; it is usually due to a patent processus vaginalis but may be due to trauma or infection. It appears as a soft, usually painless mass on the testicle. It is not harmful and has no serious long-term complications.

191. A: Graves disease is one of the most common causes of hyperthyroidism, causing tremor, unintentional weight loss, palpitations, goiter, hypertension, fatigue, nervousness, increased appetite, and exophthalmos. Addison disease is due to insufficient cortisol, causing nausea, vomiting, diarrhea, hypotension, and darkening of the skin color, making the patient look like he or she went tanning. Cushing disease is due to the presence of excessive cortisol, causing unintentional weight gain, striae, a fat pad (buffalo hump) on the posterior neck, facial swelling, and fatigue. Hashimoto disease occurs when the immune system attacks the thyroid gland, causing hypothyroidism. Signs and symptoms of hypothyroidism include bradycardia, unintentional weight gain, puffy face, fatigue, muscle weakness, hair loss, and dry skin.

192. C: The patient should be evaluated by a psychiatrist immediately and should be admitted for further observation. The patient is not a minor and does not need to have her parents notified of her hospitalization unless she requests it. Benzodiazepines are pregnancy category D medications and should not be given unless directed to do so by a psychiatrist. The patient's tetanus status should be investigated, but it is not an urgent priority.

193. B: Tetralogy of Fallot is the most common cyanotic heart defect. The classic four features of tetralogy of Fallot are ventricular septal defect, narrowing of the pulmonary outflow tract, right ventricular hypertrophy, and an overriding aorta. The classic "coeur en sabot," or boot-shaped heart, is due to the right ventricular hypertrophy. Risk factors for this condition include chromosomal abnormalities, advanced maternal age, and maternal history of alcohol abuse.

194. A: Graves disease is one of the most common causes of hyperthyroidism, causing tremor, unintentional weight loss, palpitations, goiter, hypertension, fatigue, nervousness, increased appetite, and exophthalmos. Tests to confirm the diagnosis include a thyroid function panel and an ultrasound or computed tomography (CT) scan of the thyroid if a goiter is present.

195. C: This patient is immune to hepatitis B due to prior vaccination. HBsAg (hepatitis B surface antigen) is present in active or chronic infections. In this case, it is not present. Anti-HBc (total hepatitis B core antibody) indicates previous or acute hepatitis B infection. In this case, it is not present. Anti-HBs (hepatitis B surface antibody) is present in patients with immunity to hepatitis B who are recovering from an infection or have been immunized. Because the other two laboratory test values are negative, this could only mean that the patient has been successfully vaccinated.

196. D: The drop arm test is a maneuver that can help confirm the diagnosis of a rotator cuff tear, although the only way to truly confirm the diagnosis would be an MRI. The examiner will passively abduct the patient's arm 90°, then ask the patient to slowly lower his arm. If the patient is unable to keep his affected arm abducted or it suddenly falls, the examiner should suspect a rotator cuff tear.

197. D: This patient most likely has Addison disease, which is treated with exogenous steroids, dextrose if hypoglycemia is present, and IV fluids for moderate to severe hypotension. Addison disease is due to insufficient cortisol produced by the adrenal glands, causing nausea, vomiting, diarrhea, hypotension, and hyperpigmentation. Due to the low cortisol levels, patients will generally have low sodium levels, causing them to crave salty foods.

198. B: The patient has diabetes and should be advised to modify his diet and maintain an active lifestyle. A patient without diabetes should have an HbA1c of less than 6.5. Because this patient's HbA1c is 6.7, his BMI is normal, and he has no other past medical problems, his diabetes may be manageable with dietary modifications. His BMI is normal, so losing weight would not help. If his HbA1c does not normalize in the next 2-3 months with dietary modifications, starting antihyperglycemic medications would be recommended; he would not require insulin yet.

199. D: Finasteride (Proscar) is used to treat benign prostatic hypertrophy; it is also used to treat baldness (under the brand name Propecia). Levitra, Cialis, and Viagra are all used to treat erectile dysfunction. These three medications increase the level of nitrous oxide, which allows for vasodilatation of the blood vessels. With increased vasodilatation, the penis will stay erect longer and help reverse the symptoms of erectile dysfunction.

200. C: This patient has a negative PPD. No further intervention is required. A patient who has a normal immune system and no underlying disease, is not a healthcare worker, and doesn't have regular contact with tuberculosis-positive patients would need an induration of 15 mm to have a positive PPD test. Because the patient has no medical issues and works as a librarian, the size of her induration is considered to be a negative test result. An induration of 2 mm in any patient is considered a negative PPD test result. An induration of 5 mm or more is considered positive in any patient that is immunocompromised. Healthcare workers, or those who work in close contact with people who have tuberculosis, would need to have 10 mm or greater induration to have a positive PPD test.

201. C: In sexually active males, the causative organisms are likely to be gonorrhea (GC)/chlamydia. This patient most likely has been getting epididymitis due to GC/chlamydia from unprotected sex. Drinking plenty of fluids is general advice given to those who suffer from sickle cell disease or nephrolithiasis, and those who get persistent urinary tract infections (UTIs). Fluid hydration would not help prevent epididymitis. Avoiding red meat, alcohol, and seafood are recommendations generally given to those with gout or cardiovascular disease. Epididymitis is also commonly caused by *E. coli*. If he did not have a history of having unprotected sex, *E. coli* would be the more likely causative organism, and so a urology referral might be recommended.

202. B: Diverticulosis is the presence of pockets in any organ or fluid-filled cavity. The potential for developing this condition increases with age. Development of these pockets does not cause symptoms. If an infection develops within the diverticula, then this condition is called diverticulitis. Mallory-Weiss tears are usually found in the esophageal junction. They are commonly seen in alcoholic patients, caused by persistent episodes of vomiting; however, any pathologic process that causes forceful coughing or vomiting may cause a Mallory-Weiss tear. Celiac sprue is an immune reaction that damages the lining of the small intestine and prevents it from absorbing important nutrients. It presents with nausea, vomiting, diarrhea, and abdominal pain, which occur after ingesting gluten products. Intussusception is when one part of the bowel folds in on itself and causes an obstruction. This is common in children. Symptoms include nausea, vomiting, lethargy, and "red currant jelly" stools.

203. A: The most common causes of transudative pleural effusions in the US are CHF and cirrhosis. They are caused by increased permeability of the capillaries in the lung. Unless the effusion is large or symptomatic (then perform a thoracentesis), no intervention is warranted other than to diurese and correct the underlying cause. Rule out other causes of pleural effusions.

204. C: This patient likely has cor pulmonale caused by his COPD. Signs of right ventricular failure are fluid retention, chronic cough, shortness of breath, enlarged liver, and congestion. An echocardiogram is the best initial diagnostic test for evaluating this condition.

205. B: Herpes zoster (shingles) is a viral disease characterized by a painful skin rash with blisters along a dermatome. The chicken pox virus remains latent in the body after initial infection. Advancing age, stress, trauma, or infection can cause reactivation of the virus; this is called herpes zoster. Antiviral medications, if given early enough, can shorten the course of illness. Pain medications should also be given.

206. B: Prednisone is a common medication used to treat polyarteritis nodosa. Polyarteritis nodosa is a vasculitis that affects small and medium-sized arteries, causing a large range of nonspecific symptoms. There is no known cause, but its incidence is higher in men than women, and people with hepatitis B have a higher incidence of developing this disorder. Treatment includes steroids and possibly plasmapheresis and antivirals. The prognosis is poor without treatment.

207. C: This patient has pulseless ventricular tachycardia. Epinephrine would be the drug of choice according to Advanced Cardiovascular Life Support (ACLS) protocol. Amiodarone and magnesium sulfate could be given during a code involving a patient with pulseless ventricular tachycardia, but they would be given after administration of epinephrine. Atropine is used for symptomatic bradycardia.

208. D: Ramipril is an antihypertensive medication and is not used in the treatment of benign prostatic hypertrophy. Proscar, Cardura, and Rapaflo are all medications used to treat benign prostatic hypertrophy. α-blockers such as Cardura and Rapaflo help the muscle in the prostate to relax so it does not impinge on the urethra. Medications such as Proscar, which is a 5-α reductase inhibitor, help slow the growth of the prostate.

209. D: Antiplatelet medications or anticoagulation therapy should never be given to a suspected stroke patient until a CT scan of the brain shows that there is no hemorrhage present. Although 80% of strokes are ischemic, the remainder are hemorrhagic strokes. If the patient has a hemorrhagic stroke, these medications can exacerbate the bleeding and can potentially kill the patient.

210. A: *Clostridioides difficile* (*C. difficile*) colitis is a common nosocomial (hospital-acquired) infection. It is caused by the alteration of one's normal gastrointestinal (GI) flora, usually caused by long-term antibiotic usage. Vancomycin by mouth is one of the treatments for *C. difficile* colitis. The other medications used are PO metronidazole or PO fidaxomicin. Clindamycin is one the antibiotics that runs an increased risk of causing *C. difficile* colitis. Azithromycin plays no role in the treatment of *C. difficile* colitis. Vancomycin IV cannot be used in the treatment of *C. difficile* because insufficient amounts of it reach the colon to have any effect.

211. C: Status epilepticus describes a patient who continuously seizes. Phenytoin is an antiseizure medication, and lorazepam is used for sedation; both medications are used to help treat status epilepticus. Levetiracetam is also used for the treatment of seizure disorders. Lomotil helps to treat diarrhea. Linezolid is an antibiotic. Phenylephrine is an α-1 agonist for hypotension. Neither Lomotil nor linezolid plays any role in the treatment of status epilepticus.

212. B: The Virchow triad comprises hypercoagulability, endothelial injury, and stasis (hemodynamic changes) that increase one's risk of thrombosis. The Beck triad is the combination of distended jugular veins, hypotension, and muffled heart sounds. It occurs as a result of pericardial effusion. The Charcot triad is the combination of jaundice, fever, and right upper quadrant abdominal pain. It occurs as a result of ascending cholangitis. The Cushing triad is a clinical triad defined as hypertension, bradycardia, and irregular respirations. It suggests rising intracranial pressure due to intracranial pathology such as hemorrhage.

213. B: This patient may have a Lisfranc fracture. A Lisfranc fracture is the fracture and dislocation of one or more of the metatarsals. A Monteggia fracture is a fracture of the ulna and dislocation of the radius. A Colles fracture is a fracture and dorsal displacement of the distal radius. It is commonly referred to as a "dinner-fork deformity" on x-ray. A Le Fort fracture is a fracture of the maxilla; this type of fracture has 3 categories based on severity (I: horizontal; II: pyramidal; III: craniofacial disjunction).

214. B: Amiodarone is an antiarrhythmic medication used for diseases such as atrial fibrillation. It plays no role in the treatment of cystic fibrosis (CF), nor does it prevent complications that may be associated with CF. Nonsteroidal anti-inflammatory drugs (NSAIDs) such as Motrin help decrease inflammation, which can help with infections and prevent airway damage. Mucinex helps thin out the copious mucus that collects in the airways of those with CF. By thinning out the mucus, the patient is able to expectorate it more easily, which helps prevent infection. Albuterol is a bronchodilator that opens up the airways and makes it easier to breathe for those with pulmonary diseases such as CF, asthma, and chronic obstructive pulmonary disease (COPD).

215. D: Pott disease is caused by the spread of tuberculosis to the spine. Signs and symptoms may include night sweats, anorexia, back pain, and lower extremity weakness. Parkinson disease destroys dopamine-producing neurons in the substantia nigra, and it causes motor symptoms (dyskinesia, tremor, and rigidity) as well as cognitive symptoms. Hashimoto disease occurs when the immune system attacks the thyroid gland, causing hypothyroidism. Signs and symptoms of hypothyroidism include bradycardia, unintentional weight gain, puffy face, fatigue, muscle weakness, hair loss, and dry skin. Cushing disease is due to the presence of excessive cortisol, causing unintentional weight gain, striae, a fat pad (buffalo hump) on the posterior neck, facial swelling, and fatigue.

216. A: Fibromyalgia is a diagnosis of exclusion. Patients often complain of generalized body aches and pains with no known cause found during a workup. It is linked to anxiety and depression in many cases. Polyarteritis nodosa is a type of vasculitis with unknown cause. Signs and symptoms of this disease may include painful red bumps on the skin, myalgia, fever, arthralgia, and weakness. It is diagnosed through a variety of lab tests and a biopsy. Osteoarthritis is a degeneration of one or more joints from overuse, usually diagnosed by x-ray. Polymyalgia rheumatica is a type of rheumatoid disease that usually affects the larger joints, such as the shoulders and hips. It is diagnosed by a variety of lab tests, which show the presence of inflammation, as well as by physical examination.

217. D: Paroxetine is an SSRI used to treat generalized anxiety disorder, depression, posttraumatic stress disorder, and other psychiatric conditions. Prednisolone is a type of steroid used to treat inflammatory reactions, such as localized skin reactions and asthma. Promethazine is used to treat and prevent nausea and vomiting. It is also used for motion sickness. Permethrin is used to treat infections caused by scabies.

218. A: This patient has cataracts, which are sclerotic lesions on the lens that slowly obstruct vision. They become more common with age. Conditions such as diabetes, hypertension, tobacco, and alcohol abuse predispose people to developing cataracts. Surgical intervention alleviates symptoms.

219. B: Doppler ultrasound is the imaging of choice in diagnosing deep venous thrombi. It is very sensitive and exposes the patient to the least amount of radiation. CT and MRI scans are usually reserved for tissue, muscular, or ligamentous injuries or pathologies. They are also good in diagnosing infections or fluid collections. X-rays are not used because they only show radiopaque structures like bones. They do not clearly show muscles, ligaments, tissues, or blood vessels.

220. A: Mallory-Weiss tears occur in the esophageal junction and are usually seen in alcoholic patients; they are caused by persistent episodes of vomiting. However, any pathologic process that causes forceful coughing or vomiting may cause a Mallory-Weiss tear. In Crohn disease, the colon wall may have a "cobblestone" appearance due to the intermittent pattern of affected and nonaffected colonic tissue. Ulcerative colitis usually affects continuous stretches of the colon and rectum. Whipple disease is a rare, chronic disease caused by bacterial infection. The affected bowel is usually swollen with raised, yellowish patches.

221. D: This patient most likely has a venous thrombus caused by her recent hip surgery. Patients with venous thrombi have a positive Homan sign in approximately one-third of the cases. A positive Homan sign may be elicited if a patient has pain with dorsiflexion of his or her foot while the leg is extended. Osteomyelitis and septic arthritis are unlikely because they are involved with infection of a joint or joints rather than presenting with muscular pain and swelling. Osgood-Schlatter disease is the swelling of the tibial tubercle due to microavulsion fractures, which commonly occurs in pubescent and prepubescent children.

222. A: Mitral regurgitation is occurring on the 2D echo. The mitral valve permits blood flow from the left atrium into the left ventricle. If the valve does not close properly, mitral regurgitation will occur. Pulmonic regurgitation is the backflow of blood from the pulmonary artery into the right ventricle. Tricuspid regurgitation is the backflow of blood from the right ventricle into the right atrium. Aortic regurgitation is the backflow of blood from the aorta into the left ventricle.

223. C: Pulseless ventricular tachycardia (VT) is treated with immediate defibrillation. You would also give 1 mg of epinephrine IV every 3-5 minutes (OR sometimes 40 units of vasopressin × 1 could be used). Epinephrine would be the first drug of choice, according to Advanced Cardiovascular Life Support (ACLS) protocol. Amiodarone would be the next medication administered after epinephrine if the patient is still in VT.

224. D: This patient has gynecomastia, which is the appearance of breasts in males due to enlarged mammary glands. This is commonly due to hormonal changes in puberty (also in newborns) or may be due to obesity, endocrine abnormality, or underlying disease. This condition usually resolves on its own in a pubescent patient with no significant past medical history.

225. A: The child has otitis media, which is an infection of the middle ear. Mastoiditis is an infection of the mastoid bone of the skull. It is generally a complication of inner ear infections. Symptoms may include fever, ear pain, ear discharge, swelling behind the ear (where the mastoid bone is located), hearing loss, headache, and erythema. Imaging studies such as magnetic resonance imaging (MRI) and computed tomography (CT) scans can make a definitive diagnosis. Otitis externa is an infection of the outer ear. Signs and symptoms may include pain with palpation of the tragus and otorrhea. These patients avoid tugging at their ear due to the pain. Acoustic neuromas are tumors of the acoustic nerve. They are much more common in adults than in children. Symptoms include gradual hearing loss, dizziness, headache, tinnitus, facial droop, and ataxia.

226. C: Ankylosing spondylitis is a type of arthritis that primarily affects the spine (axial skeleton), causing chronic pain (even at night). The inflammation leads to stiffness and bony fusion in the spine, and a kyphotic appearance. The hallmark feature of ankylosing spondylitis is the involvement of the sacroiliac joints. This appears more often in men 20-40 years old.

227. A: A boxer's fracture is the fracture and possible displacement of the fourth or fifth metacarpal, usually following a trauma with a closed fist. A Colles fracture is a fracture and dorsal displacement of the distal radius. It is commonly referred to as a "dinner-fork deformity" on x-ray. A Monteggia fracture is the fracture of the proximal ulna with dislocation the radial head. A buckle fracture is bone break resulting from a bend in the bone. The bend causes a raised bump on one side of the bone.

228. D: This patient has respiratory acidosis. The pH is low (normal value 7.35 to 7.45), and the $PaCO_2$ is high (normal value 35 to 45). To interpret an arterial blood gas test, first look at the pH. If it is low, acidosis is present. If the pH is high, alkalosis is present. Next, look at the $PaCO_2$; if it is low, alkalosis is present. If it is increased, acidosis is present. If the $PaCO_2$ explains the change of pH, then it is a respiratory disorder. If it does not, look at the HCO_3. The normal range is 22 to 26. If the HCO_3 is increased and the pH is high, then it is metabolic alkalosis. If the pH is low and the HCO_3 is low, then it is metabolic acidosis.

229. C: Nursemaid's elbow describes the dislocation of the elbow commonly due to pulling up on a child's extended forearm while holding the child's hand. It most commonly occurs in children under the age of 6 due to their hyperflexible joints and growing bones. Children usually have little to no pain and hold their affected extremity in a flexed and pronated position. Function returns, usually immediately, after it is reduced.

230. A: This patient has anorexia nervosa. It is an eating disorder much more common in girls than boys, and it is most common in adolescents. It is characterized by purposely starving oneself. Bulimia nervosa is an eating disorder much more common in girls than boys and most common in adolescents. It involves periods of bingeing followed by periods of purging. Generalized anxiety disorder is a psychiatric disorder in which a person feels anxious or nervous most or all of the time with no known cause. Bipolar disorder is a psychiatric disorder in which a person has episodes of mania, or extreme happiness and energy, followed by periods of depression.

231. B: This patient has generalized anxiety disorder. Generalized anxiety disorder is a psychiatric disorder in which a person feels anxious or nervous most or all of the time, for more days than not for ≥6 months, with no known cause. Persistent depressive disorder (dysthymia) is a milder form of major depressive disorder. Posttraumatic stress disorder (PTSD) is when a person has intrusive nervous or anxious feelings due to a known cause such as rape or a near-death experience, witnessing someone's death, or being involved in a disturbing event such as a school shooting or terrorist attack. A phobia is a feeling of intense fear about a particular stimulus that is usually nonthreatening to most people (i.e., being afraid to go outside or being afraid of water).

232. C: This patient has metabolic alkalosis. The pH is high (normal is 7.35-7.45), the $PaCO_2$ is normal (normal is 35-45), and the HCO_3 is high (normal is 22-26). To interpret an arterial blood gas test, first look at the pH. If it is low, acidosis is present. If the pH is high, alkalosis is present. Next look at the $PaCO_2$; if it is low, acidosis is present. If it is increased, alkalosis is present. If the $PaCO_2$ explains the change of pH, then it is a respiratory disorder. If not, look at the HCO_3. If the HCO_3 is increased and the pH is high, it is metabolic alkalosis. If the pH is low and the HCO_3 is low, it is metabolic acidosis.

233. C: This patient has normal pressure hydrocephalus (NPH) and should undergo a ventricular peritoneal shunt (VPS) if he or she is not a high-risk patient. There is no other way to correct NPH. An MRI scan of the brain may help diagnose NPH and reveal its cause, but it is not a treatment of NPH. A repeat lumbar puncture is not useful. Once a patient has one lumbar puncture and his or her symptoms improve, the diagnosis is made. Performing an EEG may help rule out other etiologies that are causing the patient's symptoms, but it is not a treatment of NPH.

234. D: This patient has a phobia disorder. A phobia is feeling extremely nervous or scared about a particular stimulus that is usually nonthreatening to most people (e.g., being afraid to go outside or being afraid of water). Generalized anxiety disorder is a psychiatric disorder in which a person feels anxious or nervous most or all of the time, for ≥6 months, with no known cause. Posttraumatic stress disorder (PTSD) is when a person has intrusive nervous or anxious feelings due to a known cause such as rape or a near-death experience, witnessing someone's death, or being involved in a disturbing event such as a school shooting or terrorist attack. Persistent depressive disorder (dysthymia) is a milder form of major depressive disorder.

235. A: Inherited genetic mutations are the most common cause of hypertrophic cardiomyopathy. Hypertrophic cardiomyopathy is an abnormal thickening of the cardiac fibers. The thickening of these fibers impairs the heart's ability to fill with blood and its ability to pump out blood to the rest of the body. This condition is diagnosed by an echocardiogram. Surgery, implantation of a pacemaker, and medications (e.g., β-blockers) may help alleviate the complications this condition may cause.

236. B: Chorea is not a minor manifestation of acute rheumatic fever according to the Jones criteria.

Major manifestations of acute rheumatic fever include the following:

- Erythema marginatum: raised, nonpruritic pink rings on the trunk and inner surfaces of the limbs
- Carditis: inflammation of the heart muscle
- Chorea: rapid, uncontrolled body movements
- Subcutaneous nodules: painless, firm collections of collagen fibers over bones or tendons
- Polyarthritis: temporary migrating inflammation of the large joints

Minor manifestations of acute rheumatic fever include the following:

- Fever (101 °F to 102 °F)
- Arthralgia: joint pain without swelling
- Elevated ESR or C-reactive protein (CRP)
- Leukocytosis
- Prior episode of rheumatic heart disease or rheumatic fever
- Heart block seen on an electrocardiogram (ECG)

237. D: Tricuspid regurgitation is the backflow of blood from the right ventricle into the right atrium. Aortic regurgitation is the backflow of blood from the aorta into the left ventricle. The mitral valve permits blood flow from the left atrium into the left ventricle. If the valve does not close properly, mitral regurgitation will occur. Pulmonic regurgitation is the backflow of blood from the pulmonary artery into the right ventricle.

238. D: Atropine, epinephrine, dopamine, and transcutaneous pacing are used for patients with symptomatic bradycardia. Atropine is used to increase the heart rate. In ventricular fibrillation, the heart rate is already abnormally fast, so atropine would only exacerbate this arrhythmia. Epinephrine, vasopressin, amiodarone, lidocaine, and magnesium sulfate are all medications that have been used in pulseless ventricular fibrillation or pulseless ventricular tachycardia. For pulseless ventricular fibrillation, Advanced Cardiovascular Life Support (ACLS) currently recommends defibrillation, then 1 mg epinephrine every 3-5 minutes, and then adding amiodarone.

239. B: This patient has respiratory alkalosis. To interpret an arterial blood gas test, first look at the pH. If it is low, acidosis is present. If the pH is high, alkalosis is present. Next look at the $PaCO_2$; if it is low, alkalosis is present. If it is increased, acidosis is present. If the $PaCO_2$ explains the change of pH, then it is a respiratory disorder. If it does not, look at the HCO_3. The normal range is 22 to 26. If the HCO_3 is increased and the pH is high, it is metabolic alkalosis. If the pH is low and the HCO_3 is low, it is metabolic acidosis.

240. B: The patient has horizontal nystagmus, which is common after acute drug or alcohol intoxication. It is an involuntary, oscillating eye movement that occurs bilaterally and resolves once the toxins are out of the body. Entropion is the inward turning of the upper or lower lid toward the eye. Exotropia is a condition in which one eye is normal and the other eye deviates laterally/outwardly. Conjunctivitis is the inflammation of the conjunctiva from an infection, allergy, or irritant, causing pain, blurry vision due to discharge, conjunctival erythema, and crusting of the lids and/or lashes.

241. B: This patient has right bundle branch block. This conduction arrhythmia has a widened QRS complex and two R waves or "bunny ears" best seen in V1-V3. Torsades de pointes means "twisting of the points" around the isoelectric baseline of an ECG, which describes this polymorphic ventricular tachycardia. Atrial fibrillation is a type of tachycardia with irregularly irregular QRS complexes and no P waves. Sinus tachycardia is defined as a heart rate greater than 100 beats per minute with regular QRS complexes preceded by P waves.

242. D: A transient ischemic attack (TIA) is the sudden onset of focal neurologic deficits that spontaneously resolve (usually within an hour). It is important to rule out a hemorrhage/ cerebrovascular accident (CVA).

Diffusion-weighted MRI of the brain is the best diagnostic test for evaluating possible CVAs, but is not always available. A non-contrast head CT with CT angiography is a good method to evaluate the brain tissue and vasculature in suspected TIA patients. Antithrombotic therapy should be started in TIA patients (once a hemorrhage is ruled out) since there is an increased risk of stroke post-TIA.

243. C: Although all medical professionals are bound by the Health Insurance Portability and Accountability Act (HIPAA), which ensures patient privacy, there are instances in which a medical professional may share a patient's information. If a patient threatens to injure themselves or others, a medical professional may reach out to local authorities or family members to warn them of the patient's potential plans in order to ensure the safety of the patient and others.

244. A: The patient has entropion, or the inward turning of the lid toward the eye. This may cause excessive tearing or irritation of the eye; if it is severe enough, the patient may develop a corneal abrasion. Exotropia is the outward deviation of the eye. Ectropion is the outward turning of the lid away from the eye. Esotropia is the inward deviation of the eye.

245. D: This patient has oppositional-defiant disorder (ODD), which is an emotional and psychiatric disorder that causes patients to have labile moods and have problems getting along with and listening to authority figures. There is no one cause; sometimes it runs in families. Adjustment disorder is when a patient has a problem adjusting to or getting used to new life events or circumstances. Persistent depressive disorder (dysthymia) is a milder form of major depressive disorder. Attention-deficit/hyperactivity disorder is when a patient has a high level of energy and a short attention span.

246. A: Colchicine is used for the treatment of acute gout. Phlebitis is the presence of a superficial irritation of a vein (sometimes associated with a thrombus) in an extremity (most commonly in the leg), which can cause pain, swelling, and erythema. Patients may be given antibiotics if a secondary infection is present. They may be given anticoagulation medications depending on their risk factors and past medical history. Typically, phlebitis can be treated on an outpatient basis, using analgesics such as NSAIDs, warm compresses, and compression stockings.

247. D: Testicular carcinomas present as a hard, painless, fixed, solid testicular lesion. A CBC would provide little value in confirming the diagnosis. LDH, AFP, and HCG are all tumor markers. The levels of AFP and HCG can also help providers tell which type of testicular cancer it might be. The LDH level is nonspecific, but high levels may indicate whether widespread cancer is present.

248. B: Frovatriptan is a tryptamine-based medication that helps prevent and treat migraine headaches. Other medications that may be used to treat migraines include NSAIDs, aspirin, narcotics, and β-blockers. Fluoxetine is used to treat anxiety and depression. Fexofenadine is an antihistamine used to treat seasonal allergy exacerbations. Fluvastatin is part of the statin drug class, which is used to treat hyperlipidemia.

249. D: The initiation of insulin is the first initial step in management for a gestational diabetic patient who has failed conservative measures (sometimes metformin has been used off-label before insulin is started; pregnancy category B). Regular insulin is a pregnancy category B medication. The thiazolidinediones, such as pioglitazone, are pregnancy category C medications. The patient has no evidence of diabetic ketoacidosis and does not need an endocrinologist at this point.

250. B: Tourette disorder is first noticed in childhood and is characterized by involuntary verbal sounds and/or motor movements. It does not cause cognitive impairment, although it may be seen in the presence of cognitive disorders. Alzheimer disease is a progressive cognitive decline; the underlying cause is not fully understood, but it is known to exhibit amyloid deposits and neurofibrillary tangles in the brain. Motor skills are much less affected until late stages of the disease. Multiple sclerosis is a demyelinating disease that may present with progressive ataxia, muscle spasms, dizziness, trouble with coordination of fine motor movements, urinary frequency, incontinence, nystagmus, and depression. Huntington disease is a progressive neurologic disorder caused by an autosomal-dominant chromosomal abnormality, and usually occurs in the third or fourth decade of life. Signs include progressive decline in cognitive function; ataxic gait; and uncoordinated, jerky body movements.

251. A: Spirometry is the best test to aid in the diagnosis of COPD. Spirometry measures airflow by testing lung volume and lung capacity (COPD shows decreased FEV1, decreased FVC). A chest x-ray may show pathologic changes that accompany COPD, but the x-ray may be normal. It is not a diagnostic test for COPD. Auscultation with a stethoscope may reveal wheezing and diminished breath sounds, but they can occur with many different conditions. Breath sounds may even be normal in someone with COPD. An ECG is the least helpful diagnostic aid; it generally is used to help diagnose cardiac-related abnormalities.

252. B: A Texas catheter should be applied. tPA is a very strong clot-busting medication given to patients with stroke or acute myocardial infarctions. After being given this medication, patients generally should not receive blood thinners, antiplatelet medications, or lines/indwelling catheters for 24 hours because their risk of bleeding is very high. This patient is a fall risk and should not ambulate while in the tPA window.

253. D: Aspergillosis is a fungal pneumonia commonly occurring in those who are immunocompromised. The classic radiological finding is a fungus ball (aspergilloma) seen on chest x-ray or a CT scan of the chest. Aspergillomas may also be found in the nasal sinuses. Sarcoidosis is a disease with an unknown cause in which granulomas can form in the organs or the skin. It is not a fungal disease. Cystic fibrosis is an autosomal-recessive lung disorder in which mucus in the lungs and digestive tract becomes abnormally thick, causing chronic lung infections and GI complications. Pneumoconiosis, or "miner's lung," is a lung disease caused by long-term exposure to coal or coal-related products.

254. C: Autism spectrum disorders are neurodevelopmental disorders affecting cognition and social skills. Signs may appear as early as the first year of life to as late as school age. Classic signs of this disorder are cognitive and social impairment and persistent repetitive behaviors. There is no known cause or cure. Speech therapy, behavioral therapies, psychiatric medications, and special education programs are the mainstays of treatment. Oppositional-defiant disorder is an emotional and psychiatric disorder causing patients to have labile moods and have problems getting along with and listening to others. There is no one cause; sometimes it runs in families, sometimes it is seen in children of parents who abuse alcohol or drugs, and sometimes it is seen in children whose parents have psychiatric disorders. In some cases, there is no known cause. Attention-deficit/hyperactivity disorder is when a patient has a high level of energy and a short attention span. Adjustment disorder is when a patient has a problem getting used to new life events or circumstances.

255. C: No intervention is needed if both the mother and baby are Rh positive. The Rh factor is an antigen that may or may not be attached to the red blood cells. People with a positive blood type (A+, B+, O+, AB+) have the antigen. People with Rh-negative blood do not have the antigen; problems typically arise in an Rh-negative mother after the first pregnancy with an Rh-positive baby. If a mother is Rh negative, RhoGAM is administered at 28 weeks' gestation. RhoGAM is an injection that suppresses the mother's immune response to an Rh-positive baby, which can help prevent hemolytic disease of the newborn or miscarriage. If the newborn baby is found to be Rh positive at delivery, another injection of RhoGAM is given within 72 hours of delivery. Antibiotics are unnecessary because it is a blood incompatibility, not an infection. An ultrasound would not be useful regarding Rh factor.

256. C: Labor should be induced immediately after the patient is stabilized (give magnesium sulfate to treat seizures). Eclampsia is the development of hypertension, proteinuria, and seizures that develop any time after 20 weeks' gestation through the postpartum period. The only cure for eclampsia is delivery. Blood transfusions play no role in the treatment or cure of eclampsia if the complete blood count is normal.

257. A: This patient has a pleural effusion, which is a pathologic fluid collection due to his COPD. If the effusion is large enough, it will present with blunting of the costophrenic angle on chest x-ray. Aspergillosis is a fungal pneumonia commonly occurring in those who are immunocompromised. The classic radiological finding is a fungus ball seen on chest x-ray or CT of the chest. Pneumoconiosis, or "miner's lung," is a lung disease caused by long-term exposure to coal or coal-related products. The classic chest x-ray findings are small cystic radiolucencies that look like honeycombs. Pneumothoraxes will appear as a black space on a chest x-ray with no lung markings. If they are small enough, the chest x-ray may appear normal.

258. D: If the pneumothorax is small (typically less than 10%), the chest x-ray may appear normal. A moderate-sized pneumothorax (typically one that is larger than 10% in size) will appear as a black space on chest x-ray with no lung markings. Pneumoconiosis, or "miner's lung," is a lung disease caused by long-term exposure to coal or coal-related products. The classic chest x-ray findings are small cystic radiolucencies or honeycombs. CT is also a good imaging study for this. Sarcoidosis is a disease with an unknown cause in which granulomas can form in one's organs or the skin.

259. A: Graves disease is an autoimmune disease that causes hyperthyroidism, which would promote weight loss, not weight gain. Untreated hypothyroidism may contribute to obesity because the thyroid plays a role in metabolism. If the thyroid is functioning more sluggishly than normal, weight gain may occur due to the slowing down of metabolism. Cushing disease is due to the presence of excessive cortisol, causing unintentional weight gain, striae, a fat pad (buffalo hump) on the posterior neck, and facial swelling. Women going through menopause are at an increased risk for gaining weight due to the various hormonal changes they are going through, as well as a redistribution of body fat that commonly occurs during that time.

260. C: Allergic rhinitis is caused by sensitivity to an allergen (something in the environment). It is not a bacterial infection. Antibiotics are not prescribed for allergic rhinitis unless there is a secondary infection present. Decongestants help reduce the amount of fluid and mucus that accumulates in the airways. Antihistamines are used to alleviate inflammation and pruritus. Corticosteroids help treat inflammation commonly caused by an overactive immune system, and they help reduce swelling.

261. D: Phobia disorder is a specific type of anxiety disorder. Although general anxiety disorder may not have a particular trigger or reason for the onset of symptoms, phobias are caused by a particular person, place, or thing. A phobia is a feeling of being extremely nervous or scared about a particular stimulus that is usually nonthreatening to most people (e.g., being afraid to go outside or being afraid of water). Xanax is a benzodiazepine, which will cause mild sedation. It is commonly used in those with anxiety, insomnia, and alcohol withdrawal. Metoprolol is a β-blocker that helps lower blood pressure and heart rate. It is most commonly used in the treatment of hypertension and cardiac arrhythmias, but it may also be used in patients who suffer from phobias and stage fright. Lexapro is a selective serotonin reuptake inhibitor (SSRI) used in the treatment of anxiety and depression. Ritalin is a psychostimulant used to help increase attention span and concentration; it is commonly used in patients who suffer from attention-deficit/hyperactivity disorder. It does not play a role in someone who suffers from phobias.

262. B: Naloxone (Narcan) is an opiate antidote used to treat potential or confirmed narcotic overdoses. It is not used in the treatment of alcohol withdrawal. There is no one treatment for alcohol withdrawal. Treatment is based on the symptoms displayed by the patient. Thiamine (helps prevent Wernicke encephalopathy and Wernicke-Korsakoff syndrome), magnesium, and folic acid are frequently administered to alcoholic patients because they are usually chronically malnourished and suffer from electrolyte imbalances due to their addiction. Zofran is an antiemetic medication that prevents and alleviates nausea and vomiting. Ativan is a benzodiazepine that causes mild sedation. It is usually given to alleviate symptoms such as delirium tremens.

263. C: This patient has submandibular/sublingual cellulitis called Ludwig angina that progresses rapidly. It involves a bacterial infection under the tongue, causing swelling, a sensation of choking, erythema, dysphonia, dysphagia, and fever. The classic physical finding is when patients sound like they have a "hot potato in their mouth." It may occur spontaneously, but it is commonly preceded by a dental infection. It is an ENT emergency. Oral leukoplakia is the presence of white plaques in the mouth caused by chronic irritation such as from chewing tobacco or alcohol use. It does not cause dysphagia, dysphonia, tongue displacement, neck swelling, or erythema. Acute pharyngitis is an infection of the pharynx that may cause dysphagia, dysphonia, and fever, but it does not commonly cause neck swelling and does not cause displacement of the tongue. Aphthous ulcers are sores that occur on the lips, gums, or tongue. The cause is unknown. They appear as gray, white, or yellow sores on an erythematous base. They may cause dysphagia, but they are superficial, so they do not cause dysphonia, fever, neck swelling, or tongue displacement.

264. A: Irrigation of the eye would generally be ineffective and is not used in the treatment of a blowout fracture. A blowout fracture is a fracture of the walls and/or floor of the orbital bone, most commonly caused by trauma. Antibiotics are always warranted as prophylaxis against infection. Steroids are used to help decrease swelling. Surgery may be warranted depending on the severity of the fracture.

265. D: A Le Fort fracture is a fracture of the maxilla; this type of fracture has 3 categories based on severity (I: horizontal; II: pyramidal; III: craniofacial disjunction). A boxer's fracture is a transverse fracture of the fourth and/or fifth metacarpal bones, usually as a result of trauma with a closed fist. A Lisfranc fracture is the fracture and dislocation of one or more of the metatarsals. A Colles fracture is a fracture and dorsal displacement of the distal radius. It is commonly referred to as a "dinner-fork deformity" on x-ray.

266. D: The number one cause of pelvic inflammatory disease (PID) is venereal disease, most notably, gonorrhea and chlamydia. Untreated sexually transmitted diseases may lead to PID, which is the primary preventable cause of infertility. Approximately 10% to 15% of PID cases are caused by illnesses such as appendicitis or pelvic procedures such as dilation and curettage, abortion, or childbirth. PID may be caused by a pelvic procedure, such as the removal of an ectopic pregnancy, or PID may cause an ectopic pregnancy to occur.

267. D: Esomeprazole is a proton pump inhibitor that causes the stomach to produce less acid. The reduction of acid production means that less acid is released into the esophagus, which will alleviate or partially alleviate symptoms and the damage done to the esophageal mucosa. Metronidazole is an antibiotic used in treating anaerobic bacterial infections; it is also an amebicide and antiprotozoal medication. Ketoconazole and fluconazole are antifungal medications.

268. A: A diverticulum is an outpouching of an organ or fluid-filled cavity. Meckel diverticulum is a remnant of the omphalomesenteric duct, and it is 3 times more common for boys to have symptoms (diverticulitis) from it. Meckel diverticulum is usually 2 inches long and found approximately 2 feet from the ileocecal valve. Two years of age is the most common presentation for those with a complication (hemorrhage) involving Meckel diverticulum. Approximately 2% of the population has this condition, although the majority of patients are asymptomatic.

269. B: Zollinger-Ellison syndrome is caused by tumors in the small intestine and pancreas that secrete gastrin, which can cause gastroesophageal reflux disease (GERD)-like symptoms, abdominal pain, hematemesis, and diarrhea. Celiac disease (sprue) is an immune reaction that damages the lining of the small intestine and prevents it from absorbing important nutrients. A diagnosis can be made by an upper endoscopy with biopsy. Whipple disease is rare chronic disease caused by a bacterial infection. The affected bowel is usually swollen with raised, yellowish patches. This can usually be seen during sigmoidoscopy or colonoscopy. In Crohn disease, the colon wall may have a "cobblestone" appearance due to the intermittent pattern of affected and nonaffected colonic tissue. This can usually be seen during sigmoidoscopy or colonoscopy.

270. B: The patient may have a rotator cuff tear. X-rays may be negative because they can only visualize bones, not muscles, ligaments, or tendons. MRI can definitively determine whether or not a tear is present. Not treating the patient is not appropriate, especially if he or she has a significantly limited range of motion. Not all rotator cuff tears require surgery, but further evaluation of the injury is warranted because the patient has a significantly decreased range of motion. EMG is used to help diagnose the cause of muscle and nerve disorders. It would not be particularly helpful in this case because the patient has a known history of injury. The patient's nerves and muscles are normal; the problem is with the tendon.

271. C: This patient likely has compartment syndrome. Although calling a vascular consult and administering IV fluids for the rhabdomyolysis are important interventions, the initial step should be to remove the splint to alleviate some of the pressure on the affected extremity.

272. B: Ordering a serum calcium test is ineffective in the workup of lactose intolerance. The test can be normal, yet a patient may have lactose intolerance. Lactose intolerance is the body's inability to digest lactose. The undigested lactose can cause flatulence, abdominal cramping, and diarrhea. It is a largely clinical diagnosis, but the other choices given may be ordered to confirm the suspected diagnosis.

273. A: This patient is displaying signs of inflammatory breast cancer referred to as peau d'orange, a French term meaning "skin of an orange." It is caused by impaired lymphatic drainage and edema caused by advanced inflammatory breast cancer. An abscess is a localized area of erythema and tenderness with induration and/or fluctuance caused by a collection of pus underneath the skin. Gynecomastia is the overgrowth of breast tissue in males, most commonly occurring in adolescence. A fibroadenoma is a firm, rubbery, benign breast mass. It does not cause overlying skin changes.

274. D: The patient developed supraventricular tachycardia, likely caused by her supratherapeutic digoxin level. The Valsalva maneuver can sometimes terminate this cardiac arrhythmia. An electrophysiology study is useful in establishing the diagnosis and pathway of complex arrhythmias such as supraventricular tachycardia.

275. C: If possible, this patient should have early morning surgery. Metformin should not be given the morning of surgery due to NPO status since it may cause possible renal function issues or hypoglycemia. However, it is important to maintain good glycemic ranges (generally 140-180) during the perioperative and postoperative periods, so starting an insulin infusion to be closely monitored during pre-anesthesia care is generally advised. General pre-op care includes discontinuing long-acting insulins (e.g., glargine) 2-3 days prior to surgery. Also, biguanides (e.g., metformin) and thiazolidinediones (e.g., rosiglitazone) and sulfonylureas (e.g., glipizide) should be discontinued due to possible hypoglycemia in NPO patients.

276. B: Beriberi is caused by a thiamine deficiency and is primarily seen in developing or underdeveloped countries. Symptoms may include muscle weakness and paresthesias (stocking-glove distribution) due to damaged nerves, heart failure, pleural effusion, encephalopathy, decreased reflexes, and a multitude of other complications. Some of these complications may be permanent if the thiamine deficiency is not corrected quickly.

277. A: Osteoporosis is the presence of decreased bone mineral density in the body, which can lead to persistent pathologic fractures, depending on the severity of the disease. There are a multitude of factors that can contribute, such as vitamin D deficiency, tobacco abuse, disease, and being immobile for long periods. A diet rich in calcium and vitamin D can help prevent or at least slow the development of osteoporosis.

278. B: This patient has a postoperative ileus, as evidenced by the hypoactive bowel sounds and history. The mainstays of therapy are bowel rest, nasogastric tube, antiemetics, bowel regimen, and IV fluids. Also discontinue opioids and other medications that cause constipation.

279. C: Placental abruption (abruptio placentae) is the separation of the placenta from the uterine wall (either partial or complete), causing bright-red vaginal bleeding, abdominal and/or back pain, and severe contractions. Endometriosis is the presence of uterine cells/uterine lining in other areas of the body, causing dysmenorrhea, pain with intercourse, and infertility. Premature rupture of the membranes is when a woman's water breaks prior to the onset of labor. Placenta previa commonly presents with painless, bright-red vaginal bleeding in the second or third trimester. It is due to a low-lying placenta that is near or over the cervical os. As the uterus enlarges, a small part of the placenta may tear, resulting in bright-red bleeding. However, the condition usually resolves as the uterus enlarges, thus moving the placenta away from the cervical os. If it doesn't move away, deliver by C-section.

280. A: In vitro, the ductus arteriosus is a blood vessel in which blood travels from the heart to the lungs. It normally closes a few days after birth, but in patients in which it does not, it is called patent ductus arteriosus (PDA). A continuous murmur is heard. Tachypnea, poor feeding, failure to thrive, shortness of breath, and diaphoresis are signs and symptoms with those who have moderate to severe PDA. PDAs often close on their own. Indomethacin may be used to help close PDAs. Surgical closure of this cardiac defect is generally reserved for those with large, symptomatic defects.

281. C: A Galeazzi fracture is a fracture of the middle or distal radius and dislocation of the radioulnar joint. A Le Fort fracture is a fracture of the maxilla; this type of fracture has 3 categories based on severity (I: horizontal; II: pyramidal; III: craniofacial disjunction). A Colles fracture is fracture and dorsal displacement of the distal radius. It is commonly referred to as a "dinner-fork deformity" on x-ray. A Monteggia fracture is a fracture of the ulna and dislocation of the radius.

282. D: Preeclampsia is the most concerning medical issue that puts the patient at risk for preterm labor. Advanced maternal age also puts her at risk, but the risk is lower than the risk from preeclampsia.

283. C: A completed abortion is when the miscarriage has occurred and the products of conception (POC) have left the body. Abdominal pain and vaginal bleeding may occur in a threatened abortion, but the fetus is still viable. It may be a sign that a miscarriage may occur. However, a woman who experiences a threatened abortion may still deliver a healthy, full-term child. A missed abortion is when the pregnancy is lost and POC are still present. An incomplete abortion is when the body has expelled only some of the POC. Measures must be taken to remove the remaining POC to prevent infection. Dysmenorrhea is painful or uncomfortable menses.

284. B: Paget disease is the abnormal reabsorption and formation of bone, which may be localized or may affect multiple areas in the body. This may cause pain, bony deformities, and pathologic fractures. There is no cure, but zoledronic acid can slow the progression of the disease and help minimize complications. In older patients with more extensive disease, as described in this scenario, a zoledronic acid infusion is preferred to bisphosphonates. These patients must be closely followed due to an increased risk of developing cancer.

285. A: Furosemide is not an appropriate treatment because, as a diuretic, its job is to remove fluid from the body, which would only accelerate the development of dehydration. Giardiasis, also known as "traveler's diarrhea," is caused by protozoa found in infected water supplies. Signs and symptoms may include watery, sometimes explosive diarrhea, which may be greasy, as well as nausea, vomiting, abdominal cramping, bloating, flatulence, and fever. The main concern is dehydration, so the patient must be advised to keep hydrated. Other remedies may include ondansetron to prevent nausea and loperamide to alleviate the diarrhea. Metronidazole treats the infection.

286. D: Irritable bowel syndrome (IBS) is the presence of bowel disturbances without the presence of disease or pathology. Abdominal pain must occur at least 1 day/week for 3 months, and there are two of the following: pain on defecation, change in stool frequency, or change in stool appearance. Usually symptoms improve after defecation. Dietary changes—such as eliminating carbonated beverages, and eliminating certain vegetables including cabbage, broccoli, and cauliflower, as well as raw fruits—may help alleviate symptoms. Taking antidiarrheal medications, osmotic laxatives, and fiber supplements may also provide relief. IBS medications (e.g., hyoscyamine) can also help.

287. D: A serum beta human chorionic gonadotropin (β-HCG) test should be ordered to monitor the progression of choriocarcinoma and its response to therapy. Choriocarcinoma is an abnormal overgrowth of the cells that normally cover the placenta. It may occur after an ectopic pregnancy, a normal pregnancy, or a planned or spontaneous abortion. Because the placenta produces β-HCG, serial β-HCG levels help monitor the progression or regression of the disease. If β-HCG remains, chemotherapy may be needed. A complete blood count is nonspecific and ineffective at monitoring choriocarcinoma. Bence Jones proteins are found in the urine and may be diagnostic of multiple myeloma. A CT scan may help show the size of the tumor and whether metastases are present, but ordering several of them would be unwise because it exposes the patient to a significant amount of radiation.

288. C: Antibiotics do not play a role in treating leiomyomas, or uterine fibroids. Fibroids are benign growths of smooth muscle that may cause dysmenorrhea, menorrhagia, dyspareunia, abdominal cramping, and urinary frequency. NSAIDs can alleviate symptoms of dysmenorrhea and abdominal pain or cramping. Birth control pills can help regulate hormones and alleviate dysmenorrhea and menorrhagia. Iron supplements help prevent anemia that may be caused by menorrhagia.

289. C: Chemotherapy does not play a role in treating leiomyomas, or uterine fibroids. Fibroids are benign uterine tumors that may cause dysmenorrhea, menorrhagia, pain with sexual intercourse, abdominal cramping, and urinary frequency. Risk factors include African American race, obesity, family history, and vitamin D deficiency.

290. A: New-onset AF can spontaneously revert to sinus rhythm, especially if this is the first episode. Many patients are discharged from the ER after episodes of AF that resolve, so ICU admission is not warranted. Evaluating for a cause such as heart failure, pulmonary issues, or hyperthyroidism could be warranted. AF is rarely the only sign of a myocardial infarction (MI), so unless other signs exist, cardiac catheterization is not indicated.

291. D: Tissue plasminogen activator (tPA) should be initiated within 4.5 hours of the onset of stroke symptoms if the patient is a candidate. The patient's embolic stroke was likely caused by the atrial fibrillation. Heparin and warfarin are a treatment alternative when not using tPA. Dabigatran is more effective than warfarin for embolic stroke prevention in atrial fibrillation, with less risk of intercranial hemorrhage, and it starts working faster. Dabigatran (like all anticoagulants) should not be started until at least 24 hours after tPA administration. Antiplatelets (e.g., ASA, clopidogrel) are not started for stroke prevention until 24 hours after tPA.

292. A: Antibiotics do not play a role in treatment of a small-bowel obstruction, unless there is an infection present. If it is a partial obstruction, conservative management is attempted first. Patients are kept in nothing-by-mouth (NPO) status and placed on IV fluid hydration. A nasogastric tube is placed to help decompress the bowel, and antiemetic medications such as Zofran are given as needed for nausea and vomiting.

293. B: Cervical cancer is caused by the human papillomavirus (HPV). Limiting one's sexual partners can decrease one's exposure to HPV and decrease the risk of developing cervical cancer. Regular Pap smears and gynecological examinations can help detect any anomalies early. Long-term use of oral contraceptives, multiparity, tobacco use, history of chlamydia, immunosuppression, and family history are other risk factors for cervical cancer.

294. B: Benign paroxysmal positional vertigo (BPPV) causes patients to feel dizzy in certain positions, or when they readjust positions too quickly, due to a disturbance in the inner ear canal. BPPV develops when small crystals of calcium carbonate break free and end up in the semicircular canal of the inner ear. The Epley maneuver and lifestyle changes are the mainstays of treatment. Cerumen impaction does not affect balance. Parkinson disease is a neurologic movement disorder. An acoustic neuroma is a slow-growing tumor that usually presents with hearing loss on one side.

295. D: Celiac disease, or celiac sprue, is an immune reaction that damages the lining of the small intestine and prevents it from absorbing important nutrients. It presents as nausea, vomiting, diarrhea, and abdominal pain, which occur after ingesting gluten products. The mainstay of treatment is to maintain a gluten-free diet to help prevent future exacerbations.

296. A: Spondylolisthesis is a condition in which the vertebra slips out of place, causing pain or discomfort. The primary cause for this condition is a congenital defect, but it may also be caused by degenerative disease, or trauma. Most treatments include conservative measures such as pain medication, physical therapy, and supportive braces. For severe symptoms or significant disk displacement, surgery may be warranted.

297. C: The withdrawal method involves the male partner pulling out prior to ejaculation. This method has a higher failure rate than the use of intrauterine devices, birth control pills, and condoms, even when it is performed consistently. It is believed that some semen enters the vagina prior to ejaculation, which can result in unwanted pregnancy.

298. D: Methotrexate is an antimetabolite used to treat cancer, to treat autoimmune disorders such as lupus or rheumatoid arthritis, and for medical abortions. Metronidazole is an antibiotic used in treating anaerobic bacterial infections; it is also an amebicide and antiprotozoal medication. Meropenem is a strong broad-spectrum antibiotic used to treat anaerobic, gram-positive, and gram-negative bacteria. Metformin is an antihyperglycemic medication used in the treatment of diabetes.

299. B: Though the exact cause of osteoarthritis is unknown, it is related to aging and degenerative disease. Cartilage is a rubbery substance that helps cushion and protect bones. As cartilage gets worn away with age and overuse, the bones begin to rub against each other, causing pain and inflammation. Strenuous activity, multiple fractures, and obesity also play roles in the development of osteoarthritis.

300. A: Kyphosis is an abnormal curvature of the spine, usually due to degenerative disease, although it may also be due to trauma, bony diseases such as spina bifida or Paget disease, and tumors. If the curvature is severe enough, surgery may be warranted, but usually the treatment is conservative management. Cauda equina syndrome can be caused by disease, trauma, or infection. It is caused by severe compression of the nerve roots below the termination of the spinal cord (below L1), which can cause motor dysfunction, urinary retention, and saddle anesthesia, among other neurologic issues. This can be a surgical emergency. Avascular necrosis occurs when there is insufficient blood flow or complete lack of blood flow to the bone, causing death of the bone cells. Patients may complain of a painful joint. The sciatic nerve runs down the lower back and down each of the legs, providing sensation to the lower extremities. The nerve can become inflamed or impinged (sciatica) due to degeneration of the spine, disease, or trauma. It does not cause an abnormal curvature of the spine.

PA Practice Test #2

To take this additional PA practice test, visit our bonus page:
mometrix.com/bonus948/pance

How to Overcome Test Anxiety

Just the thought of taking a test is enough to make most people a little nervous. A test is an important event that can have a long-term impact on your future, so it's important to take it seriously and it's natural to feel anxious about performing well. But just because anxiety is normal, that doesn't mean that it's helpful in test taking, or that you should simply accept it as part of your life. Anxiety can have a variety of effects. These effects can be mild, like making you feel slightly nervous, or severe, like blocking your ability to focus or remember even a simple detail.

If you experience test anxiety—whether severe or mild—it's important to know how to beat it. To discover this, first you need to understand what causes test anxiety.

Causes of Test Anxiety

While we often think of anxiety as an uncontrollable emotional state, it can actually be caused by simple, practical things. One of the most common causes of test anxiety is that a person does not feel adequately prepared for their test. This feeling can be the result of many different issues such as poor study habits or lack of organization, but the most common culprit is time management. Starting to study too late, failing to organize your study time to cover all of the material, or being distracted while you study will mean that you're not well prepared for the test. This may lead to cramming the night before, which will cause you to be physically and mentally exhausted for the test. Poor time management also contributes to feelings of stress, fear, and hopelessness as you realize you are not well prepared but don't know what to do about it.

Other times, test anxiety is not related to your preparation for the test but comes from unresolved fear. This may be a past failure on a test, or poor performance on tests in general. It may come from comparing yourself to others who seem to be performing better or from the stress of living up to expectations. Anxiety may be driven by fears of the future—how failure on this test would affect your educational and career goals. These fears are often completely irrational, but they can still negatively impact your test performance.

> **Review Video: 3 Reasons You Have Test Anxiety**
> Visit mometrix.com/academy and enter code: 428468

Elements of Test Anxiety

As mentioned earlier, test anxiety is considered to be an emotional state, but it has physical and mental components as well. Sometimes you may not even realize that you are suffering from test anxiety until you notice the physical symptoms. These can include trembling hands, rapid heartbeat, sweating, nausea, and tense muscles. Extreme anxiety may lead to fainting or vomiting. Obviously, any of these symptoms can have a negative impact on testing. It is important to recognize them as soon as they begin to occur so that you can address the problem before it damages your performance.

> **Review Video: 3 Ways to Tell You Have Test Anxiety**
> Visit mometrix.com/academy and enter code: 927847

The mental components of test anxiety include trouble focusing and inability to remember learned information. During a test, your mind is on high alert, which can help you recall information and stay focused for an extended period of time. However, anxiety interferes with your mind's natural processes, causing you to blank out, even on the questions you know well. The strain of testing during anxiety makes it difficult to stay focused, especially on a test that may take several hours. Extreme anxiety can take a huge mental toll, making it difficult not only to recall test information but even to understand the test questions or pull your thoughts together.

> **Review Video: How Test Anxiety Affects Memory**
> Visit mometrix.com/academy and enter code: 609003

Effects of Test Anxiety

Test anxiety is like a disease—if left untreated, it will get progressively worse. Anxiety leads to poor performance, and this reinforces the feelings of fear and failure, which in turn lead to poor performances on subsequent tests. It can grow from a mild nervousness to a crippling condition. If allowed to progress, test anxiety can have a big impact on your schooling, and consequently on your future.

Test anxiety can spread to other parts of your life. Anxiety on tests can become anxiety in any stressful situation, and blanking on a test can turn into panicking in a job situation. But fortunately, you don't have to let anxiety rule your testing and determine your grades. There are a number of relatively simple steps you can take to move past anxiety and function normally on a test and in the rest of life.

> **Review Video: How Test Anxiety Impacts Your Grades**
> Visit mometrix.com/academy and enter code: 939819

Physical Steps for Beating Test Anxiety

While test anxiety is a serious problem, the good news is that it can be overcome. It doesn't have to control your ability to think and remember information. While it may take time, you can begin taking steps today to beat anxiety.

Just as your first hint that you may be struggling with anxiety comes from the physical symptoms, the first step to treating it is also physical. Rest is crucial for having a clear, strong mind. If you are tired, it is much easier to give in to anxiety. But if you establish good sleep habits, your body and mind will be ready to perform optimally, without the strain of exhaustion. Additionally, sleeping well helps you to retain information better, so you're more likely to recall the answers when you see the test questions.

Getting good sleep means more than going to bed on time. It's important to allow your brain time to relax. Take study breaks from time to time so it doesn't get overworked, and don't study right before bed. Take time to rest your mind before trying to rest your body, or you may find it difficult to fall asleep.

> **Review Video: <u>The Importance of Sleep for Your Brain</u>**
> Visit mometrix.com/academy and enter code: 319338

Along with sleep, other aspects of physical health are important in preparing for a test. Good nutrition is vital for good brain function. Sugary foods and drinks may give a burst of energy but this burst is followed by a crash, both physically and emotionally. Instead, fuel your body with protein and vitamin-rich foods.

Also, drink plenty of water. Dehydration can lead to headaches and exhaustion, especially if your brain is already under stress from the rigors of the test. Particularly if your test is a long one, drink water during the breaks. And if possible, take an energy-boosting snack to eat between sections.

> **Review Video: <u>How Diet Can Affect your Mood</u>**
> Visit mometrix.com/academy and enter code: 624317

Along with sleep and diet, a third important part of physical health is exercise. Maintaining a steady workout schedule is helpful, but even taking 5-minute study breaks to walk can help get your blood pumping faster and clear your head. Exercise also releases endorphins, which contribute to a positive feeling and can help combat test anxiety.

When you nurture your physical health, you are also contributing to your mental health. If your body is healthy, your mind is much more likely to be healthy as well. So take time to rest, nourish your body with healthy food and water, and get moving as much as possible. Taking these physical steps will make you stronger and more able to take the mental steps necessary to overcome test anxiety.